NURSING RESEARCH
DESIGNS AND METHODS

DEDICATION

We wish to dedicate this book to special people in our lives with mention of the following: Harry Watson, George Davidson, Trish, Gowain and Saoirse McKenna, Jonathan, Rebecca and James Cowman, Jessica and Christopher Keady.

Commissioning Editor: Steven Black
Development Editor: Gill Cloke, Fiona Conn
Project Manager: Christine Johnston
Designer: Charles Gray
Illustration Manager: Merlyn Harvey
Illustrator: David Gardner

NURSING RESEARCH
DESIGNS AND METHODS

Edited by

Roger Watson BSc PhD RGN CBiol FIBiol FHEA FRSA FAAN
Professor of Nursing, School of Nursing and Midwifery, University of Sheffield, UK
Editor-in-Chief, Journal of Clinical Nursing

Hugh McKenna PhD DipN(Lond) AdvDipEd RGN RMN RNT FRCN
Dean, Faculty of Life & Health Sciences, University of Ulster, UK

Seamus Cowman MSc PhD PGCEA DipN(Lond) RGN RNT RPN FFNMRCSI
Professor of Nursing and Head of Department, Faculty of Nursing & Midwifery, Royal College of Surgeons
in Ireland, Dublin, Republic of Ireland

John Keady PhD CertHEd RMN RNT
Professor of Older People's Mental Health Nursing, The University of Manchester/Bolton, Salford and
Trafford Mental Health NHS Trust, UK
Co-editor Dementia: the International Journal of Social Research and Practice

Forewords by

Patricia Benner PhD RN FAAN FRCN
Professor, University of California San Francisco School of Nursing,
San Francisco, USA

Shake Ketefian EdD RN FAAN
Professor and Director of International Affairs,
University of Michigan School of Nursing,
Ann Arbor, USA

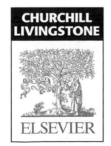

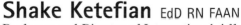

Edinburgh   London   New York   Oxford   Philadelphia   St Louis   Sydney   Toronto 2008

CHURCHILL
LIVINGSTONE
ELSEVIER

CHURCHILL LIVINGSTONE
An imprint of Elsevier Limited

First published 2008

ISBN-13: 978-0-443-10277-6

British Library Cataloguing in Publication Data
A catalogue record for this book is available from the British Library

Library of Congress Cataloging in Publication Data
A catalog record for this book is available from the Library of Congress

Notice
Neither the Publisher nor the Editors assume any responsibility for any loss or injury and/or damage to persons or property arising out of or related to any use of the material contained in this book. It is the responsibility of the treating practitioner, relying on independent expertise and knowledge of the patient, to determine the best treatment and method of application for the patient.

The Publisher

ELSEVIER your source for books,
journals and multimedia
in the health sciences

www.elsevierhealth.com

Working together to grow
libraries in developing countries

www.elsevier.com | www.bookaid.org | www.sabre.org

ELSEVIER BOOK AID International Sabre Foundation

The publisher's policy is to use paper manufactured from sustainable forests

Printed in China

Contents

Section 1 **Approaches to Research**

Section 2 **The Process of Research**

Section 3 **Research Designs**

Section 4 **Data Collection and Analysis**

Contributors

Shona Agarwal BA(Hons) MSc
Research Associate, Department of Health Sciences,
University of Leicester, UK
http://www.hs.le.ac.uk/group/bge/staff/agarwal.html

Ian Atkinson BSc(Hons) PhD RGN RMN PGCLT
Senior Lecturer, School of Health & Social Care,
University of Teesside, Middlesbrough, UK
http://www.tees.ac.uk/schools/SOH/index.cfm

Rachel Baker BA PhD
Lecturer in Health Economics, Institute of Health and
Society, Newcastle University, Newcastle-Upon-Tyne, UK
http://www.ncl.ac.uk/ihs/people/profile/r.m.baker

Cecily Begley MSc MA PhD RGN RM RNT FENRCSI
FTCD
Director of School of Nursing and Midwifery, Trinity
College Dublin, Republic of Ireland
http://www.tcd.ie/Nursing_Midwifery

Heeseung Choi DSN MPH RN
Assistant Professor, College of Nursing, University of
Illinois at Chicago, USA
http://uic.edu

Linda Clare MA MSc PhD CPsychol
Reader, School of Psychology, University of Wales,
Bangor, UK
http://staff.psychology.bangor.ac.uk

Seamus Cowman MSc PhD PGCEA DipN(Lond) RGN
RNT RPN FFNMRCSI
Professor of Nursing and Head of Department, Faculty of
Nursing & Midwifery, Royal College of Surgeons in
Ireland, Dublin, Republic of Ireland

John Cutcliffe BSc(Hons)Nrsg PhD RN RGN RMN RPN
'David G Braithwaite' Professor of Nursing,
University of Texas, Tyler, USA; Adjunct Professor
of Psychiatric Nursing, Stenberg College, Vancouver,
Canada; Visiting Professor, University of Ulster, UK

John Daly BA MEd PhD RN
Head, School of Nursing, College of Health & Science,
University of Western Sydney, Australia
http://www.uws.edu.au/about/acadorg/schools/nursing

Patricia Davidson BA MEd PhD RN
Associate Professor of Nursing, Director Nursing
Research Unit, School of Nursing, University of Western
Sydney, Australia
http://www.uws.edu.au/about/acadorg/schools/nursing

Mary Dixon-Woods BA MSc DPhil DipStat
Reader in Social Science and Health, University of
Leicester, UK
http://www.hs.le.ac.uk/staff/profiles/dixon-woods.html

Gerard M Fealy PhD, MEd, BNS, RGN, RPN, RNT
Dean of Nursing and Head of School, School of Nursing,
Midwifery & Health Systems, University College Dublin,
Republic of Ireland
http://www.ucd.ie/nmhs/staff/fealy_gerard.htm

Carol Haigh BSc MSc PhD RN
Senior Lecturer in Research, Salford Centre for Nursing,
Midwifery and Collaborative Research, University of
Salford, UK
http://www.ihscr.salford.ac.uk/SCNMCR/

Ingalill Rahm Hallberg PhD RN RNT FEANS
Professor in Health Care Science, Lund University;
Director of the Swedish National Institute for Health Care
Sciences, Sweden
http://www.research.med.lu.se

Kevin Hope BSc(Hons) MA PhD CertEd RGN RMN
RNT
Senior Lecturer, School of Nursing, Midwifery and Social
Work, The University of Manchester, UK
http://www.nursing.manchester.ac.uk/staff/KevinHope

Charlotte Humphrey MSc PhD
Professor of Health Care Evaluation, Florence
Nightingale School of Nursing and Midwifery, Kings
College London, UK
http://www.kcl.ac.uk

Debra Jackson PhD RN
Leader, NFORCE Research Group, School of Nursing,
College of Health & Science, University of Western
Sydney, Australia
http://www.uws.edu.au/about/acadorg/schools/nursing

David R. Jones BA MSc PhD DipHE CStat CMath
Professor of Medical Statistics, Department of Health
Sciences, University of Leicester, UK
www.hs.le.ac.uk/group/bge/staff/jones.html

Pauline Joyce BNS MSc RGN RM RNT FFNMRCSI
Director of Academic Affairs, International School of
Healthcare Management, Royal College of Surgeons in
Ireland, Dublin, Ireland
http://www.rcsi.ie

John Keady PhD CertHEd RMN RNT
Professor of Older People's Mental Health Nursing,
The University of Manchester/Bolton, Salford and
Trafford Mental Health NHS Trust, UK
http://www.nursing.manchester.ac.uk/staff/JohnKeady/

Sinead Keeney BA(Hons) MRes PhD
Senior Lecturer, Institute of Nursing Research, University
of Ulster, UK
http://www2.ulster.ac.uk/staff/sr.keeney.html

Mi Ja Kim PhD RN FAAN
Professor and Dean Emeritus, College of Nursing,
University of Illinois at Chicago, USA
http://www.uic.edu/

Debbie Kralik MN PhD RN
Director of Research, Research Unit, Royal District
Nursing Service, South Australia, Australia
http://www.rdns.net.au/research_unit/research_focus.shtml

Tanya McCance BSc(Hons) MSc DPhil RN
'Mona Grey' Professor of Research & Development,
Belfast Health and Social Care Trust and
University of Ulster, Belfast, UK
http://www2.ulster.ac.uk/staff/tv.mccance.html

Geraldine McCarthy PhD MSN MEd DipNursing RGN
RNT
Professor and Head of School, Catherine McAuley School
of Nursing & Midwifery, National University of Ireland,
Cork, Republic of Ireland
http://www.ucc.ie/acad/nursing/

Sonja Mcilfatrick BSc(Hons) MSc PhD PGDipNursEd
RGN RNT
Lecturer in Nursing, Institute of Nursing Research,
University of Ulster, Belfast, UK
http://www2.ulster.ac.uk/staff/sj.mcilfatrick.html

Hugh McKenna PhD DipN(Lond) AdvDipEd RGN RMN
RNT FRCN
Dean, Faculty of Life & Health Sciences, University of
Ulster, UK

Zena Moore MSc RGN FFNMRCSI
HRB Clinical Nursing and Midwifery Research Fellow,
Faculty of Nursing and Midwifery, Royal College of
Surgeons in Ireland, Dublin, Republic of Ireland
http://www.rcsi.ie

Paul Murphy BA, MLIS
Deputy Librarian, Royal College of Surgeons in Ireland,
Dublin, Republic of Ireland
http://www.rcsi.ie/library

Rob Newell PhD RGN RMN RNT ENB 650
Professor of Nursing Research & Director of
Postgraduate Research, School of Health Studies,
University of Bradford, UK
http://www.bradford.ac.uk/health/nursing/staff.php?
showstaff=newell_rj#research

Mike Nolan MA MSc BEd PhD RGN RMN
Professor of Gerontological Nursing, Sheffield
Institute for the Study of Ageing, University of
Sheffield, UK
http://www.shef.ac.uk/sisa/

Ian Norman BA MSc PhD RN RNT CQSW
Head of the Mental Health Section & Head of
Graduate Research Studies, Florence Nightingale
School of Nursing & Midwifery, King's College
London, UK
http://myprofile.cos.com/I124021NOs

Ruth Northway MSc PhD CertEd(FE) RNLD FRCN
Professor of Learning Disability Nursing,
Faculty of Health, Sport & Science, University of
Glamorgan, UK
http://udid.research.glam.ac.uk/rnorthway

Jane Noyes MSc PhD RGN RSCN
Noreen Edwards Chair in Nursing Research, School of
Healthcare Sciences, University of Wales, Bangor, UK
http://www.bangor.ac.uk/healthcaresciences/research/
disabled_child.php.en

Dawn O'Sullivan BSc RN
Research Assistant, Catherine McAuley School of
Nursing & Midwifery, National University of Ireland,
Cork, Republic of Ireland
http://www.ucc.ie/acad/nursing/

Kader Parahoo BA(Hons) PhD RMN
Professor of Nursing and Health Research, University of
Ulster, UK
http://www2.ulster.ac.uk/staff/ak.parahoo.html

Catherine Quinn BSc(Hons) MSc
Research Psychologist, School of Psychology, University
of Wales, Bangor, UK
http://www.psychology.bangor.ac.uk/

Graeme D. Smith BA PhD RGN
Senior Lecturer in Nursing Studies, School of Health in
Social Science, University of Edinburgh, UK
http://www.ed.ac.uk

Alex J. Sutton BSc MSc PhD
Reader in Medical Statistics, Department of Health
Sciences, University of Leicester, UK
http://www.hs.le.ac.uk/group/bge/staff/sutton.html

Carl Thompson BSc(Hons) PhD RN
Senior Lecturer, Department of Health Sciences,
University of York, UK
http://www.york.ac.uk/healthsciences/gsp/
staff/cthomp.htm

David R. Thompson BSc MA PhD MBA RN FRCN
FESC
Professor of Cardiovascular Nursing, Department of
Health Sciences, University of Leicester, UK
http://www.hs.le.ac.uk/

Antonia M. van Loon MN PhD DipAppSc(CIIN) RN
Senior Research Fellow, Research Unit, Royal District
Nursing Service, South Australia, Australia; Adjunct
Faculty, Flinders University, Adelaide, Australia
http://www.rdns.net.au/research_unit/research_projects.
shtml

Heather Waterman BSc(Hons) PhD OND DipN RGN
Professor of Nursing & Ophthalmology, School of
Nursing, Midwifery and Social Work, The University of
Manchester, UK
http://www.nursing.manchester.ac.uk/staff/
HeatherWaterman

Roger Watson BSc PhD RGN CBiol FIBiol FHEA
FRSA FAAN
Professor of Nursing, School of Nursing and Midwifery,
University of Sheffield, UK
http://www.youldpublicationsltd.com

Richard Whittington BA PhD CPsychol AFBPsS PGCert
Reader, School of Health Sciences, University of
Liverpool, UK
http://www.liv.ac.uk/haccru/

Anne Williams BA MA PhD RGN RN
RCN Professor of Nursing Research, Nursing,
Health & Social Care Research Centre, Cardiff
University, UK
http://www.cardiff.ac.uk/nursing/research

Sion Williams BA(Hons) PhD CertHEd RGN RNT
Lecturer in Nursing, School of Healthcare Sciences,
University of Wales, Bangor, UK
http://www.bangor.ac.uk/healthcaresciences/
index.php.en

Bridget Young BA(Hons) PhD
Senior Lecturer and Director of Communication Skills,
Division of Clinical Psychology, University of
Liverpool, UK
http://www.liv.ac.uk

Renzo Zanotti MEd PhD RN DAI FEANS
Professor of Nursing Research, School of Medicine,
Director of International Institute of Nursing Research,
University of Padova, Italy
http://www.unipd.it/en/index.htm

Foreword

The editors and authors of the chapters in this introduction to nursing research have put together an accessible and scholarly international guide to nursing research. The book will be excellent for beginners in nursing research, but will also be a great reference work for all levels of researchers who often need a guide to the current state of the art textbook on nursing research. There are useful and creative assignments at the end of the chapters to guide the reader's understanding and use of the knowledge presented in the chapter.

The authors and editors provide the reader with a rigorous and well-reasoned guide to: (1) Approaches to nursing research, (2) the process of research, (3) research designs, (4) data collection and analysis. The beginning researcher can be assured of a well-ordered introduction to nursing research specific to the nursing discipline, but also relevant to medical research and the social and natural sciences as well. The book is accessible, while remaining interesting to all levels of researchers. For example, Section 2 introduces the importance of asking research questions, demonstrating the intellectual work of framing the research question at the appropriate level for the current development of the research area. From well-investigated and developed questions, come the decisions as to what research approach, processes and designs will be most effective in answering the question(s).

The authors and editors put to rest the invidious debates over the relative value of qualitative and quantitative research approaches. Both qualitative and quantitative research designs and strategies for data collection and analysis are included. The authors maintain that, in isolation, neither qualitative nor quantitative research approaches will be sufficient for answering all nursing research questions. Where fitting and feasible, a research design that includes both quantitative and qualitative methods is highly desirable to address both understanding and explanation.

The editors also include practical and accessible chapters on: research governance and ethics, developing the research proposal, managing a research project, supervising research students, publishing and disseminating the research. The relevance and critical review of the open internet are included in all aspects of research approaches, processes, interpretation and analysis.

Accessing, synthesising, and evaluating the relevant literature are central to doing good research and writing effective research proposals. The authors and editors have done an exceptional job of presenting state-of-the-art information technology database searches and meta-analyses relevant to nursing research. They offer strategies that will help the reader to organise and synthesise a comprehensive literature search. This section will serve all nurses who need to learn how to find and evaluate the relevant evidence to guide their nursing practice. This is an added value to a comprehensive and well-written introduction to nursing research.

I enthusiastically commend this research text for both undergraduate and graduate nurses, as well as researchers and practising nurses.

Patricia Benner
San Francisco, USA
October 2007

Foreword

Nursing research has come of age worldwide. Evidence of this maturity can be noted in the number of nursing research journals in many countries, providing a multitude of forums for an increasing number of nurse investigators. This maturity can also be seen in the number of books on nursing research, addressed to audiences from novice students to experienced investigators.

This book is a most valuable addition to the growing library of text and reference books on nursing research. It is highly readable, with chapters prepared by authors with expertise in their assigned topic. The coverage of topics and themes is broad and comprehensive, though not exhaustive. Sections deal with approaches to research, the processes of research, designs, and analytic techniques. They cover the traditional as well as the more recent designs and analyses. A review of chapters indicates a highly intelligent and useful organisation that helps to structure the content in a meaningful way, rendering the book appropriate for use by beginning students of nursing research, and as a reference for more experienced investigators. Complex and technical material is explained in a clear and understandable way, focusing on concepts rather than the 'how to' aspects.

The authors are drawn from Australia, Canada, Ireland, Italy, Sweden, the UK and the USA; this broad representation of authors assures the reader/ user that multiple perspectives, traditions and orientations are recognised and included, further enhancing the value of the book. An important feature of most chapters is that they are accompanied by exercises and study questions that can help users in delving into greater depth on the topics. This is a welcome addition for those who use the book as a text, both from a student or teacher perspective.

The editors and authors are to be congratulated for their excellent collaborative work in producing a book of high quality and utility.

Shaké Ketefian
Ann Arbor, USA
October 2007

Preface

There are many books available on nursing research – so what is different about this one? First, we hope it is as good as any of the others that are commonly used in nurse education at all levels, but we also hope that it adds a new dimension. The book is neither a manual of research methods nor a treatise on nursing research; it is a book about nursing research by people who are expert in the aspects of research in which they are writing. Second, the book is truly international with contributions from Europe, Australia and the United States – as such, we believe this accords the book a special status in the literature, upon library shelves and in day-to-day reference.

In commissioning authors for this book we considered carefully their contribution to the field and reputation for delivering high quality work. Whilst we have aimed for consistency in the presentation of material throughout the book, by way of including 'end of chapter' exercises for instance, we have tried not to constrain authors in this process. We appreciate, for example, that not every topic listed in this book lends itself to an 'examples and exercises'

format and, indeed, some authors may find such an approach an unnecessary obstacle to presenting work on their topic area. Therefore, whilst we hope that you appreciate the consistently high standard of writing throughout the book, please do not expect to find each chapter exactly the same in style and format; this is a cohesive text but not, necessarily, a textbook.

It has been a pleasure and a privilege to edit this book and our thanks go to all contributors who delivered their material on time and who attended swiftly to the inevitable queries and who accepted our editorial changes gracefully. We would also like, especially, to thank Dinah Thom, Stephen Black and Gill Cloke of Elsevier who responded so positively to all our suggestions and who kept the project going through to publication.

Roger Watson
Hugh McKenna
Seamus Cowman
John Keady

Section 1

Approaches to Research

Chapter 1

The Nature and Language of Nursing Research

Roger Watson and John Keady

- What is nursing research?
- What is nursing research for?
- The language of research
- Conclusion

What is nursing research?

In the UK the origins of nursing research are often ascribed to Doreen Norton, who developed a system of grading pressure sores – the Norton Score (Goldstone & Goldstone 1982). Other small pieces of research either about nursing or involving nurses from about that time are also credited as being foundational. We are sure that in each country where this is read there will be pieces of nursing research of similar importance. However, although some nurses in the UK were involved in research, it has to be said that these pieces of research were rarely independent of the medical profession, and it was not until the Briggs report (Briggs 1972) that nursing research became codified in the sense that this report called for the development of nursing as a research-based profession in the UK. The Briggs report was published in the 1970s yet nursing had, after a considerable struggle, been in the university sector, admittedly on a small scale, since the early 1960s after the University of Edinburgh became the first European university to incorporate it (Weir 1996). Academic nursing has a much longer tradition in North America and, likewise, nursing research (Polit & Hungler 1995).

What is nursing research for?

Research serves many purposes: at one end of the continuum it serves to generate new knowledge purely for the sake of doing so; at the other end of the continuum, research serves to solve problems. Arguably, research that is designed to solve problems is useful to more people than just the person carrying out the research; on the other hand, research that is not designed to solve a problem but merely to generate new knowledge is probably most useful to that person and less so, especially in the short term, to others. This consideration of the apparent usefulness of research is not abstract; it has very tangible implications for nursing research, especially in the UK. Research in nursing sponsored by public money and administered by government bodies, such as research funding bodies and the UK Department of Health, commonly has to state what the purpose of the research is in terms of its application to the services delivered by nurses and, especially, to patients (Department of Health 2006).

For the purposes of this chapter, we will look at what nursing research is for under the following headings:

- solving clinical problems;
- evaluating practice;
- evaluating policy;
- generating and testing theory.

Solving clinical problems

Actually, there can have been very few clinical problems in nursing that have been solved by research; nevertheless, it was precisely how one of us (Watson) came to be involved in nursing research. In the area of urinary incontinence it was clear that some older men with dementia reached a stage where preventing the incontinence became unrealistic and, indeed, interventions aimed at alleviating incontinence became more distressing for the older men than managing the urinary incontinence (Watson 1989, Watson & Kuhn 1990). Clinical experience with urinary sheaths was varied and there were also several products on the market being offered at varying prices. We were able to demonstrate the superiority of one product and also that, despite its greater unit cost, it was better and proved to be cheaper to use as fewer sheaths were required and

patient comfort and safety were increased (Watson 1989, Watson & Kuhn 1990).

The feeding difficulty of older people with dementia proved to be a more intractable problem to 'solve' by research. The literature on feeding difficulty in older people with dementia was reviewed and an assessment instrument to measure feeding difficulty was designed. This body of work is well published and the instrument is known as the EdFED Scale (Watson 1996).

Evaluating practice

In a different vein from research aimed at providing solutions to specific problems, nurses also carry out research to evaluate their practice. This may be done to see if some change in clinical practice that has been implemented is working or to find out, based on current practice, if any changes are required. Clearly, such research may help to identify problems in clinical practice that need to be solved by further research. In fact, this is not uncommon – research rarely provides answers; it usually provides more problems.

Closely related to research that evaluates practice is the use of audit, a key feature of UK NHS clinical governance (Knight & Hostick 2004), and many are confused about the distinction between audit and research. One way of looking at audit is to consider it as a means of evaluating, for the purposes of management, agreed and standard aspects of clinical practice. On the other hand, if data are being gathered to evaluate clinical practice based on someone's hypothesis that a particular result may be found and that the result may merit further investigation to seek improved practice, then this is definitely research. It should be noted that audit and research are not distinguished by the methods employed to carry them out – audit should be as rigorous as research.

Evaluating policy

Policy and practice are not entirely distinct as a great deal of practice stems from policy. However, policy often arises for purely political reasons and it is common for policy changes to be implemented prior to any research being conducted to inform that policy change. Thus, policies need to be evaluated after their implementation. Whereas investigating changes in clinical practice may involve a very limited range of colleagues, policy evaluation commonly involves a wider range because practice implications, economic implications and social implications may all need to be included in the evaluation.

A word of caution is required to those who would become involved in policy evaluation. Due to the political nature of most policy, there is a preconception by those who have implemented the policy and also commissioned the evaluation, that the policy is good and that the changes implemented as a result of it are beneficial. This leads to the possibility of bias in the research and also to difficulty in publishing negative results. Cadet nurses were reintroduced on a national scale in England following the publication of *Making a Difference* (Department of Health 1999) with the aim of widening access to the study of nursing and widening the ethnic and socio-economic background of the nursing workforce. However, an evaluation of this policy showed mixed results and it is unclear what the future of cadet nursing programmes will be (Watson et al 2005).

Generating and testing theory

The purpose of research is to generate knowledge and insights into our world. However, the nature of the inquiry will vary depending upon the stance that we take to view the world and our understanding of 'truth' as being either universal or context-specific. For example, if we see the world as being 'external and concrete', then to generate and test theory based on this belief structure, quantitative approaches will be used to measure representations of universal truth. On the other hand, if we view the world as 'fluid and plural', then qualitative approaches will be used to represent/generate theory within a version of the 'truth' that is context-specific and located within a meaning that the event has for individual human beings.

At its most fundamental level, randomised controlled trials (RCTs) are used as a vehicle to establish the existence of a fixed (universal) truth and this is operationalised through the generation and testing of hypothesis. Here, objectivity and distance are the watchwords of theory production. The hypothesis is worked up by the research team to logical deduction (e.g. using the findings of previous research studies), samples of similar characteristics are then recruited into the study and divided (blindly) into experimental and control groups, the measures agreed, bias neutralised and the interventions conducted in a randomised, rigorous and blind manner with the impact then measured (objectively) and compared across and between groups. In this approach, should the interventions in the experimental group be found to have a demonstrably positive impact (in contrast to results from the control group) derived via scores from the agreed measures, then the resulting evidence is seen to symbolise a universal 'truth' that is replicable in all similar situations.

Theory generated and tested in this manner is seen as a 'gold standard' and actively promoted as the evidence base necessary to advance health care professions and underpin clinical decision-making. Accordingly, the search for high quality RCTs pervades the discourse on reliability in evidence-based health care and is promoted as such through organisations such as the Cochrane Collaboration (www.cochrane.org).

Distilling the production (and, with certain data analysis styles, the testing) of qualitative research down to a few lines is challenging to say the least as comprehensive and weighty handbooks, spread over several volumes, have been dedicated to the subject (Denzin & Lincoln 1994, 2000, 2005). However, it is probably safe to assume that qualitative research approaches, such as phenomenology, grounded theory or ethnography, whilst differing in their epistemology, are held together by a representation of human experience that is grounded in the individual and their subjective interpretation of events and the meaning that it holds. Therefore, producing theory from individual experience that holds as a truism, or a reality, for all representations of human experience makes little conceptual sense. In following a qualitative research approach, fieldwork is (generally) conducted in naturalistic settings and, as Field and Morse (1985) stated in an early and influential text on nursing research through qualitative approaches, with the aim of seeing 'research as a process that builds theory inductively, over a period of time, step by step' (p. 11).

Of the existing qualitative approaches, it is grounded theory (Glaser & Strauss 1967) that makes the claim of developing testable qualitative research. Whilst Cutcliffe in this book (Chapter 21) develops this argument and position further, it is important to acknowledge that grounded theory stands alone in developing mid-range (qualitative) theories that seek to explain and predict phenomena under study. Indeed, the central ideas and philosophy delineated in Glaser and Strauss' (1967) seminal text *The Discovery of Grounded Theory: Strategies for Qualitative Research* were only ever meant to be a beginning. This was especially evident in the development of 'theory as process' (p. 9) and in the strategic method of comparative analysis, which Glaser and Strauss (1967) saw as a general approach 'just as statistics exist for the experimental methods' (p. 21), with the addendum that both approaches use the logic of comparison. Grounded theories exist to 'take hard study of much data' and Glaser and Strauss (1967 p. 3 slightly abridged) believed that the interrelated role of theory within sociology was to:

- enable prediction and explanation of behaviour;
- be useful in theoretical advance in sociology;
- be usable in practical applications – prediction and explanation should be able to give the practitioner understanding and some control of situations;
- provide a perspective on behaviour – a stance to be taken toward data; and;
- guide and provide a style for research on particular areas of behaviour.

As such, Glaser and Strauss (1967) saw the role of theory in sociology as a strategy for handling data in research which provided modes of conceptualisation for describing and explaining. Thus, in conducting grounded theory the researcher attempts to give the data a more general sociological meaning, as well as to account for, and interpret, what has been found.

Glaser and Strauss (1967) believed that, by making theory generation a legitimate enterprise, they would be able to free research from the 'rigorous rules' of objective verification, assimilating verification instead into the ongoing process of generating theory. Accordingly, the canons of the deductive approach exist in grounded theory not only as tests of the generalisability of the study, but also as a method for theory modification. Whilst the approach to generating grounded theory may have developed over the years, it is important not to lose sight of this important separation of grounded theory from the mainstream of other qualitative approaches which are described elsewhere in this book.

The language of research

When we first encounter research, our first impression is often that we do not understand much, if anything, that is being said. This is usually the fault of the lecturer, the writer or the presenter. Either they are trying to impress you with their superior knowledge – a vice shared by many researchers – or they simply have not taken the time to explain the terms they are using. For example, neither 'phenomenological hermeneutics' nor 'structural equation modelling' trip of the tongue or convey much about what they actually mean – yet they may both be encountered in the same issue of a nursing research journal. Therefore, while researchers should strive to express themselves clearly and comprehensibly, both in writing and when speaking, it is also essential that those entering the world of research – whether to undertake their own research or to make use of research – should learn something about the language of research.

What is research?

What is it that unites the – somewhat stereotyped – white-coated scientist in the laboratory and the person conducting interviews with a group of people when both claim to be 'doing research'? One, the scientist, is carrying out research where the conditions are created and controlled to make sure that what is being investigated may be demonstrated (or disproved). The other, the interviewer, is working in the 'real world' having to deal with the differences between people and the different situations in which they may be interviewed. Both researchers are likely to claim that they are investigating their chosen areas for research in a systematic way: they set out with clear aims and objectives and they follow a pattern of activity which should be reproducible by someone else. Both would claim to be trying to find something out about the world we live in, either by creating new knowledge or by seeking to repeat research done by someone else. To some extent, a definition of research arises as discussed above: research is systematic and aims to create new knowledge or verify existing knowledge. Most research textbooks will contain a variation on this theme as a definition of research.

Such a definition is useful and a good starting point to consider the language of research. However, as evidenced by the range of articles published in nursing journals, there are considerable differences between research projects. Methods differ widely, but also sample sizes, in human research, and the aims and objectives and the importance of the subject being studied. The question arises as to where the line is drawn between what is and what is not considered to be research. This is why it is important to have at least a working knowledge of the language of research.

The language of investigation

Research is usually based around projects or programmes; a programme of research usually refers to a long-term engagement (10 years or more) with an area of research. An excellent and topical example of this would be the programme of research aimed at sequencing the human genome. However, a programme of research may have more than one aim. A programme of research will usually consist of several projects and these projects will usually be relatively short term (1 to 3 years) and highly focused. The importance of research projects is that they are planned with a starting and end point and with clear aims and objectives. Research requires resources to be dedicated to it, and the submission of proposals in which a project is described in detail is the way funding is obtained. Most research begins with a research question, a clear statement of what the research is aiming to address, and this topic will be covered in Chapter 7.

In qualitative research, there has been a recent trend to involve service users in the setting of research questions and aims, tailoring research investigation and its dissemination to the language of the community it represents, and also to the involvement of the population under study in conducting part of the research process (Burr & Nicholson 2005, Lowes & Hewlett 2005). The language of investigation is therefore changing in qualitative research, from a position of 'researcher objectivity' (where the researcher is the sole 'expert' who collects and interprets respondent data) to a place of 'co-researcher', where the research act is viewed as a shared enterprise with those whose experience is being explored. Here, the values of participation, collaboration and involvement are instilled throughout the research inquiry.

The language of methods

The range of research methods is wide, as exemplified by the contents of this book, and the 'golden rule' regarding the application of any research method is that it should be suitable for the problem that is being investigated. Research methods fall broadly into two areas and nurse researchers will, generally, describe themselves as being either a 'quantitative' or 'qualitative' researcher. In doing so they are indicating which of a range of methods of investigation they tend to use. However, with some exceptions, it is very rare to find researchers who adhere exclusively to one set of methods or another and the application of 'mixed methods' is common in research projects, often by the same person.

Quantitative and qualitative methods have their roots in different philosophical perspectives on the world. Quantitative methods, as the name suggests, are concerned with measurement and, therefore, come from a perspective (sometimes described as 'positivist') which considers that the world around us, and the people in it, are amenable to study by measurement of, for example, anatomical and physiological parameters or by measuring psychological parameters using questionnaires. Quantitative research methods, therefore, try to provide an objective viewpoint of the world and, in so doing, tend to eschew subjective views of the world. Quantitative research methods, therefore, are concerned with 'variables' which can be measured and manipulated.

In contrast, qualitative methods are usually interactive and seek to obtain the opinions, experiences and meanings of those whose perspective on the research topic is being sought. Interviews are by far the most common form of qualitative research method and in themselves can be conducted in a variety of ways, such as face to face, over the telephone or in small groups, for instance if interviewing a family over their way of adapting and coping with a young child who has had learning difficulties since birth. The quality, depth and insights gained from the interview will usually depend upon the skills and reflexivity of the researcher. Arguably, it is this inherent application of communication and interpersonal skills that makes qualitative research methods appealing to nurses as they are embedded within the culture of nursing care and symbolise 'good' nursing practice. As we will see later in the book (Chapter 27), the format of interviews can be structured, non-structured or, more commonly, semi-structured.

The language of research designs

The different approaches to research lead to different research designs. The prime example of the quantitative research genre is the experiment where one variable (a dependent variable) is measured while another variable (an independent variable) is manipulated; the RCT, whereby drugs are tested on human beings, is an example of an experiment. In the RCT the independent variable, the drug being tested, is manipulated and the dependent variable, the effect of the drug, is measured. Manipulation, in this case, would involve providing one group of people with the drug being tested and another group of people with another drug, or a placebo (e.g. an identical looking substance to the one being tested but which has no active ingredients) so that the effect of the drug being tested can be measured. The experiment has many variations, to be described in Chapter 18, as it is not always possible where people are involved to carry out a true experiment for ethical reasons.

The remaining methods that fall under the quantitative umbrella can all be described as survey methods, and there are many different types of survey. What defines a survey from an experiment is that there is no manipulation of variables; variables are simply gathered, usually from large numbers of people, and the relationships between the variables are analysed. It is not always as clear in a survey which is a dependent variable and which is an independent variable. For example, we may wish to look at the relationship between health status and income. If we find that there is some relationship then we cannot say that one variable is causing the other as poor health status is as likely to lead to low income as low income is to lead to poor health status.

In qualitative research the language of the research design is 'softer' in focus and is geared towards participative methods of inquiry. As we discussed earlier, qualitative research is context-specific and does not make claims over the universality of 'truth'; therefore, the 'truth' will only be represented by the experiences and values of those who take part in the study. This is both a strength and a weakness. Certainly, one of the limitations of qualitative research is lack of representativeness and, at times, this is not helped by the difficulties encountered in sample recruitment. The quality and representativeness of the data is a manifestation of the study sample, and if those in vulnerable or excluded groups, for example, are unable, or unwilling, to participate, then their experiences will be lost from the final report.

In recent years, the qualitative field has constructed a new language around consumer involvement, partnerships and participation in research design and conduct (Burr & Nicholson 2005, Lowes & Hewlett 2005). This development is discussed in greater detail in this book by Northway (see Chapter 3) and provides exciting new avenues for methodological development and dissemination.

Research tools

Linked to research designs, especially quantitative designs, are a variety of research tools or research instruments and this language has been borrowed from laboratory research where tools and instruments are commonly used. In nursing research, which falls largely within the social as opposed to laboratory sciences, tools and instruments refer to the means whereby information or data are gathered. Commonly, research tools refer to schedules or inventories on which data from a research project can be entered and stored for later analysis. Such tools take many forms from paper to electronic and a common format is the questionnaire. The common features are that these tools must be designed in advance of the data collection and the design of such research tools involves a great deal of detailed work, which will be described in Chapter 17. However, it is important to remember that, in qualitative research, the researcher is also a research 'tool' and their reflexivity – accounting for themselves – is central to the conduct, and eventual product, of the research.

The language of validation

In the development of research tools a great deal of effort is expended – or should be – on validation. In fact, it is common to read research papers and to hear conference papers that are solely concerned with the validation of research instruments; for some, this is an end in itself, leaving others to apply the instrument in their research. To know if an instrument is valid it is necessary to understand the language of validation and the two key words are 'reliability' and 'validity'. Reliability refers to the extent to which a tool will make the same measurement each time it is used; validity refers to the extent to which an instrument measures what it purports to measure. Again, the language is borrowed from the physical sciences and in the social sciences it is even more essential to investigate and establish the properties (sometime called psychometric properties) of any instrument. The purpose of a research instrument is to measure something about what people think or how they behave and many factors may influence this. The point behind measuring traits in humans is to measure differences between them and this can only be done with instruments that are well designed.

To understand the concept of reliability, consider a ruler marked off in 12 sections which are described as inches but, in fact, are longer and the total length of the ruler is 13 inches. Each time this ruler is used it will provide the same measurement: it will be completely reliable even if it is informing you that 13 inches is really 12 inches. However, while the ruler is absolutely reliable it is not valid. To be valid, each of the sections marked off as inches should actually measure one inch and the total length of the ruler should be 12 inches; thereafter the ruler will be valid as well as reliable. Note the relationship between reliability and validity: to be valid an instrument has to be reliable; an unreliable instrument cannot be valid. Validity is quite a complex subject and will not be covered in more detail here, but readers are referred elsewhere for comprehensive consideration of all the different types of validity such as content, discriminant, convergent and construct validity (Bowling 2004).

In qualitative studies, the terms validity and reliability are translated into 'truth value'. In other words, validity is about accounting for the way the study has been conducted to ensure its truthfulness and consistency of approach. On this latter point, it remains essential, as Flick (1998) commented, to ensure that the researcher's constructions are grounded in the constructions of those he or she has studied and 'how far this grounding is transparent to others' (p. 225). Transparency of approach and clear and coherent documentation of the research audit trail are essential components in distilling the 'truth value' of the reported qualitative research. Arguably, it is this quest for transparency and the valid representation of the 'truth value' that is currently fuelling the involvement of interviewees in the conduct of qualitative research, from data collection through to data analysis and the subsequent reporting/dissemination of the research findings.

The language of analysis

A research project does not end with gathering data; they need to be analysed and this is, perhaps, one of the areas where the language of research becomes most complex. In the same way that research methods, research designs and research tools follow one another logically, analysis does likewise. This book does not cover the whole range of analytical methods because there are too many and it would be difficult here to give a comprehensive understanding of all the language used. Nevertheless, it is possible to simplify what analysis is about so that your understanding improves and so that you can get a better understanding of what a researcher is describing in a paper or a conference presentation. In quantitative research, analysis is concerned with relationships between variables and there are really only a limited number of ways in which variables can be related: variables can change relative to one another (e.g. increase dose of analgesic and get reduced pain) and this is called correlation; the same variable can be different between a treatment group and a control group (one that has not received the treatment) in an RCT or differ in the same group before and after a treatment. Essentially, therefore, all quantitative analysis is concerned with associations between variables or differences between variables. However, there are many complex analyses, for example factor analysis, that look at the association between large numbers of variables at the same time or analyses such as co-variance analysis which look at the differences between some variables while taking into account the effect of confounding variables which may be associated (i.e. correlated) with either

of the variables in the analysis. A range of common statistical analyses used for quantitative research will be covered in Chapter 35.

In qualitative research the analysis of the data is dependent upon the methodological approach that has been adopted to guide the study process. However, a common bond between the methodologies (i.e. phenomenology, narrative, grounded theory, ethnography) is in the methods that are employed to collect the data, one such method being an interview. Taking this example further, if interviews are conducted and permission has been sought, and granted, to tape-record the words of the interviewee, then at the end of the interview the recording will be transcribed in readiness to be analysed. It is at this time that the interview data are searched, coded and formed into patterns that adhere to the 'rules' of the guiding methodology. For example, in a Glaserian grounded theory study, the constant comparative method (Glaser & Strauss 1967, Glaser 1978) will be used to search for properties of process that begin to account for, and explain, the phenomenon under study.

It is also important to emphasise that, in qualitative data analysis, scrutiny of the transcripts by others with an interest in the study (with permission of course), and consensus agreement over the meaning of words and patterns in the data, will give an added 'truth value' to the coding phase and the eventual transferability (Lincoln & Guba 1985) of the reported study. Member checking, i.e. returning to the field to 'verify' the analysis with the contributors to the study, will also give the reported analysis a heightened meaning and claims on transferability.

Conclusion

This chapter has introduced the language of nursing research methods and approaches and has addressed both qualitative and quantitative approaches. The remainder of the book is aimed at developing and extending salient points from this chapter to broker a more complete understanding of the research process.

EXERCISE

This exercise is set simply to begin to familiarise you with how the concepts discussed in this chapter are used within the reporting of research. It is not meant to represent a detailed critique of a research paper, simply an appreciation of its component parts and how the pieces – and research language – begin to fit and work together.

1. Select an original research paper from a recent issue of a nursing journal such as *Journal of Advanced Nursing* or *International Journal of Nursing Studies*. Carefully and slowly read through the paper and make personal notes on:

   ■ The study title – does this capture the essence of the article?
   ■ The author(s) and their qualifications/work location.
   ■ The composition and succinctness of the abstract: does it tell you what you want to know?
   ■ The scope, applicability and depth of the supporting research literature.
   ■ If the research question/aims flow from the literature review and how they are constructed.
   ■ The methodological approach being adopted in the reported study (e.g., qualitative or quantitative).
   ■ How the sample was gained and reported.
   ■ How ethical issues were addressed by the author(s), and the safeguarding of research participants.
   ■ The structure and composition of the research findings and if they adhere to the chosen/selected/discerned methodology.
   ■ How the issues of reliability and validity (as currently understood) have been addressed in the paper.
   ■ If the Discussion section applies the findings of the reported study within a relevant and contemporary context.
   ■ What financial funding was used to support the study and if this was acknowledged.

2. Make a note on any words/phrases/symbols that are used in the paper but are not immediately understood. Use this book to find out more about this specific subject area, or consult another resource should more specialist information be required.

References

Bowling A 2004 Measuring Health: A Review of Quality of Life Measurement Scales, 3rd edn. Open University Press, Buckingham

Briggs A 1972 Report of the Committee on Nursing (Cmnd. 5115). HMSO, London

Burr J, Nicholson P 2005 Researching Health Care Consumers: Critical Approaches. Palgrave, London

Denzin N K, Lincoln Y S 1994 Handbook of Qualitative Research. Sage, London

Denzin N K, Lincoln Y S 2000 Handbook of Qualitative Research, 2nd edn. Sage, London

Denzin N K, Lincoln Y S 2005 Handbook of Qualitative Research, 3rd edn. Sage, London

Department of Health 1999 Making a difference. Department of Health, London

Department of Health 2006 Best research for best health. Department of Health, London

Field P A, Morse J M 1985 Nursing Research: The Application of Qualitative Approaches. Chapman & Hall, London

Flick U 1998 An Introduction to Qualitative Research. Sage, London

Glaser B G 1978 Theoretical sensitivity. Sociology Press, Mill Valley, CA

Glaser B G, Strauss A L 1967 The Discovery of Grounded Theory: Strategies for Qualitative Research. Aldine, Chicago

Goldstone L A, Goldstone J 1982 The Norton score: an early warning of pressure sores? Journal of Advanced Nursing 7: 419–426

Knight S, Hostick T 2004 Accountability in NHS Trusts. In: S Tilley, R Watson (eds) Accountability in Nursing and Midwifery, 2nd edn. Blackwell, Oxford: 77–86

Lowes L, Hewlett I 2005 Introducing Service Users in Health and Social Care Research. Routledge, London

Polit D F, Hungler B P 1995 Nursing research: principles and methods, 5th edn. Lippincott, Philadelphia

Watson R 1989 A nursing trial of urinary sheath systems. Journal of Advanced Nursing 14: 467–470

Watson R 1996 Mokken scaling procedure (MSP) applied to feeding difficulty in elderly people with dementia. International Journal of Nursing Studies 33: 385–393

Watson R, Kuhn M 1990 The influence of component parts on the performance of urinary sheath systems. Journal of Advanced Nursing 15: 417–422

Watson R, Norman I J, Draper J, et al 2005 NHS cadet schemes: do they widen access to healthcare study? Journal of Advanced Nursing 49: 276–282

Weir R 1996 A Leap in the Dark. Jamieson Library, Penzance

Chapter 2

Approaches to Research

Cecily Begley

Introduction

The four main branches of academic work – the sciences, social sciences, health sciences and humanities – use various different approaches and methods to gather information and conduct research. The sciences, sometimes called the natural sciences, use predominantly laboratory-based techniques and positivist, quantitative methods. Much medical research draws on natural sciences and is laboratory-based, but quantitative experimental and descriptive work is also carried out with patient/client involvement and, to a lesser extent, some qualitative work as well. The humanities use a range of approaches, depending on discipline, and the social sciences tend towards the qualitative approach. Nursing and midwifery research can choose from a wide variety of approaches, drawn from the disciplines of sociology, psychology, anthropology, philosophy and natural sciences, as well as newer methods devised and developed within the two professions.

This chapter gives a concise introduction to theoretical perspectives, methodologies and methods and an overview of ways of approaching research, including primary and secondary research, either to confirm theories or to explore topics of interest. A brief description of the two main research traditions, qualitative and quantitative, is given, and will demonstrate that they are not coming from two opposing backgrounds but may be used in conjunction with each other to increase the breadth, depth and rigour of one's work. The use of mixed methods is advocated and future directions for progress in terms of developing collaborative research teams and conducting systematic reviews are discussed.

Approaching research

It is best to keep an open mind on which research methodology to use until you have decided on your main research question and on your guiding theoretical perspective. Bear in mind that the focus might change as you progress through the planning stages of your study, but prior to data collection you need to have your exact research question identified. For that reason, please try Exercise 1 now (p. 19), in order that you will have a research question in mind before you start to read about the various research approaches available to you.

Primary and secondary research

The first practical consideration in conducting research is to know whether or not the study is necessary and, if necessary, whether or not you need to collect new data. Primary research is the term used when data are collected specifically for the study in question. It may be exploratory or confirmatory and may stem from quantitative or qualitative paradigms (or both). Secondary research is the name given to studies where previously collected data are used (i.e. retrospective studies) or previous published research findings are gathered together and presented (i.e. as a systematic review). At the preliminary stages of your study, you will conduct a comprehensive literature review, during which you will discover whether primary or secondary research is needed to answer your research question. For this reason, secondary research is discussed here first.

Secondary research

Secondary research is a valid method of conducting research and should be used if sufficient primary research has already been conducted. It should be borne in mind that it may be unethical to conduct a further study in the same area if there is already ample evidence available to answer the research question.

Retrospective studies

Retrospective studies can be very useful in demonstrating what is happening, thus drawing our attention to issues that one perhaps would otherwise not be fully aware of. For example, O'Farrell et al's (2004) retrospective study, in one health board region in the Republic of Ireland, of emergency hospital admissions of people with a diagnosis of acute alcohol intoxication, found that the rate of admissions with this diagnosis increased significantly over the 5-year period 1997–2001; this increase mirrored the national increase in alcohol consumption over the same time period, suggesting that increased alcohol consumption nationally may lead to an increase in hospital admissions due to acute alcohol intoxication. The study used figures collected routinely under the Hospital In-Patient Enquiry (HIPE) data collection system and merely analysed and presented them in statistical form.

Systematic reviews

Systematic reviews are mainly based on quantitative studies, usually randomised trials, and may use meta-analysis techniques to present an aggregate view of the results of all studies, thus presenting what may be assumed to be the definitive statement of the best evidence available on that topic at that time. The Cochrane Library, which is free via the internet to everyone in the UK and Ireland (and many other countries), is a unique source of reliable information on the effects of interventions in health care, based on systematic reviews of all international literature (The Cochrane Collaboration 2005). The Cochrane Database (considered in Chapter 10), which is published quarterly, at present holds 2524 systematic reviews, each of which is updated as new evidence accumulates (Clarke 2004). More recently, some authors have undertaken systematic reviews of qualitative studies, but this technique is still being developed (Lloyd Jones 2004, Meadows & Morse 2001, Walsh & Downe 2005). As more systematic reviews are published in future, it will be necessary to conduct reviews of reviews.

Primary research

Primary research may be either exploratory or confirmatory.

Exploratory research

Exploratory research is conducted when you are not aware of any other studies in this area, or there is no definitive answer as to the best care, despite previous work. You will (usually) start with a literature review and/or a systematic review, which, if no authoritative answer can be found, remains in the realm of exploratory work. Further exploratory work, if deemed necessary, is usually conducted using qualitative methods, although quantitative questionnaires and scales may be used. One example of this is the study conducted in Ireland by Matthews et al (2005), which explored the conditions important in facilitating the empowerment of midwives, as judged by 95 practising midwife respondents. A survey approach was used, and four factors important for the empowerment of midwives were isolated: control, support, recognition and skills.

Confirmatory research

Confirmatory research is conducted when a theory has already been propounded and one is trying to confirm (or refute) that theory. It most usually uses a quantitative approach, such as a randomised trial to test a hypothesis or closed-ended questions in a survey, but qualitative methods may also be used. One example is the work of Templeton and Coates (2004); in their study in Northern Ireland, half of a group of 55 men with prostate cancer who were on hormonal manipulation therapy were randomly assigned to receive an education package, testing the hypothesis that such education would result in improvements in quality of life and coping. The results showed that those who received the education package had increased knowledge and improved quality of life and satisfaction with care, but there was no beneficial effect on coping.

Conclusion

From the above you will see the importance of preliminary thought and reflection before deciding on a particular research approach. The next section describes the main theoretical research perspectives from which your chosen methodologies will be drawn. Before reading on, please try Exercise 2 (p. 19), in order that you may refine your 'practice' research question, write outline aims and decide whether or not your research needs to be primary or secondary and whether it is exploratory or confirmatory. In addition, it may be useful to read Chapter 7 at this stage, to assist you in developing your research question.

Theoretical perspectives

Methodological choices made by researchers (i.e. whether research is to be experimental, survey, phenomenological, grounded theory, action and so on) are guided by their theoretical and philosophical positions. There are a number of theoretical perspectives from which all research stems, including positivism, postpositivism, interpretivism, critical enquiry, feminism, postmodernism and poststructuralism (Crotty 1998). Positivists believe there is a truth that can be found and that one's goal in research is to find, study and report that truth usually by testing a theory through quantitative studies and inferential tests, and drawing conclusions that can be generalised to a stated population. Some qualitative work claims to take a positivist stance also, through the search for one substantiated theory (Johnson 1999), although this is strongly debated (Glaser 2002). While positivism appears to be objective and scientific, it is important to acknowledge that no study of humans and their world can possibly be completely free of the researcher's influence (Koch & Harrington 1998, Payne et al 2003). Postpositivists realise that one can never reach one truth, but endeavour to capture as much of reality as is possible, using multiple methods to do so (Racher & Robinson 2002).

Interpretive researchers assume that gathering knowledge about a particular population can only be done through shared consciousness, meanings and language and believe that it is not possible to separate the researcher from the research in any objective manner (Racher & Robinson 2002). The research approach used tends to be qualitative in nature; for example, Dunniece and Slevin's work on palliative care nursing, where a hermeneutic approach was used to explore the lived experience of seven nurses working in the palliative care field (Dunniece & Slevin 2002). Critical researchers believe that the ability of people to alter their economic and social circumstances is hindered by the power and control exerted by social, political and cultural influences. The main aim of critical research is to empower and emancipate those who are the focus of the research (Fontana 2004) and is thus similar, in many respects, to feminist research. Research approaches would include participatory action research and gender-focused studies, such as the work on men and masculinities undertaken by the CROME group in Europe (The CROME Network 2004).

In critical theory, binary oppositions are identified, such as the perceived higher status of male versus female, and a reversal of the opposition is attempted. Post-structuralism also identifies and challenges these hierarchies, but does not privilege one partner over another (Francis 2000).

Deciding which theoretical perspective to guide your study will influence your choice of methodology and research methods. In general, all methodologies lie within one or other of two main research approaches, qualitative or quantitative.

Qualitative and quantitative approaches to research

These two research approaches are often portrayed as though they opposed one another, whereas in fact they can be used to supplement and balance each other. Some research methods use aspects from both approaches, and many researchers are now using both approaches in the same study in the process of triangulation (Adami & Kiger 2005).

Qualitative approaches to research

In general, qualitative approaches gather verbal or observational data, are concerned with how people understand their experiences and are said to present the uniqueness of each participant's individual situation (idiographic). They concentrate more on explaining and understanding people's experiences, thus taking an insider (emic) perspective, in the process of which researchers acknowledge and use their subjectivity (Morgan & Drury 2003). Qualitative research techniques include:

- in-depth interview;
- focus group interview;
- observation;
- diaries;
- written records.

Qualitative methods are described as inductive and exploratory (Janesick 2000) and require a purposive sample, i.e. one that is chosen with a purpose (Patton 2002), in order to describe the phenomenon under scrutiny.

Quantitative approaches to research

In contrast, quantitative research is based on numerical data, or quantities, and is concerned with the detection of general laws (nomothetic) and the examination of aggregated views. It tends to focus on control and prediction of events and takes an outsider (etic) position, claiming to be objective (Punch 2005). Quantitative methods include:

- randomised trial;
- survey;
- observation (using pre-formulated check sheets).

Quantitative approaches are said to use deductive methods (Punch 2005), often testing hypotheses and deducing the result using inferential tests; because of this, quantitative researchers must use correctly-calculated random samples of their population (Devane et al 2004) and are thus able to generalise from their findings.

Conclusion

The above brief descriptions conform to the stereo-typical versions of these two research approaches, as depicted in Table 2.1, but this is, necessarily, a narrow view. Quantitative approaches can also be used for exploratory work and the generation of hypotheses, and qualitative methods, in conjunction with quantitative methods, may be used to test hypotheses and theories (Miles & Huberman 1984, Punch 2005). The important factor to be considered in every research study is the overall purpose of the research and therefore what combination of approaches should be taken in order to ensure that the best possible study will be conducted to answer the question.

The academic debate on qualitative and quantitative approaches

The debate between nursing and midwifery academics on the relative merits of qualitative and

Table 2.1 – *Stereotypical characteristics of quantitative and qualitative approaches*

Quantitative approaches	Qualitative approaches
Gather numerical data	Gather verbal or observational data
Use measurement	Illuminate and provide meaning
Explain and predict	Understand and interpret
Use a representative sample	Use a purposive sample
Can be used to generalise	Cannot be used to generalise
Exclude context	Provide context
Are said to be deductive	Are said to be inductive
Test previously set hypotheses	Are usually exploratory
Claim to be objective	Acknowledge and use subjectivity

quantitative approaches has been raging for dec-ades, with considerable time and energy expended. It could be stated that there is not much difference between the two approaches, as all research is some-what quantitative, because even verbal responses can be counted and measured, and all research is somewhat qualitative, because answers to basic questions, no matter how quantifiable the answers may be, are based on individuals' interpretations of the question. So the real difference between qualita-tive and quantitative lies not so much in the method, but in the researcher's philosophical stance.

For example, quantitative methods stem from positivism and qualitative methods, many would argue, do not. And yet, when a grounded theorist carries out interview after interview until the data are saturated, they are collecting data until a valid and firm theory has been produced, which in itself suggests that some may believe in one 'truth', or as near as one can arrive to that state. Similarly, the 'bracketing' propounded by Husserl (Lowes & Prowse 2001) is an attempt to be objective, which is the antithesis of the usual qualitative researcher's stance of acknowledging and, indeed, valuing (Morgan & Drury 2003) subjectivity.

Despite these similarities, the debate in the litera-ture continues today. Quantitative approaches have recently been described as the only acceptable 'scien-tific' way of conducting research (Watson 2003), though this view was hotly contended (Draper & Draper 2003, Payne et al 2003). Qualitative researchers promote the benefits and credibility of this approach and discuss and support ways of ensuring the integ-rity of their research (Cutcliffe & McKenna 2004, Mea-dows & Morse 2001). Johnson (1999) critiques some qualitative researchers for what he calls 'uncritical verificationism' (Johnson 1999, p. 70), where studies are conducted with a clear intent to verify previously developed theories. He suggests that this will bring qualitative methods into disrepute (Johnson 1999).

Conclusion

A continued argument as to which approach, qualitative or quantitative, is the better is invidious;

both have their benefits and both their weaknesses. Neither one is better than the other, they are merely two ways of obtaining data, one of which might be more useful than the other in any given situation. Both approaches have strengths and weaknesses, and it is incumbent upon all researchers to try to strengthen every study that they undertake, by whatever means possible. For many studies, a combination of the two approaches might be best, to achieve confirmation and completeness of findings (Adami & Kiger 2005, Begley 1996a).

Choosing a research approach

When starting a research study, it is best to identify clearly what goal you wish to attain and then to think out the best way of achieving it. It does not make sense to limit one's choices by forming non-essential philosophical boundaries around them, or by deciding in advance that you are 'not able to do' or 'don't like doing' one type of research or method of data collection. All research approaches are possible, manageable and, once you have learnt how to do them, just as easy or difficult to use as any other method. Perceived difficulties such as 'not liking maths' do not mean that you cannot undertake quantitative research, as statisticians exist to assist you with such endeavours.

It is, ultimately, the research question that chooses the design or approach to be used, not the researcher, as it becomes obvious during the initial stages of your research planning that a particular approach or methodology is the best, although in practice experienced researchers often have expertise in a particular method and tend to phrase their research questions to favour their expertise. As your research question becomes more refined during your initial planning stages, so too will your research approach become more obvious. The main pitfall to avoid at this stage is what Janesick describes as 'methodolatry', that is: 'a preoccupation with selecting and defending methods to the exclusion of the actual substance of the story being told' (Janesick 2000, p. 390).

The following section provides an outline of triangulation, or the use of mixed methods, which will assist you to do this. A more detailed description of this technique is presented in Chapter 21. Before you read on, try Exercise 3 (p. 20), so that you will have your main research approach selected and can then decide whether or not you wish to add some subsidiary methods.

Using mixed methods

The depth and extent of your study can be improved by using more than one research approach, or by using within-method triangulation, which will provide a more inclusive view of the participants' world. Triangulation is not merely the combination of dissimilar methods of study, however, and it is recommended that researchers should consider using one or more of the five other less common types of triangulation (considered in Chapter 26), i.e. data, investigator, theoretical, unit of analysis and triangulation of communication skills (Begley 1996b, Tobin & Begley 2002). It may also be more effective for some studies to use qualitative and quantitative methods sequentially, rather than simultaneously. In all mixed method studies, one approach tends to take precedence over the other, in terms of the philosophy driving the research (Foss & Ellefsen 2002).

Combining methods in this way helps to prevent oversimplification of conclusions and assists researchers to move away from narrow, uniform beliefs. However, research development is not about planning to gather lots of data in different ways, and putting all the findings together in the hope that a more coherent picture may emerge. Planning your research is the most important step in the whole research process, and your choice of approaches and methods should stem directly from your final question. Regardless of what approach is undertaken, the study should be conducted with the utmost rigour (Arminio & Hultgren 2002), with a commitment to excellence through the use of the 'triangulation state of mind' (Miles & Huberman 1984, p. 235) and the search for 'goodness' throughout the study

(Tobin & Begley 2004). Awareness of the importance of rigour transcends any minor differences between research approaches.

Collaborating in research

There is a need for an increase in collaborative research in the health sciences, which might involve having a team of researchers educated in different disciplines, each with their own unique perspective on the topic. In addition, collaboration with patients or clients at the planning, implementation and analysis stages of research will improve your findings. Evaluation research, in particular, should be based on qualitative views of respondents first (Patton 2002). Participatory action research, which is driven predominantly by the need to create positive social change (Hughes & Seymour-Rolls 2000), is an inherently collaborative model and should be considered, in particular, when change is desired.

Collaborative research does require active management of projects and considerable insight into the strengths and weaknesses of one's own and others' disciplines. It is worth working hard at developing research partnerships as collaborative research is, where feasible, the optimum research approach (Smith & Katz 2000). As a final assessment of learning throughout this chapter, try Exercise 4 (p. 20), to see if you can improve your research plan by using additional methods or different approaches, or by the inclusion of other researchers.

Conclusion

Planning your study is the most important phase of research and should not be rushed. It is important that the research approach used matches the research question and stems from your theoretical perspective. The method or methods should then be chosen by their ability to answer the research question, and must be rigorous. Collaboration in research, with patients/clients and with members of other disciplines, is recommended where possible as the optimum research approach.

EXERCISES

1. *Getting ideas.* On your own, or as part of a group, pick a topic that interests you, challenges you or concerns you in your work as a health professional. Now brainstorm possible research questions from that idea, by asking yourself 'who, where, what, why, when, how?' [Example: It concerns you that patients/clients wait for three hours in your outpatient clinic. Questions derived from this concern might include: Who are they waiting to see? Where do they have to sit? Why do we keep them waiting for so long? How do they feel about this long wait?]

   Some of these questions can be answered by present knowledge, a search of present records or from superficial observation (Who are they waiting to see? Dr White), (Where do they have to sit? Rows of plastic chairs). Keep generating questions until you have succeeded in identifying a number that cannot be answered so easily. Select one and write it as a meaningful 'practice' research question, with one or more aims and objectives to guide your study. [Example: 'Why do we keep them waiting for so long?' might become: What are the multiple reasons for delay of patients/clients in the waiting area of the outpatients department? Your aim might then be: To identify the causes of delay of patients/clients in the waiting area of the outpatients department.]

2. *Refining your question.* Refine your research question and rewrite your aims. [Example: Regarding the question above, you might need an aim setting out your intention to ascertain the actual waiting times. You might also decide that it was not enough merely to identify the causes of delay, but you would like to improve the situation. This could happen automatically, once you give your findings to the hospital/clinic manager, but you might also wish to include it as an aim.]

Continued

EXERCISES—Cont'd

Your aim(s) might thus alter to:

- To measure the time spent waiting in the outpatients department.
- To identify the causes of delay of patients/clients in the waiting area of the outpatients department.
- To implement measures to reduce the time spent waiting in the outpatients department.]

3. *Selecting your research approach.* On your own, or as part of your group, discuss, debate and decide on a research approach, or number of approaches to answer your question. [Example: 'To measure the time...' requires a quantitative approach, but could be done in different ways. 'To implement measures...' could also be done in many ways, but you might decide to take an action research approach that, through collaborative involvement of clinic staff, would ensure that changes were implemented as part of the research process.]

4. *Considering the addition of other methods, approaches or researchers.* On your own, or as part of your group, discuss and debate how your study might be improved by the use of additional methods or different approaches either simultaneously or sequentially. Consider how other researchers from different backgrounds/disciplines might be included in the team. Decide on your final preferred approach, method and team.

References

Adami M F, Kiger A 2005 The use of triangulation for completeness purposes. Nursing Research 12: 19–29

Arminio J L, Hultgren F H 2002 Breaking out from the shadow: The question of criteria in qualitative research. Journal of College Student Development 43: 446–456

Begley C M 1996a Using triangulation in nursing research. Journal of Advanced Nursing 24: 122–128

Begley C M 1996b Triangulation of communication skills in qualitative research interviews. Journal of Advanced Nursing 24: 688–693

Clarke M 2004 Systematic reviews and the Cochrane Collaboration. Online. Available: http://www.cochrane.org/docs/whycc.htm 13 Nov 2005

Crotty M 1998 The Foundations of Social Research. Meaning and Perspective in the Research Process. Sage, Thousand Oaks

Cutcliffe J R, McKenna H P 2004 Expert qualitative researchers and the use of audit trails. Journal of Advanced Nursing 45: 126–133

Devane D, Begley C M, Clarke M 2004 How many do I need? Basic principles of sample size estimation. Journal of Advanced Nursing 47: 297–302

Draper J, Draper P 2003 Response to Watson's Guest Editorial 'Scientific methods are the only credible way forward for nursing research'. Journal of Advanced Nursing 44: 546–547

Dunniece U, Slevin E 2002 Giving voice to the less articulated knowledge of palliative nursing and practice: An interpretive study. International Journal of Palliative Nursing 8: 13–20

Fontana J S 2004 A methodology for critical science in nursing. Advances in Nursing Science 27: 93–101

Foss C, Ellefsen B 2002 The value of combining qualitative and quantitative approaches in nursing research by means of method triangulation. Journal of Advanced Nursing 40: 242–248

Francis B 2000 Poststructuralism and nursing: uncomfortable bedfellows? Nursing Enquiry 7: 20–28

Glaser B G 2002 Constructivist grounded theory? Forum: Qualitative Social Research 3(3). Online. Available: http://www.qualitative-research.net/fqs-texte/3–02/3–02glaser-e.htm 30 Dec 2005

Hughes I, Seymour-Rolls K 2000 Participatory action research: getting the job done. Action Research E-Reports 4. Online. Available: http://www.fhs.usyd.edu.au/arow/arer/004.htm 26 Nov 2005

Janesick V J 2000 The choreography of qualitative research design. In: Denzin N K, Lincoln Y S (eds) Handbook of Qualitative Research, 2nd edn. Sage, Thousand Oaks, CA: 379–399

Johnson M 1999 Observations on positivism and pseudoscience in qualitative nursing research. Journal of Advanced Nursing 30: 67–73

Koch T, Harrington A 1998 Reconceptualizing rigour: the case for reflexivity. Journal of Advanced Nursing 28: 882–890

Lloyd Jones M 2004 Application of systematic review methods to qualitative research: practical issues. Journal of Advanced Nursing 48: 271–278

Lowes L, Prowse M A 2001 Standing outside the interview process? The illusion of objectivity in phenomenological data generation. International Journal of Nursing Studies 38: 471–480

Matthews A, Scott P A, Gallagher P et al 2005 An exploratory study of the conditions important in facilitating the empowerment of midwives. Midwifery Online. Available: doi:10.1016/j.midw. 2005. 08.003 13 December 2005

Meadows L M, Morse J M 2001 Constructing evidence within the qualitative project. In: Morse J M, Swanson J M, Kuzel A J (eds) The Nature of Qualitative Evidence. Sage, Thousand Oaks, CA: 187–200

Miles M B, Huberman A M 1984 Qualitative Data Analysis. Sage, Thousand Oaks, CA

Morgan A K, Drury V B 2003 Legitimising the subjectivity of human reality through qualitative research method. The Qualitative Report 8(1) Online. Available: http://www.nova.edu/ssss/QR/QR8–1/morgan.html 13 Nov 2005

O'Farrell A, Allwright S, Downey J et al 2004 The burden of alcohol misuse on emergency in-patient hospital admissions among residents from a health board region in Ireland. Addiction 99: 1279–1285

Patton M Q 2002 Qualitative Research and Evaluation Methods, 3rd edn. Sage, Thousand Oaks, CA

Payne S, Seymour J, Ingleton C 2003 Response to Watson's Guest Editorial 'Scientific methods are the only credible way forward for nursing research'. Journal of Advanced Nursing 44: 547–548

Punch K F 2005 Introduction to social research: quantitative and qualitative approaches, 2nd edn. Sage, Thousand Oaks, CA

Racher F E, Robinson S 2002 Are phenomenology and postpositivism strange bedfellows? Western Journal of Nursing Research 25: 464–481

Smith D, Katz J S 2000 HEFCE fundamental review of research policy and funding collaborative approaches to research. Final Report. A joint project with the Higher Education Policy Unit (HEPU), University of Leeds and the Science Policy Research Unit (SPRU) University of Sussex. Online. Available: http://www.sussex.ac.uk/Users/sylvank/pubs/collc.pdf 30 Dec 2005

Templeton H, Coates V 2004 Evaluation of an evidence-based education package for men with prostate cancer on hormonal manipulation therapy. Patient Education and Counseling 55: 55–61

The Cochrane Collaboration 2005 Online. Available: http://www3.interscience.wiley.com/cgi-bin/mrwhome/106568753/HOME 28 Dec 2005

The Critical Research on Men in Europe (CROME) Network 2004 Men and Masculinities in Europe. Whiting & Birch, London

Tobin G A, Begley C M 2002 Triangulation as a method of inquiry. Journal of Critical Inquiry into Curriculum and Instruction 3: 7–11

Tobin G A, Begley C M 2004 Methodological rigour within a qualitative framework. Journal of Advanced Nursing 48: 388–396

Walsh D, Downe S 2005 Meta-synthesis method for qualitative research: a literature review. Journal of Advanced Nursing 50: 204–211

Watson R 2003 Scientific methods are the only credible way forward for nursing research. Journal of Advanced Nursing 43: 219–220

Chapter 3

Participative Approaches to Research

Ruth Northway

Introduction

Tetley and Hanson (2000) suggest that a definition of participatory research 'remains elusive'. However, for the purpose of this chapter, it will be defined as a continuum of research approaches which recognise that, traditionally, some groups of people have tended to be marginalised and powerless within the research process and that this can be oppressive. In order to change such a situation participatory research thus seeks to promote and facilitate the active involvement of such groups (often referred to as 'the community') at all stages of the research process. It is concerned with both changing power relations within the research process and with producing knowledge which can be used to bring about wider change and transformation. Action and education are integral parts of participatory research.

The context of participatory research

The origins of participatory research are said to lie in Tanzania in the 1970s (Hall 1992) and the first meeting of the International Participatory Research Network produced a definition of such research (Hall & Kidd 1978) emphasising its focus on promoting the active participation of powerless groups at all stages of the research process. The term participatory action research is also sometimes used but whilst Park (1999) acknowledges that this may be a more accurate reflection of the action component of participatory research, it can lead to some confusion with action research in which a professional researcher directs the research. Khanlou and Peter (2005) argue that action research and participatory research differ in terms of ideological beliefs, the training of researchers, and the context in which they work. The former is grounded in clinical and social psychology and management theory whereas the latter is usually undertaken by community organisers and adult educators, being informed by sociology, economics and political science (Khanlou & Peter 2005).

A further term encountered is 'emancipatory research'. Such terminology is often found in the disability literature where some authors (such as Stalker 1998) argue that participatory and emancipatory research are used interchangeably. Others (e.g. Chappell 2000) draw a clear distinction, arguing that whilst participatory research aims to increase the participation of disabled people, emancipatory research transforms the material and social relations of research such that disabled people control all aspects of the research process. Yet other authors (e.g. Beresford 2005, Finn 1994, Northway 2003) argue that participatory research is best viewed as a continuum in which there are increasing levels of participation on the part of those who have traditionally held less powerful positions and in which they are enabled to take control over the research process. INVOLVE (2004) suggest that on such a continuum a distinction can be made between user consultation, collaboration and control. In this chapter, the term 'participatory research' will be used as an umbrella term for a range of research approaches which seek to shift control from powerful to less powerful groups within the research process by consultation, collaboration and facilitating control.

Whilst traditional approaches to analysing participation have tended to concentrate on the level of involvement (as above), the focus has now shifted to include examination of the 'ideological underpinnings' of the differing approaches to participation (Beresford 2005). The driving forces for increased participation of marginalised groups in research can broadly be labelled 'top down' (policy driven) and 'bottom up' (service user driven).

INVOLVE (2004) note that, since 1997, a range of health policy documents in the United Kingdom have emphasised the importance of public participation. In addition, some research funders stress the importance of service user involvement. Ross et al (2005) thus note that the drive for consumer involvement in their project came from both policy and the research commissioning process. Service user pressure for increased participation in, and control over, research can be seen from the disability movement in the United Kingdom, who have criticised the negative and oppressive nature of much disability research (see, for example, Oliver 1992) and who have called for control of the research process to lie with disabled people themselves.

It is evident, however, that these two dimensions of participatory research both need to be considered (Fig. 3.1) since the primary motivation for undertaking a project may be to respond to policy but the outcome of the research may be to devolve maximum control to service users. Alternatively the impetus for research may arise from a service user group but they may not wish for full participation or control at every stage of the project. Furthermore, the level and nature of participation may vary from stage to stage.

The nature of participatory research

Some authors (such as Soltis-Jarrett 2004) suggest that participatory research is a qualitative approach whilst others (such as Macaulay et al 1999) argue that it can be both quantitative and qualitative. Seng (1998) thus states that participatory research cannot be recognised as 'one particular method or design'. Instead it is more helpful to view it in terms of how the research should be conducted rather than in terms of data collection techniques (Henderson 1995) since it addresses how the research process should proceed (Huang & Wang 2005). Four key features (Box 3.1) will be discussed.

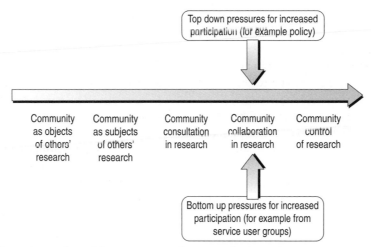

Figure 3.1 – *The dimensions of participatory research approaches.*

- A focus on countering oppression
- Promoting participation at all stages of the research process
- The production of 'useful' knowledge to promote change
- A different role for the researcher

Countering oppression

Some groups have been marginalised within the research process and are often relatively powerless due to the fact that their views are not heard (Stoeker & Bonacich 1992). This position is oppressive and participatory research seeks to counter such oppression by promoting active participation at all stages of the research process.

A key feature of participatory research is the involvement of a 'community' (Park 1999), but such communities are often disempowered in diverse ways. Whilst participatory approaches in the context of health research have often been viewed as synonymous with service user involvement in research, Beresford (2005) argues that both service users and practitioners should be considered in this.

Participation at all stages of the research process

A key feature of participatory research is that the community actively engage as fully as possible at all stages of the research process (Park 1999). Since the emphasis is on shifting power and increasing community control Stoeker (1999, p. 850) has identified six key points at which decisions need to be made:

- 'defining the research question;
- designing the research;
- implementing the research design;
- analysing the research data;
- reporting the research results;
- acting on the research results.'

Participatory research can be cyclical, with action leading to the identification of further research questions. However, whilst participation at all stages is an 'ideal' model, the community may not wish for such involvement and, even where participation has been agreed, it may not be continuous or predictable (Cornwall & Jewkes 1995). Roles, responsibilities and contributions may thus shift as a project progresses (Macaulay et al 1999).

Within participatory research the research question or issue to be explored should be identified by the community themselves. However, Park (1999) acknowledges that the deprivation often experienced by such communities can militate against their initiating research.

Community members may have limited knowledge of the research process and require support in understanding the various research methods and their implications. The researcher may thus be required at act as a resource person at the research design stage (Drevdahl 1995). However, the community members can provide an important perspective on how the use of proposed methods may be experienced by participants. It is important that data collection methods which give community members a voice are explored (Tetley & Hanson 2000).

Data analysis is perhaps one of the most complex stages of the research process and this can give rise to some difficulties in participatory research projects. For example, Schneider et al (2004) note that, due to the cognitive difficulties associated with schizophrenia, participants in their study experienced problems with this stage of the research, particularly as they found it difficult to concentrate for long periods.

Beresford (2005) suggests that data analysis raises questions as to who is best placed to undertake this task, particularly when the data gathered are concerned with the experiences of those who use services. Are the service users themselves best placed or should professionals and academics undertake such a role since they can 'claim distance' from the experiences (Beresford 2005)? One of the strengths of participatory research is that members of the research team each bring to the project differing experiences and this can enrich the process of data analysis. For example, Koch et al (2002) note that, in their participatory research involving groups of community nurses, shared meanings emerged as the projects progressed, facilitated by the fact that participants were able to compare and contrast their own interpretations against those of other group members.

Reporting the research findings can take several forms from the traditional development and publication of papers for publication in academic and professional journals through to other forms of dissemination such as theatre presentations (Schneider et al 2004). Where papers are written for publication, ideally, they should be written in a collaborative manner (Ham et al 2004, Northway et al 2001, Schneider et al 2004). However, if findings are disseminated only in professional and academic contexts there is a danger that the people whose lives are the focus of the research will not gain access to information which could help them. Findings should be disseminated more widely and in formats that are accessible to service users.

The nature of the action to be taken will inevitably differ from project to project and hence it is difficult to be prescriptive. One example involved making theatre presentations to health care staff concerning communication with people with mental health problems which resulted in some health professionals reporting a change in their perceptions and practice (Schneider et al 2004). In the study reported by Ross et al (2005), consumers involved in the project became involved in decision-making meetings with the Primary Care Trust. The nurses involved in one of the studies reported by Koch et al (2002) developed a video concerning the prevention of workplace violence which, combined with feedback from educational activities and discussion with management, resulted in the development of a model for best practice. What each of these examples has in common is that they each seek to address issues of concern to the community and to enhance quality of life.

The nature of knowledge produced

Khanlou and Peter (2005) argue that participatory research values 'useful knowledge', namely that which has some practical use. Park (1999) identifies three different forms of knowledge (representational, relational and reflective), each of which he suggests are typically developed in the course of a successful participatory research project.

Representational knowledge has two different forms – functional and interpretive. The former is concerned with the linking of variables and seeks to investigate cause and effect. The latter is concerned with understanding the meanings that humans give to events and experiences. Representational knowledge can thus be seen to encompass both quantitative and qualitative elements.

Participatory research, however, goes beyond these forms of knowledge typically generated in other research approaches. Members of the research team work together over a period of time and seek to investigate the conditions that shape their lives. As a result they come to know each other and their communities better. Park (1999) refers to the knowledge gained by such processes as *relational knowledge*, arguing that, whilst it is not a form of knowledge which is explicitly pursued, it is an outcome that is often valued by participants.

Park (1999) argues that participatory research is motivated by a vision of what should be. *Reflective knowledge* is thus that which results from people's critical reflections concerning the difference between what is, what should be, and hence what needs to change. It is knowledge which motivates people to take action to produce such change.

Each of these three forms of knowledge 'reinforce and interact with one another' (Park 1999, p. 149). They can also operate at a variety of different levels. For example, the process of working together with others in the course of a participatory research project can lead researchers to reflect upon their own motivations, values and performance and take action to bring about personal change (Northway 1998b, Wahab 2003).

A different role for the researcher

Traditionally, researchers have been encouraged to take a detached and objective role. However, this is not the case in participatory research. Instead the researcher is expected to be a committed participant (Hall 1979), to challenge those processes which separate the researcher from the researched (Finn 1994); it has been suggested that being a participatory researcher is a vocation rather than a job (Park 1999).

Seng (1998) notes that, being accountable in the usual ways (e.g. to research funders and employers), participatory researchers are also directly

accountable to the community with whom they are undertaking the study. The potential for tensions between these differing lines of accountability can thus be seen.

Stoeker (1999) has identified four key roles that may be required of the participatory researcher: animator (assisting people to develop a sense of important issues), community organiser (planning and organising the research activity), popular educator (facilitating learning during the research process) and participatory researcher. The demands placed upon the researcher will vary according to the stages of the research and according to the needs and abilities of the community. They thus need to demonstrate a high level of self awareness and reflexivity since such critical self-reflection enables them to examine their own values, motivations and actions (Northway 1998b) and hence to assume the most appropriate role at each stage.

Other requirements of the participatory researcher include good communication skills (Finn 1994, Koch et al 2002, Ross et al 2005), the need for confidence and good organisational skills (Tetley & Hanson 2000), the ability to tolerate ambiguity (Finn 1994) and facilitation skills (Koch et al 2002). Given this wide range of demands, it is not surprising Drevdahl (1995) suggests the 'enormity' of such work can exhaust a lone researcher – physically and mentally. The need for 'novice' participatory researchers to receive mentorship has thus been suggested (Tetley & Hanson 2000).

The relevance of participatory research to nursing

Papers concerning participatory research have been published by nurses from several countries: Australia (Koch et al 2002, Soltis-Jarrett (1997, 2004)), the United States (Drevdahl 1995, Henderson 1995, Seng 1998), the Philippines (Corcega 1992), Taiwan (Huang & Wang 2005), Canada (Khanlou & Peter 2005) and the United Kingdom (Northway (1998b, 2000a, 2003), Richardson (1997 & 2000), Ross et al 2005, Tetley & Hanson 2000). These papers address people with mental health problems (Northway et al 2001, Soltis-Jarrett 2004), older people (Ross et al 2005), people with learning disabilities (Ham et al 2004, Northway 1998b and 2003), Richardson (1997, 2000)), female drug users (Henderson 1995), community nurses (Koch et al 2002) and community health development (Corcega 1992, Huang & Wang 2005). Therefore, there is evidence of international participatory research in nursing across a period of at least 14 years working with a wide variety of groups.

Participatory research offers one way to close the theory–practice gap and to develop evidence that is relevant to practice. Throughout the participatory research process there is an emphasis on combining research, education and practice (Khanlou & Peter 2005) and hence the distinction between research and practice is 'overtly rejected' (Henderson 1995). Finally the emphasis within participatory research on taking action as a key outcome means that the understanding of a practice issue gained as a result of the research can directly change such practice where this is required.

Key issues to be considered by the participatory researcher

The challenges involved in participatory research are major (Beresford 2005, Wahab 2003) and should be considered before commencing a project and regularly reviewed as work progresses. Here they will be considered under the headings of resources and ethical issues (see Box 3.2 and Table 3.1). It should be noted, however, that as with many aspects of participatory research, these issues are interrelated. For example, a lack of appropriate

Box 3.2 – *Key ethical considerations in participatory research*

- Membership of the research 'team'
- Who benefits from the research?
- Negotiating and reviewing the terms of working together
- Recognising the potential for harm
- Ending the research

attention to resource considerations could have negative ethical implications.

Resources

The key resource within any participatory research project is the people involved. This includes both the participatory researcher and the community (or co-researchers). Careful consideration of the *human* resource issues is thus imperative.

The need for participatory researchers to receive appropriate support and mentoring has already been noted (Tetley & Hanson 2000). However, whilst they often come to the research project with some research experience, for the community this may not be the case. It is not enough to provide opportunities for participation in research: support may also be required for participation to be meaningful (Beresford 2005). The community may not be aware of the methodological options available, of the implications of using such approaches, or possess the skills and confidence to undertake such tasks as data collection, data analysis or making conference presentations. The participatory researcher needs to be able to discuss possible options and to provide training where necessary (Park 1999).

Cornwall and Jewkes (1995) note many health care professionals are ill prepared to undertake participatory research since the training of 'medical researchers' can make it difficult for them to relinquish control given that such training is rooted in notions of objectivity. Participatory researchers are, however, working in a different context of changed relationships which challenge traditional research approaches (Ross et al 2005). There is thus a need to consider the research education of all nurses and for individual participatory researchers to identify their own learning needs in the context of specific projects.

Other forms of support which may be required include the provision of written materials in different languages or in accessible formats. It may be necessary to provide information in Braille or on a tape for those with visual impairments. Some members of the community may require the support of a personal assistant both to prepare for, and to attend, meetings.

Table 3.1 – *Resource issues to be considered by those undertaking participatory research*

Human resources	■ Training and support of both the participatory researcher and the community
	■ Support to facilitate participation
Environmental resources	■ Accessibility of meeting venues
	■ Layout of meeting rooms
Time resources	■ Time for the development of trusting relationships and shared decision-making
	■ Existing time commitments of both the researcher and the community
	■ The relationship between the desired level of participation, the scope of the research and the time available
Financial resources	■ Payment of community members for participation
	■ Potential difficulties with securing funding

Environmental considerations also need to be taken into account. For example, the venue for meetings may need to be carefully chosen to ensure access for wheelchair users or those with limited mobility, and to ensure that it is accessible via public transport for those without cars. Both the venue for meetings and the layout of meeting rooms can convey a sense of unequal power and it may be important to consider whether a meeting should be held at a community venue or in a health service setting.

If participation is to be genuine it is important not to underestimate the *time* required to undertake a participatory research project (Northway 2000a). Relationships are central to such research and these can take a long time to develop to the point where there is mutual trust. Where decisions are shared and meanings are jointly constructed, this can also take much longer than a principal researcher undertaking a leading role throughout the research project.

The time needed to undertake a participatory research project may be greater than a researcher is able to commit (Macaulay et al 1999). However, as Beresford (2005) notes, those who use services may also have limited time. It is important to acknowledge the relationship between the time available for a project, the desired level of participation, and the scope of the project (Northway 1998b) and for this to be discussed prior to the project commencing.

Participatory research may require the provision of training and additional support, and particular environmental supports, and it may take longer than other forms of research. The *financial* implications thus need to be considered.

Participatory researchers will normally be paid for their research work as it is undertaken as part of their normal role. However, where community members are invited to participate actively in a research project, the question of payment needs to be addressed. Thomas and O'Kane (1998) gave payment of £10 to the children who participated in the activity day 'to reflect the value ... placed on their work' (p. 341). Similarly, consumer participants in the study undertaken by Ross et al (2005) received expenses and an honorarium for their time; although they noted an unwillingness to accept personal payment, some panel members preferring to donate their payment to charity. It is important to consider the implications for any members of the community who are receiving state aid. Further helpful guidance is provided by INVOLVE (2005).

Macaulay et al (1999) state that funding agencies are increasingly recognising that the potential benefits of participatory research outweigh its potential costs and, as has already been noted, some funding agencies require evidence of service user involvement in the development of bids for funding. However, in a recent study of the experience of service user controlled research, Turner and Beresford (2005) found the 'strongly held view' that it is difficult to secure funding for such research and that it does not compete on equal terms. Furthermore, these difficulties are compounded by additional resource requirements. Some progress has been made but further work is required. Researchers seeking to undertake participatory research should not underestimate the resource requirements and the consequent financial costs but the potential benefits need to be stressed to funders.

Ethical issues

Whilst the inclusion of participatory approaches has been viewed as enhancing the ethical acceptability, reliability and validity of research (Thomas & O'Kane 1998), the huge ethical challenges posed have also been noted (Beresford 2005, Wahab 2003). This has led to the suggestion that ethics committees may require some additional guidelines to assist them with assessing participatory research studies (see Khanlou & Peter 2005).

The first issue that needs to be considered is the question of which 'community' to work with and who might be viewed as being a member of that community. The researcher may be approached by the community to undertake a specific piece of work (see, for example, Northway et al 2001); in other situations, existing relationships may facilitate the development of a research partnership (see, for example, Wahab 2003) or volunteers may be sought from a range of different sources (see, for example, Ross et al 2005). There is a danger that researchers may (inadvertently) collaborate with an unrepresentative section of the community (Macaulay et al 1999) and attention needs to be given to the issue of equal opportunities (Beresford 2005).

Participatory research involves working with marginalised groups to bring about positive change. The question of who is intended to benefit from the research is thus a key ethical issue about which researchers need to be clear (Beresford 2005, Khanlou & Peter 2005). Clearly, there is the potential for professionals and academics to benefit through, for example, gaining qualifications, publications and promotions. However, it is the community who should be the primary beneficiaries. Since both communities and participatory research projects vary widely it is not possible to be prescriptive as to what such benefits might be. The key issue, however, is that this is discussed at the early stages of the research projects and that hopes and expectations are clarified.

Within participatory research, the roles of researcher and researched are blurred and this gives rise to a number of particular ethical concerns (Khanlou & Peter 2005). There is the issue of whether members of the community are viewed primarily as co-researchers or as participants from whom data are to be gathered. Of course, these two are not mutually exclusive and, as reported by Schneider et al (2004), members of the research group both gathered data and were interviewed, hence they signed consent forms confirming their willingness to participate. In other studies, community members act as co-researchers and gather data from others (from whom consent is required). For example Ham et al (2004) describe how self advocates with learning disabilities worked alongside nurses to develop their study for ethical approval.

Whichever approach is taken, it is important that those invited to work on a research project are provided with as much information as possible. If the potential for participation and control is limited at some stages of the research process, then this should be made clear. It is also important to agree that, where there are opportunities for participation, such opportunities do not have to be taken by everybody: it is acceptable to choose not to participate actively in some stages (Ham et al 2004). Consent to work together on a participatory research project should thus be viewed as a process rather than as an event and the terms of working together should be agreed and reviewed regularly during the project (Northway 1998a).

Relationships are central to the process of participatory research and the potential for the ending of such projects to be experienced as harmful by those with limited social networks (and who may lose valued relationships at this stage) has been noted (Booth 1998). There is limited guidance in the literature concerning this stage in the research process (Northway 2000b). This may be due to the fact that participatory research is viewed as a continuous process in which one project leads to another (Park 1993), but the reality of research means that it may not be possible for the researcher, the community or both to remain involved for a long period.

As with any ethical dilemma it is important to consider that, given the choice, people with limited social networks may prefer to be involved in a research project over a fixed period rather than to miss such an opportunity for interaction (Northway 2000b). Participatory researchers thus need to be clear about the level of commitment they are able to give and to work closely with their co-researchers regarding expectations (Northway 2000b). However, since differences in perception can arise (Booth 1998, Stalker 1998), they also need to be prepared to provide a commitment over a lengthy period if this is desired (Northway 2000b). It is essential that 'ending' the research is carefully considered before the research commences.

Whilst these ethical issues can be complex they should not be viewed as providing an argument against taking a participatory approach. It should be remembered that not seeking to increase participation in research also has ethical implications.

Example – the 'ForUs' study

ForUs, a mental health service user forum, had undertaken a small-scale study which sought to investigate the views of mental health service users concerning their experiences of service provision. However, they felt that they wished to undertake a wider study and thus contacted the School of Care Sciences at the University of Glamorgan for assistance.

It was agreed that a project advisory group would be established and that one member of the ForUs group would be a full member of this group acting as a point of liaison with other ForUs group members. Decisions would thus not be taken without agreement of the wider service user group.

Some key areas of interest had already been identified by ForUs but a wider literature review was undertaken and shared with the group. From this an interview schedule was developed. Members of ForUs were involved in piloting the schedule and advised concerning its acceptability.

The interviews with people who attended day centres, day hospitals and outpatients' clinics were conducted by third year student nurses. They were provided with a day's training which a representative of ForUs was involved in.

The data were analysed by the university-based researchers and a draft report written which was then shared with ForUs for discussion and comment. A launch event was held to which mental health service users, mental health service professionals, and service commissioners were invited. Other means of dissemination involved the development of joint papers and joint conference presentations.

Following the launch, ForUs also undertook their own analysis of the findings of the research and presented these to the local joint commissioning body. As a result of this some changes in practice were forthcoming. For further information, see Northway et al (2001).

Conclusion

Participatory research can be very challenging and it is important that researchers considering using such approaches consider carefully the resource and ethical implications in order that these can be identified and effectively managed. Despite these challenges, however, participatory research can also be very rewarding to all who participate. It is thus important that nurses increase their awareness of such approaches, that they increase their confidence in using them, and that they report both the findings and process of such studies in order that others can learn from their experiences.

EXERCISES

1. Identify a research paper and, using the decision-making stages identified by Stoeker (1999), try to determine whether service users were consulted, collaborated or had control at any stage of the research process. Consider also the following:

   ■ Were there any stages where you felt participation of service users could have been increased?
   ■ What would have been the potential benefits or disadvantages of seeking to increase participation?

2. Working either as a group or as an individual, identify a practice situation where you feel change is needed. What would be the possible advantages and disadvantages of seeking to use a participatory research approach to bring about change?

3. Identify a 'community' with whom you might undertake a participatory research study. What issues would you need to consider? What problems do you feel you might encounter? How might such problems be overcome? What do you feel would be your personal support needs as a participatory researcher?

References

Beresford P 2005 Theory and practice of user involvement in research. Making the connection with public policy and practice. In: Lowes L, Hulatt I (eds) Involving Service Users in Health and Social Care Research. Routledge, London: 6–17

Booth W 1998 Doing research with lonely people. British Journal of Learning Disabilities 26: 132–134

Chappell A 2000 Emergence of participatory methodology in learning difficulty research: understanding the context. British Journal of Learning Disabilities 28: 38–43

Corcega T F 1992 Participatory research: getting the community involved in health development. International Nursing Review 39: 185–188

Cornwall A, Jewkes R 1995 What is participatory research? Social Science and Medicine 41: 1667–1676

Drevdahl D 1995 Coming to voice: the power of emancipatory community interventions. Advances in Nursing Science 18: 13–24.

Finn J 1994 The promise of participatory research. Journal of Progressive Human Services 5: 25–42

Hall B L 1979 Knowledge as a commodity and participatory research. Prospects 9: 393–408

Hall B L 1992 From margins to center? The development and purpose of participatory research. American Sociologist Winter 1: 15–28

Hall B L, Kidd R J 1978 Adult Learning: A Design for Action. Pergamon, Oxford

Ham M, Jones N, Mansell I, et al 2004 'I'm a researcher!' Working together to gain ethical approval for a participatory research study. Journal of Learning Disabilities 8: 397–407

Henderson D J 1995 Consciousness raising in participatory research: method and methodology for emancipatory nursing inquiry. Advances in Nursing Science 17: 58–69

Huang C L, Wang H H 2005 Community health development: what is it? International Nursing Review 52: 13–17

INVOLVE 2004 Involving the public in NHS, public health and social care research: briefing notes for researchers. INVOLVE, Hampshire

INVOLVE 2005 A guide to paying members of the public who are actively involved in research: For researchers and research commissioners (who may also be people who use services). INVOLVE, Hampshire

Khanlou N, Peter E 2005 Participatory action research: considerations for ethical review. Social Science and Medicine 60: 2333–2340

Koch T, Selim P, Kralik D 2002 Enhancing lives through the development of a community based participatory action research programme. Journal of Clinical Nursing 11: 109–117

Macaulay A C, Commanda L E, Freeman W L, et al 1999 Participatory research maximises community and lay involvement. British Medical Journal 319: 774–778

Northway R 1998a Oppression in the lives of people with learning difficulties: a participatory study. Unpublished PhD thesis, Bristol University

Northway R 1998b Engaging in participatory research: some personal reflections. Journal of Learning Disabilities for Nursing, Health and Social Care 2: 144–149

Northway R 2000a The relevance of participatory research in developing nursing research and practice. Nurse Researcher 7: 40–52.

Northway R 2000b Ending participatory research? Journal of Learning Disabilities 4: 27–36

Northway R 2003 Participatory research. In: Jukes M, Bollard M (eds) Contemporary Learning Disability Practice. Quay Books; Salisbury: 165–174

Northway R, Davies P, Lado A, et al 2001 Collaboration in research. Nurse Researcher 9: 75–83

Oliver M 1992 Changing the social relations of research production? Disability, Handicap and Society 7: 101–114

Park P 1993 What is participatory research? A theoretical and methodological perspective. In: Park P, et al (eds) Voice of Change: Participatory Research in the United States and Canada, Bergin and Garvey, Westport, CT: 1–19

Park P 1999 People, knowledge and change in participatory research. Management Learning 30: 141–157

Richardson M 1997 Participatory research methods: people with learning difficulties. British Journal of Nursing 6: 1114–1121

Richardson M 2000 How we live: participatory research with six people with learning difficulties. Journal of Advanced Nursing 32: 1383–1395

Ross F, Donovan S, Brearley S, et al 2005 Involving older people in research: methodological issues. Health and Social Care in the Community 13: 268–275

Schneider B, Scissons H, Arney L, et al 2004 Communication between people with schizophrenia and their medical professionals: a participatory research project. Qualitative Health Research 14: 562–577

Seng J 1998 Praxis as a conceptual framework for participatory research in nursing. Advances in Nursing Science 20: 37–48

Soltis-Jarrett V 1997 The facilitator in participatory action research: les raisons d'etre. Advances in Nursing Science 20: 45–54

Soltis-Jarrett V 2004 Interactionality: wilfully extending the boundaries of participatory research in psychiatric-mental health nursing. Advances in Nursing Science 27: 316–329

Stalker K 1998 Some ethical and methodological issues in research with people with learning difficulties. Disability and Society 13: 5–19

Stoeker R 1999 Are academics irrelevant? Roles for scholars in participatory research. American Behavioural Scientist 42: 840–854

Stoeker R, Bonacich E 1992 Why participatory research? Guest editors' introduction. American Sociologist Winter 5–14

Tetley J, Hanson␣E 2000 Participatory research. Nurse Researcher 8: 69–88

Thomas N, O'Kane C 1998 The ethics of participatory research with children. Children and Society 12: 336–348

Turner M, Beresford P 2005 User controlled research. Its meanings and potential. Shaping Our Lives and the Centre for Citizen Participation, Brunel University, Middlesex

Wahab S 2003 Creating knowledge collaboratively with female sex workers: insights from a qualitative, feminist and participatory study. Qualitative Inquiry 9: 625–642

Chapter 4

Feminist Research

Debbie Kralik and Antonia M. van Loon

- Introduction
- Feminist theory
- Feminist epistemology
- Feminist principles in research
- Case study on the use of feminist research principles
- Conclusion

Introduction

The purpose of this chapter is to explore feminist methodology in the context of nursing research. The questions posed in this chapter are: what is feminist research and how can feminism inform nursing research? To respond to these questions, we explore feminist epistemology, feminist principles, methodology (how research should proceed) and method (approach to generating data) used by feminist researchers. We demonstrate the method and methodology used in community-based research with women who were sexually abused when they were children.

Feminist theory

There are four main orientations of feminist theory: liberal, Marxist, radical and socialist feminist theory. Whilst further reading is required to understand each of these orientations, a brief overview is provided. The liberal feminist view developed during the 1800s where the focus was women's lack of rights and opportunity based on family, gender, race, religion, and unequal distribution of wealth (Chinn & Wheeler 1985). Liberal feminism focused on reform through education.

Marxist feminist theory claims women's oppression was caused by the introduction of private property which led to the development of class systems and sexism. Marxist feminists contend that the oppression of women will resolve when there is a revolution to redistribute the property to society as a whole (Chinn & Wheeler 1985).

Socialist feminist theory proposes that the patriarchal family, motherhood, housework and consumerism are the basis of women's oppression. This theory considers the oppression of poor, working class women, third world women and women of colour (Chinn & Wheeler 1985, Speedy 1991).

The principles of radical feminist theory are derived from a woman-centred world view that challenges patriarchal systems. The perspective is that the oppression of women is caused by cultural institutions and cannot be resolved by changing those institutions. For oppression to be resolved gender discrimination and gender roles must be abolished (Chinn & Wheeler 1985).

Feminist epistemology

Feminist epistemologies argue that knowledge is incomplete, situated in time and place, and embodied by cultural constructions. Feminist epistemologies identify the manner that dominant ways of knowing may be disadvantaging women and other oppressed groups, with the aim of surfacing and challenging power constructions to reshape understandings and practices, aiming to improve the situation for the oppressed group. Central to feminist epistemology is the idea of situated knowledge. The knower's perspective that situates their understanding of a topic is questioned. Feminist epistemologies contend that gender affects understanding; informing approaches to the central issue being studied and influencing social and political roles of people in the study. This impacts the values underpinning the inquiry and understanding of objectivity, consistency and authority. Consequently feminism becomes difficult to define, but a simple description by Stanley and Wise (1983, p. 55) provides a useful summary from which to start our discussion. It says feminist understanding relies on 'theoretical constructions about the nature of women's oppression and the part that this oppression plays within social reality more generally'.

It is important to recognise that there is no single way of knowing that can be described as feminist because all knowledge is context based. Thus diverse methods of understanding women's experiences are legitimate ways of knowing in feminist epistemology. Many understandings of the same subject will be reflected by the individual's location to, and relationship with, the subject under investigation. People experience the world with their body and their mind. Thus understanding personal experiences of a phenomenon is assisted by first person accounts about the lived experience of the phenomenon under study. The researcher may only know these states by interpreting signs and features, or obtaining descriptions of the study subject from the person experiencing the phenomenon. Such knowledge relies on how the person represents their experience and the emotions, values, attitudes and interests the phenomenon holds for that person. In many instances this knowledge is tacit, unspoken and highly intuitive.

Those who have more information about the phenomenon under study are likely to interact and react to the phenomenon in different ways than those who come from a position of ignorance. People will form various beliefs about the phenomenon and these will be influenced by their prior experiences, values and belief systems, and their prior knowledge of the phenomenon under study. The varying places in which the person stands in relation to other inquirers also affects their access to necessary information about the phenomenon and their capacity to communicate about the phenomena to other people. This position may have an impact upon their judgement regarding what is significant or otherwise regarding the study subject. So we can see that how a person is situated affects their understanding of their experience and/or the phenomenon under study. The incredible diversity of individual people's lives and personal experience necessitate the need for multiple and flexible approaches to research. Feminist knowledge emerges from an exploration and unpacking of each person's terms of reference, which are evolving understandings.

Feminist approaches to research enable one's personal perspectives to surface (Chinn 2003). The researcher's epistemology is shaped by the life experiences she or he brings to the research as well as the influences of the many voices and conversations within feminism. As researchers, our assumptions and values underpin the research process. It is important to identify them prior to embarking on research and during the research process. The challenge for us is 'to develop a kind of self reflexivity that will enable us to look closely at our own practice in terms of how we contribute to dominance in spite of our liberatory intentions' (Lather 1991, p. 150).

Feminism is not a set of rules, methods and ideas (Lumby 1997) but is a perspective that may inform and guide the way we live. Hence feminism challenges us to be accountable for congruence between our thought and our behaviour (Maguire 1996). Locating one's feminism, and one's personal epistemology, is a dynamic process involving reflection and a critical consciousness. Feminist research is not an intellectual exercise guided by theory, but is passionate, political, participatory and personal. Feminist principles are intimately connected to our lives; hence knowing our world through a feminist lens has implications for how we live and work, and whether we engage in feminist research (Maguire 1996).

Diverse feminist positions have evolved over time (Olesen 1994). The historical context and development of the arguments that constitute feminist theory are important for gaining a sense of where we have been and how we have arrived at this point. Theoretical history has meaning and purpose in connecting the old to the new as it allows us to record advances and lay the foundation for advancing inquiry. Many gains made for women can be attributed to the feminist movement. One example is the movement against domestic violence. Until feminism, there had been no acknowledgement of domestic violence, no legal avenues and support for women and no supported accommodation/sheltered housing. During the 1970s, feminist groups funded shelters, but the government, police, and media paid little attention to violence within the family, even though violence continues to be one of the most pervasive health and social issues facing women worldwide. In 2006 there is funded supported accommodation in our cities, improving public awareness based on long-term media campaigns

against domestic violence, reformed laws and police practices, and altered legislative strategies aimed at contesting violence against women and children.

Feminist principles in research

Common to the various feminist theoretical orientation is the notion of patriarchal power relations that oppress women where women's interests or social positions are subordinate to men (Speedy 1991). Although there are many forms of feminist thought, there are also shared aspects. A feminist worldview sensitises researchers to consider voice, that is who is being heard and who is being excluded. It is also of central importance to explore and understand the context and lives of people participating in research by understanding power relations and how those play out in individual experiences of help-seeking (Crotty 1998). In so doing, however, a feminist perspective refrains from perpetuating the view of the 'woman as victim' of their circumstances; instead it celebrates diversity and varied strengths (Maguire 1996). Chinn and Wheeler (1985, p. 76) explain this characteristic of feminist research:

A feminist perspective does not seek to romanticise or idealise these women, but rather to develop insights that allow us to appreciate their struggles, understand their limitations and see their joys and their pains as similar to ours.

The diverse feminist theories hold differing perspectives about the forces that oppress women, and consequently advocate different ways by which justice (via action and change) may be achieved (Kolmar & Bartkowski 2000). Feminist theory aims to transform women's lived experiences and women's participation in the construction of new possibilities (Smith 1991). A woman-centred approach is fundamental to feminist research, with the aim of illuminating the life context and experiences of women, grounded by their frame of reference, experiences and language (DuBois 1985, Speedy 1991). This thinking develops through a critical awareness of experiences, values, ideologies and goals. It is through this awareness that consciousness raising and action becomes possible as women learn to view the world through a critical lens and contradictions in their lives become illuminated. Some 'common threads in feminism' (Maguire 1996, p. 107) have been identified as:

- acknowledgement that women face oppression and exploitation;
- women experience their oppressions, struggles and strengths in diverse ways;
- a commitment to reveal the forces that cause and sustain oppression;
- a commitment to working *with* women (individually and collectively) towards action that will challenge and change oppressive structures and forces.

The intent of feminist principles is to encourage women to take action to develop new structures or reshape existing forces so that women can 'live out new ways of being in relationship with the world' (Maguire 1996, p. 108).

Feminist inquiry has often been conceptualised as research *for* women and *with* women rather than research *on* women (Campbell & Bunting 1991, Hall & Stevens 1991, Olesen 1994, Scharbo-DeHaan 1994, Webb 1993). Feminism focuses on the way women are represented, and the *way* in which knowledge is constructed (Griffiths 1995, Maynard & Purvis 1994). Feminist research has revealed that, while most knowledge has been generated and defined by males, the perspective they espouse is not the only one and not always appropriate (Speedy 1991). The experiences of men are not the experiences of women, nor are the experiences of women homogeneous. Feminists have challenged not only the view of the way knowledge is produced but also whose view the research represents. Feminist principles in research are political, transformative and transparent and therefore used where the aim of the research is to create change (Jackson 1997).

It is important that feminist research extends further than the creation of knowledge to have a commitment to social justice (Drevdahl 1999) and social change that will serve to enhance the lives of women (Hall & Stevens 1991).

Speedy (1991, p. 201) identified three main principles that inform feminist research. They are:

- recognition that women are oppressed, and that the reasons for oppression need to be examined so that action can be taken and changes made;
- valuing of women's experiences; and
- consciousness-raising that results in alternative views of the world from a woman's perspective.

Consciousness-raising involves the recognition of social, political, economic and personal constraints on freedom, and is the forum in which decisions of actions are made that will challenge those constraints and initiate change (Henderson 1995). Consciousness-raising allows women the opportunity to view the world in a different way.

Consciousness-raising is when:

... women experience a shared sense of reality and a shared sense of oppression; they become conscious of their problems as group problems rather than as their own individual problems (Henderson 1995, p. 63).

In feminist research, the questions that are asked and the research focus are as important as the data generated. Questions focus on exploring women's perceptions and feelings, and experiences are valued and made visible (Bowes 1996, Crowley & Himmelweit 1992, Lather 1988 and 1991, Puwar 1997). It is important that the words 'feminism' or 'feminist' are used in the research and that feminist literature is cited (Chinn 2003). The research process ensures a balance of power in the relationship between researcher and researched, and consciousness-raising is used as a methodological tool to empower women participants (Bowes 1996, Millen 1997, Punwar 1997, Webb 1993). The research is reported in a way that the reader becomes engaged with women's experiences (Chinn 2003) and the research findings are made available to those who participated in the generation of data. It is also important that the research findings are disseminated widely to women so that the findings can be incorporated into their lives (Webb 1993). Participants are involved in all aspects of the research; hence it is important that researchers consider ways of ending the research so that participants are unharmed and the benefits of the research can be sustained. It is fundamentally important that feminist research also attempts to bring about progressive change in the interests of women.

Feminist theory can guide nurses to explore issues that are relevant to women and nursing, and yet a review of the literature will reveal that in comparison with the total amount of nursing research that is published, the contribution from feminist research is relatively small. Drevdahl (1999) called for nursing research and the development of nursing theories to extend further than the creation of knowledge and have social justice as their goal. Ford-Gilboe and Campbell (1996, p. 173) were also concerned with a narrow focus of feminist nursing research:

Feminist research not only studies women and women's experience within the social context, but it also seeks to help women deal with the issues that are revealed as part of the process. Both the knowledge gained and the research process itself may serve as vehicles for creating social change that enhances lives of women.

A feminist perspective in nursing research can challenge the medical dominance over health care consumers and create a consciousness raising that is necessary to plan and implement change (Drevdahl 1999, Speedy 1991). Feminism provides a framework by which differences such as gender and culture may be incorporated into the design of nursing research. Jackson (1997) contends that feminism is an openly political and transformative process; hence feminist principles can be used in research where the aim is to catalyse changes in nursing practice.

Case study on the use of feminist research principles

The purpose of this section is to demonstrate how feminist principles (shown in italics) can guide nursing research. We illustrate using a research study that aimed to promote the capacity of adult women survivors of child sexual abuse (CSA) who had become addicted to alcohol and/or drugs and subsequently become homeless (van Loon & Kralik 2005a, 2005b and 2005c). Through the research process that spanned 2 years, women participants generated personal resources that enabled them to move into a healthier and more life-affirming future.

The intention was to develop a programme that *facilitated change through action* and to *disseminate* that programme in the form of resources that were sustainable and transferable to similar service settings. The resources *increase understanding* of the issues impacting women survivors of CSA, and those with alcohol, drug and gambling misuse problems as they transition their past and move toward self-management. The resources aim to promote personal *capacity* for this community group and service provider capacity to provide more appropriate responses to the needs that these women have identified.

Feminist research considers how the *social position of the knower* affects what and how they understand. A person's social location is culturally endorsed by such attributes as *gender*, *race*, *ethnicity*, family *relationships*, *social status*, *roles* and *positions*. These attributes are shaped into a social identity that affords the person *power* and status. This identity is subject to sociocultural norms which prescribe the responsibilities, qualities, behaviours, feelings and life-skills which the society believes are proper for that role. The women in this study on child sexual abuse experienced significant social dislocation, as this woman explains:

My Mum used to say to me, 'You've always been weird. You're strange.' The strangeness came from seeing the dislike in her face and reacting to it. I developed another identity. I did it to save myself from being hurt. I've had severe beatings and stood up and said, 'Yeah, come on, go again!' Even though it was killing me inside. I was hurting so much and crying within. It's the face you put on to pretend it doesn't matter, so you can survive emotionally. I think inside all of us there's a little grain of hope that wants to keep trying to save the relationship all the time. There's a little spark that keeps waiting and hoping to find a connection. (van Loon & Kralik 2005c, p. 38)

The groups included women from culturally diverse backgrounds: Indigenous Australians; women from fragmented families – homeless due to violence; and women struggling with addictions. These women were *positioned by society* as problematic and less worthy citizens. The women recognised their 'difference', being fully aware that they did not fit the status and roles of 'normal' members of our community. They had always felt different, as this woman illustrates:

I was very quiet. I did a lot of reading, it was my escape. I didn't get along with other kids, because I was very shy. I was often sick. No one was allowed to come to my place, not that I would have invited them anyway. I never went to anyone's house either. I didn't trust anyone because it wasn't safe to do that. I was tormented at school because I was different. . . I got used to it. . . I was everyone's scapegoat at home and at school. I was just different so I learnt to shut up so I was noticed less. I stopped speaking because that meant less trouble for me. (van Loon & Kralik 2005c, p. 39).

Most had accepted a position of 'less than' and always 'wanting'. They affirmed the norms that went with labels such as 'homeless' and 'addict', viewing themselves as incapable of changing their circumstances. They had been typecast and marginalised by mainstream society as a group who were wasting valuable resources. This common understanding and its concomitant oppressive fate had to be *challenged* if it was to be overcome, then *change* may be possible (van Loon et al 2004).

The research *partnership* was a South Australian community nursing organisation and an organisation that facilitates emergency and transitional supported accommodation, plus a range of service providers to women with complex health and social needs. The main stakeholder groups (women and services) were bought together in discrete groups between 2003 and 2005 using a *participatory action*

research process. We documented the process and articulated the outcomes, so that both would be *transferable* to other settings.

The need to work with women to develop capacity was important. Over 93% of the women coming through the supported accommodation had experienced the trauma of child sexual abuse and as a result, some had used drugs, alcohol and gambling to manage their emotional and physical suffering (van Loon & Kralik 2005a). Thus it was essential that the research method employed built capacity while providing a degree of *liberation* from this oppressive state. Feminist inquiries seek to understand oppression in social groups, and via this understanding, *transform* that situation. The commitment to feminism was one motivation for this research; thus research and action could not be separated. The unashamed goal of emancipatory inquiries is *social change* that *surfaces oppressive processes* so they can be overcome (Freire 1970). Both the research process and the research outcomes must meet this objective. Thus participatory action research was deemed the most appropriate method to meet these goals.

This research took a *feminist standpoint* by representing the experience of child sexual abuse from the perspective of the women CSA survivors, giving *epistemic privilege* and *authority* to their voices. Thus the subject matter generated remained in the *participants' control*. The *language used was theirs* so we could accurately describe and *represent the truth of their experience*. We sought to understand their current social location, role, and the *subjective identity* resulting from labels such as 'homeless', 'unemployed', 'abused', 'addict' etc. It was important to *privilege* the women's voices if we were to gain a reliable understanding of what was required to help these women transition their struggles and their oppressed social position. The goal was to understand the *realities of experiences* constructed by this particular group of women, with the emphasis being on the context in which their lives were lived. In this way, the research was grounded in the actual experiences of the women and was therefore able to *raise the consciousness* of the women who participated. Their understanding was illuminated through the processes of reflecting on and describing their lives, as this participant notes:

I have been here for six months and in that time I kind of believe the hardened shell I had around me about talking about these things has cracked a bit. It was really hard to speak about my life at first, but since the shell cracked, it has been a real release of a lot of pain and pressure within me. (van Loon & Kralik 2005c, p. 8).

These women were disadvantaged, experiencing fundamental disruption in their lives that drove them to misuse alcohol, addictive substances and/or gambling. If we only heard from the service providers' standpoint we would not understand the strengths and human potential present in these women. We would gain a superficial understanding of their experience. *Privileging the standpoint of the women* represents their understandings as socially contingent and allows the women to consider actions they can take to overcome their situation. We took the perspective that *every woman was the expert of her experience* and she knew what she needed to facilitate her healing. We believed and accepted that each woman's story was true and sought to *validate her experiences, empowering* her to work with the strengths in her story.

Our research used a *participatory* perspective where we aimed to help women *reflect* on past experiences and current issues in their lives, *making connections* between past and present in their life story. Finally, each woman was *invited to action* change that might move her toward her preferred future. We did not engineer discussion to a prefixed agenda, although we did seek clarification on discussion to unpack issues as they surfaced. This was done to facilitate understanding. We did not psycho-pathologise the women's addiction/s, or any other behaviour they may have used to cope with their life situations. Instead we viewed these as responses that enabled survival at that time. Through dialogue, perspectives shift, as these women note:

I don't think the reasons for using have disappeared; they will always be there; but the way I have storied those within my head has changed. I think what I

used to treat with contempt, rebellion and anger has changed into something else. I have become more patient and compassionate with myself and others. (Van Loon & Kralik 2005c, p. 18)

I couldn't get emotionally close to anybody. It was like my body would just switch off and I'd just be there, but you know I might as well have been doing something else. Now it's starting to feel like my body's coming back to me and all my emotions and everything's coming together in a more manageable way. (van Loon & Kralik 2005c, p. 31)

As a group, we *discussed* issues raised by the women and these were fed back in written form after each meeting for *reflection* and *considered action*. We listened for what was being said and what was not being said. We paid particular attention to *power constructions, gendered understandings*, choices – or lack thereof, and the practices and structures sustaining reactions and choices. We looked carefully for *barriers and enablers* that impacted upon each woman's capacity to act. This was their story so we tried to *faithfully represent their issues* to the service providers for their action. This service provider speaks about how that process can initiate changes to practice:

I have noticed improvement in my own approach to working with young people. I am changing the way I do assessments (actually considering CSA questions as part of assessment) since I have been partaking in this group. This is due to my heightened awareness. (van Loon & Kralik 2005c, p. 58)

Feminist research says participants are the owners of their story and as such material must be critiqued and validated by the participants. This occurred at every stage of this research process up to publication. It did add workload and expense to the project, which is a challenge in today's competitive funding environment. As researchers we did author and collate the work, but the women owned the final product with great pride as their work. They could look back on the process and see how they had shifted to a position of more personal power, as this woman notes:

What makes up you makes up me, but in different degrees. Everyone has strengths and weaknesses. With the new knowledge I gain, I can build a new sense of who I am – a new beginning each day – always changing, always becoming. I am more than the sum of what happened to me as a child. Much, much more! I am only just beginning to see the real me, and I think I like what I see! (van Loon & Kralik 2005c, p. 86)

Conclusion

Feminist research acknowledges that most women face some form of oppression and exploitation.

Women experience their oppression, struggles and strengths in various ways because of their diverse realities and their identities as women. Within this context of diversity, feminist research celebrates the practical and informs the theoretical. Understanding and knowledge gained from feminist research approaches are more than theory or description; they are based on women making sense of their own lives and facilitating collective action to change their social situation.

EXERCISES

Consider the following questions:

1. Where can feminist theory be identified or located in nursing?
2. What is 'theory'?
3. What is the subject or focus of 'feminist theory' – women? What women?
4. What are the goal(s) or role(s) of feminist theory and feminist research?

References

Bowes A 1996 Evaluating an empowering research strategy: reflections on action-research with South Asian Women. Sociological Research Online 1(1). Available: http://ideas.repec.org/a/sro/srosro/0-1-1.html 28 Sept 2006

Campbell J, Bunting S 1991 Voices and paradigms: Perspectives on critical and feminist theory in nursing. Advances in Nursing Science 13(3): 1–15

Chinn P 2003 Feminist approaches. In: Clare J, Hamilton H (eds.) Writing Research. Churchill Livingstone, London, 61–85

Chinn P. Wheeler C 1985 Feminism and nursing. Nursing Outlook 33: 74–77

Crotty M 1998 Feminism: revisioning the man-made world. In: The Foundations of Social Research. Sage Publications, London: 160–182

Crowley H, Himmelweit S 1992 Knowing Women: Feminism and Knowledge. Polity Press in Association with The Open University, Cambridge

Drevdahl D 1999 Sailing beyond: nursing theory and the person. Advances in Nursing Science 21(4): 1–13

DuBois E 1985 Feminist Scholarship: Kindling in the Groves of Academe. University of Illinois Press, Urbana

Ford-Gilboe M, Campbell J 1996 The mother-headed single-parent family: a feminist critique of the nursing literature. Nursing Outlook 44: 173–183

Freire P 1970 Pedagogy of the Oppressed (translated by Myra Bergman Ramos). Penguin Books, Melbourne

Griffiths M 1995 Feminisms and the Self: The Web of Identity. Routledge, London

Hall J, Stevens P 1991 Rigor in feminist research. Advances in Nursing Science 13(3): 16–29

Henderson D 1995 Consciousness raising in participatory research: Method and methodology for emancipatory nursing inquiry. Advances in Nursing Science 17(3): 58–69

Jackson D 1997 Feminism: a path to clinical knowledge development. Contemporary Nurse 6: 85–91

Kolmar W, Bartkowski F 2000 Feminist Theory. Mayfield, London

Lather P 1988 Feminist perspectives on empowering research methodologies. Women's Studies International Forum 56: 257–277

Lather P 1991 Getting Smart: Feminist Research and Pedagogy Within/in the Postmodern. Routledge, New York

Lumby C 1997 Bad Girls. Allen and Unwin, Sidney

Maguire P 1996 Considering more feminist participatory research: What's congruency got to do with it? Qualitative Inquiry 2(1): 106–118

Maynard M, Purvis J 1994 Researching Women's Lives from a Feminist Perspective. Taylor and Francis, London

Millen D 1997 Some methodological and epistemological issues raised by doing feminist research on non-feminist women.

Sociological Research Online, 2, (3), http://www.socresonline.org.uk/socresonline/2/3/3.html, accessed 28 Sept 2006

Olesen V 1994 Feminisms and models of qualitative research. In: Denzin NK, Lincoln YS (eds) Handbook of Qualitative Research. Sage, Thousand Oaks, CA: 158–174

Puwar N 1997 Reflections on Interviewing Women MPs. Sociological Research Online, 12, (1), http://www.socresonline.org.uk/socresonlin/2/1/4.html, accessed 28 Sept 2006

Scharbo-DeHann M 1994 Connected knowing: Feminist group research. In: Chinn P (ed) Advances in Methods of Inquiry for Nursing. Aspen, Bethesda, MD: 88–101

Smith S 1991 A feminist analysis of constructs of health. In: Neil R, Watts R (eds.) Caring and Nursing: Explorations in Feminist Perspectives. National League for Nursing, New York: 209–225

Speedy S 1991 The contribution of feminist research. In: Gray G, Pratt R (eds) Towards a Discipline of Nursing. (Churchill Livingstone, Melbourne: 191–210

Stanley L, Wise S 1983 Breaking Out: Feminist Consciousness and Feminist Research. Routledge and Kegan Paul, London

van Loon AM, Kralik D 2005a Facilitating Transition after Child Sexual Abuse. Royal District Nursing Service Foundation Research Unit, Catherine House Inc, Centacare, Adelaide

van Loon AM, Kralik D 2005b Reclaiming Myself after Child Sexual Abuse. Royal District Nursing Service Foundation Research Unit, Catherine House Inc, Centacare, Adelaide

van Loon AM, Kralik D 2005c Final Report: Promoting Capacity with Homeless Women Survivors of Child Sexual Abuse Misusing Alcohol, Drugs or Gambling. Royal District Nursing Service Foundation Research Unit, Catherine House Inc, Alcohol Education and Rehabilitation Foundation, Adelaide

van Loon AM, Koch T, Kralik D 2004 Care for female survivors of child sexual abuse in emergency departments. Accident and Emergency Nursing Journal 12(4): 208–214

Webb C 1993 Feminist research: definitions, methodology, methods and evaluation. Journal of Advanced Nursing 18(3): 416–423

Chapter 5

Historical Research

Gerard M. Fealy

Introduction

The American scholar Sandelowski (2000) observed that 'writing history is no easy task' and that 'those attempting it have ... to write against the prevailing view in nursing of worthy scholarship as exclusively "scientific" '. In this observation, Sandelowski is referring to the fact that historical scholarship in nursing may not be valued as a legitimate form of scientific inquiry, when compared with other forms of research. Thankfully, this bias is not widespread, and the increasing output of high quality historical studies in nursing is a testament to the fact that this area of scholarship is expanding and is attracting research funding.

One of the aims of this chapter is to demonstrate that, just like any form of research, historical research is a systematic and rigorous method of inquiry and that the pursuit of knowledge of history is as legitimate as the pursuit of knowledge of present-day phenomena and events in clinical practice, education or service management. It will be seen that historical research differs from other forms of research only in its subject matter, in the form that its data assume, and in its method of reportage. While the relationship between theory and method may be based on diverse assumptions about the role of the researcher and about the sourcing and interpretation of evidence, historical research demands no less scientific rigour than other forms of research. Because the theory and method of historical inquiry is itself the subject of much debate within the discipline, this chapter also aims to introduce the reader to salient aspects of this debate by reference to some seminal writers in the philosophy of history.

What is history?

For the purpose of this chapter, history is considered to be both the process and the product of scholarship, and historical research in nursing is thus one expression of 'the scholarship of inquiry' in nursing (AACN 1999). History is a systematic process of discovering evidence about the past and of providing a written account of that evidence in the form of an historical narrative. Accordingly, the process of historical research comprises a number of distinct but interrelated activities. These are: the identification, gathering and recording of historical evidence, the analysis and interpretation of that evidence, and writing the historical narrative. Writing the narrative is a fundamental element of *doing* history and is thus a part of the method of historical inquiry.

Relationship between theory and method

A rich debate concerning the nature of historical inquiry has ensued for much of the latter half of the twentieth century. According to Jenkins, this 'history debate' is concerned with whether historical knowledge can ever be obtained through objective inquiry or whether it is an interpretive, intersubjective process (Jenkins 1991). This debate is best exemplified in the views of seminal writers in the philosophy of history, such as Elton and Carr.

For Elton, the historian and philosopher of history, historical method consists of a critical examination of the available evidence, and, ideally, *only* that evidence, to reconstruct the events of history and their causes (Roberts 1998). What distinguishes history from other forms of inquiry is the role of evidence in generating, delimiting, and validating the assertions and conclusions of historians, and any interpretations of the past on the part of the historian should be permitted to emerge only from the evidence to hand. History is the rigorous pursuit of facts that are to be presented without the interpretive intrusion of the historian; governed by the evidence

of the past, historical inquiry should, therefore, be balanced and objective (Elton 1967). Elton's position is not to deny the role of the historian in the process of historical inquiry, but to caution against writing a narrative that is based on limited evidence, conjecture, and subjective bias. In this 'common sense', empiricist view of history, the facts are seen as *a priori*, separate and independent of the historian, and the interpretations and conclusions are the historian's way of presenting the facts (Carr 1987).

In his seminal book *What is History?*, Carr challenges this empiricist view of history, arguing that the historian plays a central role in the process and the product of historical inquiry:

> *When we attempt to answer the question 'What is history?' our answer, consciously or unconsciously, reflects our position in time, and forms part of our answer to the broader question what view we take of the society in which we live. (Carr 1987, p. 8)*

On the role of the historian in dealing with historical 'facts', Carr remarks:

> *It used to be said that facts speak for themselves. This is, of course, untrue. The facts speak only when the historian calls on them; it is he who decides to which facts to give the floor, and in what order or context ... The historian is necessarily selective ... The element of interpretation enters into every fact of history ... The historian ... is balanced between fact and interpretation, between fact and value. He cannot separate them (Carr 1987, pp. 11, 13 and 132).*

For Carr (1987), history is the product of the historian's interpretation of available facts; historical inquiry is imbued with the particular view of the historian, is conducted for a purpose, and is as much a representation of the historian's perspective as it is about true facts.

These perspectives reflect a type of art–science distinction that are rendered passé in a postmodern perspective, which calls into question the possibility that objective historical truth can ever exist (Rafferty 1997). Thus, from a postmodern perspective, when subjected to interpretation, the historical evidence may have multiple meanings (Brooks 2000). Moreover, as a form of thought, postmodernism rejects any kind of narrative, such as the Marxist critique of capitalism, and is antipathetic to sociological abstractions such as class, capitalism, and even society itself (Foster 1997). It rejects notions of historical determinism, denies that history is purposive and 'that it is possible to have a definitive knowledge of the origins, causes, tendencies, and fundamental constitutive elements of history' (Foster 1997, p. 185). This scepticism is extended to a rejection of the certainties of modernism, as exemplified in the scientific method of cause and effect. Within the discipline of history, postmodernism does not confine itself to disciplinary boundaries and may readily cross the boundaries of many disciplines in the pursuit of historical scholarship.

The discipline of history and nursing

Interest in history extends to all cultures, and any differences in cultural approaches to history generally occur in different historiographical traditions (Burke 2002). Burke (2002) identifies a number of propositions or 'theses', which characterise Western historical thought and which represent the sort of ideas, assumptions or emphases within the tradition. These 'peculiarities of the West' include:

- A 'linear' view of history that assumes that change through time is usually for the better.
- A view that each historical period has its own 'cultural style' and that cultural styles change over time.
- A concern with the particular as opposed to the general.
- An assumption that certain groups, such as families, religious orders, social classes, and so forth, play a role in historical events; this emphasis on 'collective agency' produces a 'history without names'.
- A preoccupation with the ways and methods for arriving at knowledge about the past.
- A concern with historical explanation; this causal approach is modelled on the natural scientific approach and assumes that there are certain

laws of history, such as laws of human behaviour, that account for historical events.
- A pride in objectivity and in the ideal of impartiality in historical inquiry.
- A tendency to describe history in quantitative terms, in such areas as population, demography and economics.

It is possible to extract some of the trends in Western historical thinking in the ways that nursing history has been conducted. For example, the first major histories of nursing written in the early years of the twentieth century characterised nursing history as a history of development and progress (Rafferty 1992). With its interest in social groups, such as social classes, the professions, religious orders and women as a distinct social group, nursing history also emphasises 'collective agency'. Nevertheless, nursing history also places great emphasis on the role that individuals played in historical events inside and outside of nursing and is a particular characteristic of nursing history.

Echoing Burke's exposition of the assumptions of Western historiography, Lynaugh and Reverby (1987) refer to the 'myths of history', or the common assumptions concerning the nature of nursing history that can give rise to problems with the quality and credibility of historical research. Among these assumptions are that historical research is about seeking a single truth or cause, that history must be about important events and important people, and that good history will arise from good facts. In cautioning against adherence to such assumptions, Lynaugh and Reverby (1987) argue that there may be multiple forms of explanation for historical evidence, some of which 'fit' better than others, and they remark:

Historical scholarship is judged by its ability to assemble the best facts and generate the most cogent explanation of a given situation or period. (Lynaugh & Reverby 1987, p. 68)

According to Connolly (2004), the two methodological paradigmatic traditions in the discipline of history in the twentieth century were 'political history' and 'social history'. The former presented history through the lens of politics and the state, important events, and 'great' people, and it represented a consensus, deterministic and somewhat celebratory approach. The latter, in contrast, emphasised the lives of ordinary people and it approached history in a more critical way using interpretive frames of reference that included gender, class, race and ethnicity. Connolly points out that, while social history was the dominant paradigm after the 1960s, the boundaries between political and social history became blurred in the 1990s, with each paradigm drawing on the contribution of the other, resulting in the emergence of a new synthesis of social and political history. Connolly contends that the broader history debates and the shifting methodological trends in the discipline are of concern to nurse historians and that the newly synthesised paradigm of political history can provide nurse historians with new subject matter and new interpretive frames of reference when studying nursing history.

Doing history

Lewinson (1999, p. 198) writes that the researcher who chooses historical methods 'must exhibit more than just a curiosity about the past, [must] ... formulate a thesis about relationships among ideas, events, institutions, or people in the past', and must engage in questioning, reasoning, probing and piecing together clues to discover meanings in the past. This suggests that history is not merely about discovering and recording facts, but involves a number of processes, including generating one or more specific research questions, focusing on evidence to be discovered, assuming a critical stance, and using analytical, interpretive and narrative skills.

The research question provides focus and direction for the entire study, while the review of literature identifies other related scholarship and can contribute to refinement of the research question(s) and the methods. The review of literature also provides the historian with a better understanding of the topic and the historical period, assists with the identification of gaps in the field and can provide information on potential methodological difficulties, such as limited sources of evidence or multiple possibilities in the interpretation of evidence (Lewinson 1999). Data collection involves a search for information on the topic of interest and this information is collectively referred to as historical primary sources (Fig. 5.1).

The 'data' of historical inquiry: archives and sources

While historical inquiry relies on reliable evidence, the historian must acknowledge that, as with all research, the evidence is finite, that interpretations and conclusions can be gleaned from 'samples' of the evidence and that the particular can be at least partially representative of the general. The evidence for historical research is located in diverse sites and is often interspersed with other archives and repositories, such as medical and institutional archives (Fealy & O'Doherty 2005, Ó hÓgartaigh 1999).

Sandelowski (2000) remarks that writing nursing history is not easy because the historian must 'read between the lines to find nurses'. Nurses are not visible partly because there is often little recorded evidence of nurses' ideas, since these were frequently transmitted in the oral rather than the written medium, and even when nurses recorded their work in nursing notes, they were doing so to support and record the work of physicians (Sandelowski 2000). Moreover, the 'voice' of nursing was seldom heard in professional debate concerning social policy and practice in health care.

The historian may have to look for evidence of nursing history to sources in which nurses and nursing were the *objects* of commentary and discourse. Such evidence may be found in the institutional minute book, the hospital annual report, the parliamentary committee report, the early textbook, or in artefacts, such as photographs and films. The historian must frequently retrieve nursing history from sources that do not appear to be related directly to nursing. In her historical study of the relationship between gender, technology and nursing, Sandelowski (2000, p. 15) crossed many disciplinary

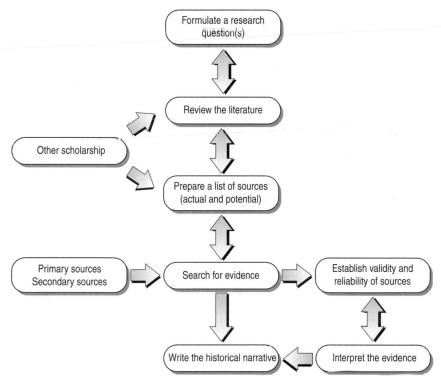

Figure 5.1 – *Historical method.*

boundaries in her quest for sources; in her own words, she used 'whatever sources were available to me to rescue and ... redeem nursing from the pages of history and technology studies.'

Fortunately for historians, people in the past were quite likely to communicate and record both the important and the mundane events in their lives. Documentary evidence is thus one of the principal sources of evidence for historians, and is found in books and treatises, official records, such as minutes of meetings and parliamentary records, reports in newspapers and journals, personal journals, diaries and letters. The voices of those who could not write because of illiteracy may be found in other narrative forms, such as the song, the story, the film or in artefacts, such as clothing and household objects.

Secondary sources refers to those historical sources that have already been discovered, analysed and interpreted by other historians and are constituted as published books, biographies, articles and

monographs, or as unpublished materials such as theses (Fealy 1999). The content of a secondary source can serve a number of important functions in the process of historical research; it can provide a good indication of the range and location of primary sources and it can provide the historian with a particular perspective on an aspect of history that can inform their study. However, while secondary sources may provide the material to construct a complete historical narrative, secondary sources by themselves are insufficient in the conduct of historical inquiry and should be used principally to assist in the construction of the narrative.

When conducting historical research, it is necessary to establish the reliability and validity of primary sources. These aspects of methodological rigour are necessary to be satisfied that evidence is authentic, generated at a particular point in time and representative of the historical period and the event or phenomenon under investigation. The validity of the evidence is determined by external criticism, which involves establishing whether it is authentic or trustworthy and not spurious. This may require further investigation to determine the original source of the evidence and the purpose of its generation.

The reliability of evidence is a measure of its capacity to illuminate the historical event or phenomenon of interest (Fealy 1999). This involves internal criticism, or examining its *content* with reference to its credibility as evidence for the event or phenomenon (Sernecky 1990). It may not be possible to establish the reliability and validity of a single source and both internal and external criticism may require corroboration of the evidence with evidence from one or more additional primary sources or two or more secondary sources (Sernecky 1990). Determining the validity of primary source evidence is often easier than determining its reliability, especially when the evidence is held in a reputable collection, such as a national or state archive (Keeling 2002).

Oral history

Oral history may be considered as both a method of data collection and a form of primary source evidence that is generated by recording the spoken words of persons deemed to hold hitherto unavailable information that is worth preserving (Church & Johnson 1995). Oral history is an important tool for historical research as it provides testimonies of those who experienced history at first hand. The testimonies of witnesses to or participants in events give unique information from the perspective of the individual who lived through the history being described. While oral testimonies represent individuals' recollections and interpretations of events, and while they are a valid source, they too need to be corroborated with other documentary evidence.

Oral testimony can provide clarification of written evidence, can provide missing evidence, and the interviewee can interpret events, personalities and relationships in ways that may otherwise be unobtainable (Biedermann 2001). However, oral history is not without its deficiencies, the most obvious being the reliability of the source, in terms of the interviewee's memory, and the likelihood of personal bias in recalling and narrating past events. However, the personal bias of the narrator may in itself constitute valid historical evidence (Everett 2006).

When recording oral testimonies, the standards of rigour and the normal ethical guidelines on research interviewing apply. Taking oral histories may involve interviewing older nurses and, in this regard, the historian should be sensitive and compassionate, not merely with the aim of eliciting good research evidence, but also of acknowledging the contribution of the interviewees to the profession and of promoting intergenerational solidarity and connectedness (Church & Johnson 1995).

Analysis and interpretation

Elton argues that all events in history happened in context, in particular conditions and circumstances of human thought and human action and that context influenced and constrained, rather than determined or directed, human thought and action (Roberts 1998). When interpreting a primary source it is, therefore, necessary to analyse it at the levels of both *content* and *context*. In the case of documentary evidence, such as a letter, the researcher needs to examine not only what was written – the text – but also the context and circumstances in which the letter was written. This may include consideration of the writer's motivation, the role of letter writing in the period in which it was written, and so forth.

Aside from the text of a documentary primary source, there may also be a subtext. The subtext represents those hidden aspects of content that can reveal or exemplify an ideological position, a political manoeuvre, or a wider social process, such as gender or class conflict. Similarly, in the case of an artefact such as a photograph, both the subject matter of the photograph and the context in which the photograph was taken need to be considered. While photography is a medium for recording images of people and events, it is also a social device that serves sub-textual functions. Frequently, photographing nurses served functions that went beyond the mere recording of the subjects' images, and could be used for a variety of purposes, including nursing recruitment or for conveying a certain image to the public about a particular institution or about the discipline of nursing itself (Fealy 2006).

In the interpretive process, the historian needs to take account of the conditions of the *particular*, to ascertain the particular *conditions* and circumstances under which an historical primary source was generated, and to develop an understanding of the social context within which the source was generated, and this will generally involve reading the work of other historians. This is particularly important when studying nursing history, since the development of nursing has always been bound up with wider social phenomena, such as gender and class relationships, the development of professions, economics, the emergence of the welfare state, technology, macropolitics, as well as the development of ideas.

In the interpretive process, it is possible to 'frame the evidence' within analytical perspectives, such as those offered by Marx and Foucault (Fealy & O'Doherty 2005). Such perspectives provide explanatory frameworks that inform interpretations of primary sources, and this framing of the evidence can offer a range of possibilities (Drudy & Lynch 1993). A good example of this framing of evidence is Hallam's historical study of the image of the nurse in popular and professional media, which she situated within the theoretical framework of feminist cultural studies (Hallam 2000). Hallam was able to draw on a range of disciplinary perspectives in such areas as sociology and media and cultural studies, and the feminist perspective also permitted self-reflexivity in the process of inquiry and narration.

For some historians, the aim is to record and relate the events of the past as a way of filling gaps in scholarship and of making visible those nurses who have not been visible in extant scholarship. Thus, in her introduction to her study of nursing, nuns and hospitals in the nineteenth century, Nelson writes:

I look closely at religious nurses, their work, and its impact, aiming to integrate the history of religious and secular nurses into the story of the emergence of professional nursing. The intention is neither critical nor celebratory ... It is historical observation. (Nelson 2001, p. 1)

Subject matter for historians

The journal *Nursing History Review* provides examples of the range of topics that are the subject of recent historical research in nursing. Topics include the professionalising of nursing in nineteenth-century London (Helmstadter 2003), a history of the Dublin Metropolitan Technical School for Nurses (Fealy 2005), nursing collaboration in a concentration camp (Benedict 2003), the tuberculosis preventorium movement in the United States (Connolly 2002), and recruitment to the Army Nursing Corps for the Vietnam War (Vuic 2006). Another subject area is the biographical study; McGann's (1992) study of eight women who influenced the development of modern nursing and Hector's (1973) comprehensive biography of Ethel Bedford Fenwick are good examples of the genre in nursing history. The development of modern hospital nursing is another rich source for nurse historians; Currie's study of fever hospitals and fever nurses (Currie 2005) and Ardern's (2002) study of some notable hospital matrons in England are good examples in this regard.

Research example

Keeling A 2004 Blurring the boundaries between medicine and nursing: Coronary care nursing, circa the 1960s. Nursing History Review 12: 139–164.

Arleen Keeling's study describes the inception and proliferation of coronary care units (CCUs) in the 1960s. The researcher draws on a range of historical primary sources, including medical and nursing journals of the period. She also uses the oral history method to record the testimonies of a number of former nurses from the Presbyterian Hospital in Philadelphia who played a central role in the development of one of the first coronary care units in the United States. Keeling describes the post-war developments in heart disease and its management and discusses the relationship between nursing and medicine at the time of the inception of coronary care units. The author provides details of the ways that nursing care and medical care were combined in the care for patients in the new clinical setting of the CCU, and through the voices of the first CCU nurses, discusses the development of a new nursing role in the period. Through her historical narrative, Keeling demonstrates how a new professional relationship between nursing and medicine developed and how the 'artificial disciplinary boundaries between medicine and nursing were blurred when nurses assumed the technological skills of cardiac monitoring and cardiac defibrillation in the early coronary care units' (Keeling 2004, p. 139).

Conclusion

Historical research is a distinct method of scientific inquiry and is an important part of the scholarship of discovery for the discipline of nursing. It is concerned with the past and, like any systematic method of inquiry, it comprises a number of distinct activities, including the formulation of a research question, a review of literature, collection, analysis and interpretation of findings, or 'evidence', and writing a report of the findings in the form of a historical narrative. The debates and trends in the wider discipline of history and concerning the nature of historical inquiry get reflected in debates and trends within nursing history. The subject matter for researching the history of nursing is rich and diverse and, to date, there is evidence of a substantial and growing body of scholarship using the methods of historical inquiry.

EXERCISES

1. Consider the views of Elton and Carr in the light of debates about the nature of scientific inquiry, and in particular, about the distinctions between qualitative and quantitative research. Consider whether there are any similarities in these debates with the history debate.
2. Consider Connolly's (2004) assertion that the new paradigm of political history provides new subject matter for nursing history, and list three topics related to political history that incorporate and/or are of relevance to the history of nursing.
3. Consider the physical environment in which you work and list any documentary materials or artefacts that might still exist to provide evidence of nursing's social history or nursing practices in the past.
4. Select a piece of published historical research and look for references to primary sources within the text. Identify three to five examples and try to identify from the author's notes on sources where these primary sources are deposited.
5. Write down three topics that you consider might be appropriate subject matter for a historical study. For example, consider an aspect of clinical practice that could be studied using historical method, or think of a nurse, practising or retired, whom you consider could be the subject of a biographical study.

References

AACN (American Association of Colleges of Nursing) 1999 Defining scholarship for the discipline of nursing. Journal of Professional Nursing 15(6): 372–376

Ardern P 2002 When Matron Ruled. Robert Hale, London

Benedict S 2003 The nadir of nursing: nurse-perpetrators of the Ravensbrück Concentration Camp. Nursing History Review 11: 129–146

Biedermann N 2001 The voices of days gone by: advocating the use of oral history in nursing. Nursing Inquiry 8: 61–62

Brooks J E 2000 Ghost of the past: capturing history and the history of nursing. International History of Nursing Journal 5(0): 00–41

Burke P 2002 Western historical thinking in a global perspective – 10 theses. In: Rüsen J (ed), Western Historical Thinking: An Intercultural Debate. Berghahn Books, Oxford: 15–30

Carr E H 1987 What is History?, 2nd edn. Penguin Books, London

Church O M, Johnson M L 1995 Worth remembering: The process and products of oral history. International History of Nursing Journal 1(1): 19–31

Connolly C A 2002 Nurses: The early twentieth century tuberculosis preventorium's 'connecting link'. Nursing History Review 10: 139–164

Connolly C A 2004 Beyond social history: new approaches to understanding the state of and the State in nursing history. Nursing History Review 12: 5–24

Currie M R 2005 Fever hospitals and fever nurses: a national service: a British social history of fever nursing. Routledge, London

Drudy S, Lynch K 1993 Schools and Society in Ireland. Gill and Macmillan, Dublin

Elton G R 1967 The Practice of History. Sydney University Press, London

Everett S E 2006 Oral history: techniques and procedures. Online. Available: http://www.army.mil/cmh-pg/books/oral.htm 16 Jan 2006

Fealy G M 1999 Historical research: a legitimate methodology for nursing research in Ireland. Nursing Review 17(1&2): 24–29

Fealy G M 2005 'A place for the better technical education of nurses': The Dublin Metropolitan Technical School for Nurses, 1893–1969. Nursing History Review 13: 27–43

Fealy G M 2006 A History of Apprenticeship Nurse Training in Ireland. Routledge, London

Fealy G M, O'Doherty M 2005 Lessons from history: Historical inquiry in Irish nursing and midwifery. In: Fealy G M (ed) Care to Remember: Nursing and Midwifery in Ireland. Mercier Press, Cork: 11–27

Foster J B 1997 In defence of history. In: Wood E M, Foster J B (eds) In Defence of History: Marxism and the Postmodern Agenda. Monthly Review Press, New York: 184–194

Hallam J 2000 Nursing the Image: Media, Culture and Professional Identity. Routledge, London

Hector W 1973 The Work of Mrs Bedford Fenwick and the Rise of Professional Nursing. Royal College of Nursing, London

Helmstadter C 2003 A real tone: professionalizing nursing in nineteenth-century London. Nursing History Review 11: 2–30

Jenkins K 1991 Rethinking history. Routledge, London

Keeling A 2002 Historical research and WOC nursing: A strange and wonderful relationship. Journal of Wound, Ostomy and Continence Nursing 29(4): 180–183

Keeling A 2004 Blurring the boundaries between medicine and nursing: Coronary care nursing, circa the 1960s. Nursing History Review 12: 139–164

Lewinson S 1999 Historical research method. In: Streubert H J, Carpenter D R (eds) Qualitative Research in Nursing: Advancing the Humanistic Imperative, 2nd edn. Lippincott, Philadelphia: 197–213

Lynaugh J, Reverby S 1987 Thoughts on the nature of nursing history. Nursing Research 36: 68–70

McGann S 1992 The Battle of the Nurses: A Study of Eight Women Who Influenced the Development of Professional Nursing. Scutari Press, London

Nelson S 2001 Say Little, Do Much: Nursing, Nuns, and Hospitals in the Nineteenth Century. University of Pennsylvania Press, Philadelphia

Ó hÓgartaigh M 1999 Archival sources for the history of professional women in late-nineteenth and early-twentieth century Ireland. Journal of the Irish Society for Archives 6(1): 23–25

Rafferty A M 1992 Historical perspectives. In: Robinson K, Vaughan B (eds) Knowledge for Nursing Practice. Butterworth-Heinemann, Oxford: 25–41

Rafferty A M 1997 Writing and reflexivity in nursing history. Nurse Researcher 5(2): 5–16

Roberts G 1998 Defender of the faith: Geoffrey Elton and the philosophy of history. Chronicon 2 R1: 1–22 Online. Available: http://www.ucc.ie/chronicon/elton.htm 14 Jan 2006

Sandelowski M 2000 Devices and Desires: Gender, Technology and American Nursing. The University of North Carolina Press, London

Sernecky M T 1990 Historiography: A legitimate research methodology for nursing. Advances in Nursing Science 12(4): 1–10

Vuic K D 2006 Officer. nurse. woman: Army Nurse Corps recruitment for the Vietnam War. Nursing History Review 14: 111–159

Chapter 6

Evaluation Research

Ian Norman and Charlotte Humphrey

- What is evaluation?
- Origins
- Evaluation and research
- Evaluating complex interventions
- Realistic evaluation
- Conclusion

What is evaluation?

There is a range of approaches to evaluation, each asking different questions, employing different methods, focusing on different aspects of the initiatives they investigate and being undertaken with different ends in view. The three key variants we summarise here are summative, illuminative and formative evaluation.

Summative evaluation

The most familiar and celebrated mode of evaluation in the health arena is the experimental study, ideally in the form of the randomised controlled trial (Chapter 18), whose purpose is to answer questions about effectiveness in respect of a specific intervention. The question at issue in such a study is, does it work? The criteria for effectiveness clearly vary according to what the intervention is intended to achieve. Evaluation may focus, for example, on the success of a treatment for head lice, or the *acceptability* to patients and staff of a new appointments system.

Sometimes interventions are compared with one another in respect of several different parameters of effectiveness at the same time. The question then is: which works better? For example, an economic evaluation study may assess the relative costs and benefits (in terms of efficacy or other desirable features) of two different modes of treatment of the same condition. A third form of evaluative question is, does it work well enough? For example, decisions about whether to offer a new screening test to a particular at-risk population group may depend on assessment of the likely health gain, taking into account the consequences of false positive and false negative results, likely level of take-up and risks associated with the test itself. In other cases, findings from evaluation studies may be used to inform decisions about how to distribute resources between different areas of care. The question then is whether the benefits gained from investing in one particular activity are sufficient to justify the opportunity costs.

In experimental studies, the outcomes of interest are specified in advance, reflecting the objectives of the intervention. However, it is increasingly recognised that interventions at any level are likely to have both intended and unanticipated effects. In some cases, the latter may prove key in deciding whether or not the intervention is worthwhile or unacceptable. Where such a possibility is anticipated, the first question may be a much more open one, simply, what are the effects of the intervention? Evaluation studies that set out to identify *all* significant outcomes of an intervention are necessarily more exploratory and descriptive, since they must collect information across a wide range of relevant parameters that may not lend themselves to formal measurement. However, all investigations designed to assess or identify impacts may be grouped in the category of *summative* or *outcome* evaluation studies. They share the aim of informing decisions, for example, whether or not an intervention or new way of working should be repeated, continued, extended or applied elsewhere. We consider the experimental approach to evaluation in more detail later in this chapter.

Illuminative evaluation

In traditional experiments the focus of attention is on specifying what is to be done and then measuring the effects. Relatively little attention is given to monitoring the actual process of implementation, since the procedures are presumed to be carried out as specified and any effects are assumed to be attributable to known events. This approach, where the process of implementation remains largely unexamined, has been called the 'black box' model of evaluation. However, in a context like health care, where interventions to improve services are often relatively complex and take place in an uncontrolled environment, such assumptions cannot so easily be made.

In these circumstances it may be unclear how or why results came about, or to what they may be attributed. In recognition of these problems, there is increasing appreciation of the benefits of tracking the implementation process in detail, checking whether what is supposed to happen at each stage actually occurs and asking if so, why so, if not, why not, so that the eventual outcomes can be better understood. This type of study is known as *illuminative* evaluation – it opens up the black box, casting light on how, why and in what circumstances particular outcomes are achieved. Such studies help specify which elements in the process are essential to achieving success and what contextual features in the environment may facilitate or obstruct progress.

Formative evaluation

Elements of both the evaluative approaches just outlined are also frequently employed during the development of an intervention or programme of work for a different purpose, which is not to make judgements about its overall value or applicability for use elsewhere, but to improve and refine the ongoing implementation process. This monitoring and scrutiny of progress is called *formative* evaluation. Its role is to inform those involved in delivering and developing the intervention about how things are going and identify what aspects need to be tweaked or more fundamentally reconsidered. While questions about the effectiveness of particular elements of the intervention may be asked, formal experiments are unlikely to be undertaken in formative evaluation, since the objective is not to determine whether something works in general, but how well it is working in the present case. For such purposes, formative evaluation is more likely to make use of reflective cycles for quality improvement such as plan–do–study act (Langley et al 1996). Methods used in illuminative evaluation, such as, for example, asking participants to make notes on their experiences of particular events, may be used in formative evaluation, to provide information and explanation about what took place, and to identify problems.

Origins

The origins of evaluation owe much to Popper (1945), who advocated 'piecemeal social engineering', that is the introduction of modest interventions to deal with social problems, together with procedures to check that these interventions are having their intended effects, and also any unintended or unwanted effects (Tilley 2000). Popper's approach was in contrast to the utopian social engineering advocated by neo-Marxists and revolutionaries of his time, of which Popper was deeply suspicious. The danger of utopian social engineering, in Popper's view, was that it was likely to produce unintended, uncontrollable consequences, which do more harm than good. In contrast, piecemeal social engineering proceeds through a process of trial and error learning whereby the theories built into well-targeted social reforms, designed to tackle particular social problems, are checked, refined and improved, through a series of social experiments. Such experiments would, according to Popper, produce measurable social benefits and contribute to the development of social science. As Popper put it:

> The only course for the social sciences is to … tackle the practical problems of our time with the help of the theoretical methods which are fundamentally the same in all sciences. I mean the methods of trial and error, of inventing hypotheses which can be practically tested, and of submitting these to practical tests. A social technology is needed whose results can be tested by piecemeal social engineering. (Popper 1945, p. 222)

Campbell, as Popper before him, saw evaluation and social reform as hand in hand. In his influential paper 'Reforms as experiments', Campbell (1969) set out the role of experimentation in evaluation studies, which was to evaluate the effectiveness of social reforms and thereby contribute to our understanding of 'what works'. This knowledge might then be drawn on to inform future social programmes to address specific problems.

These ideas were picked up wholesale by policy makers from the 1960s, helped by the US government setting aside a proportion of the budget of the many social programmes initiated at the time, for evaluation. Thus, evaluation research became an industry.

Evaluation and research

Some of the research designs discussed elsewhere in this book are methods of evaluation. The great majority of the other design, data collection techniques and methods of analysis covered in other chapters have also been used in evaluation studies, and many, such as interviews and surveys, are regularly employed. This is unsurprising, since evaluation studies need to obtain valid, reliable and trustworthy data and to draw convincing, accurate and defensible conclusions. However, the fact that evaluation studies do use research methods does not mean that all evaluation is research.

A basic definition of research is that it uses systematic procedures to generate new knowledge or build theory that has generalisable applicability. Properly conducted experimental studies are often seen as the paradigm case of research as defined in these terms. However, generalisability is often not a priority for those commissioning or undertaking evaluation. Hence many evaluation studies are not designed to deliver in this respect. One of the commonest reasons to undertake evaluation is to provide external stakeholders with evidence as to whether the initiative or programme is proceeding according to expectations. Whether the achievements are repeatable elsewhere may be of secondary concern. Another frequent purpose of evaluative work is to collect information for use in a formative way to develop the capacity of the initiative to meet its own objectives. Again, the preoccupation of the participants is likely to be merely with immediate local application of the results.

Moreover, the fact that evaluation is driven by other imperatives often means that the conditions under which it is undertaken may be less than ideal. For example, pressure for quick results may encourage premature curtailment of data collection. Concerns about reputation may impose constraints on honest reporting, especially when results are not positive. When research is not a priority, it may be difficult to allocate the time or resources to do things thoroughly enough for findings from informal formative evaluation to stand up to standards of external scrutiny.

Nevertheless, as already indicated, some forms of evaluation, such as randomised controlled trials, are specifically designed to support generalisations about effectiveness. Other approaches, such as realist evaluation (a variant of what we have referred to as illuminative evaluation), which is discussed in more detail below, are designed to generate theoretical understandings of what works, for whom, in what circumstances thereby generating theories about causative mechanisms that have the potential for broader application. Finally, evaluation studies sometimes produce outcomes of more general interest because they involve analysis of unusual data sets, or generate investigations that would not otherwise be undertaken.

The debate between advocates of summative evaluation and illuminative evaluation is particularly relevant to the evaluation of nursing services. A feature of these is that they are often 'complex' in that they comprise a number of components that act both independently and interdependently. Our aim in the remainder of this chapter is to consider the limitations of summative evaluation with respect to the evaluation of complex interventions.

Evaluating complex interventions

As described above, the 'gold-standard' approach to summative evaluation, that is establishing the effects of an 'intervention', involves experimentation, whereby the evaluator constructs equivalent experimental and control groups, applies the intervention to the experimental group alone and compares the changes that have taken place between the two groups. Ideally, there should be random allocation and sufficient numbers of subjects to ensure that there are no differences between the two groups before the intervention is applied.

Where random allocation is not practicable, quasi-experimental designs are acceptable. In such cases experimental and control communities are selected so as to be as similar as possible. In both experimental and quasi-experimental designs if the expected change occurs in the experimental, but not in the control condition, and there are no unwanted side effects associated with the experimental group, then it can be concluded that the intervention is effective and there are grounds for its more general application.

Whilst there are a variety of experimental designs, some of considerable complexity (see, for example, Portney & Watkins 1993), the basic principles described above apply.

What are complex interventions?

Summative evaluation is well suited to simple interventions, such as evaluating the efficacy of new drugs on individuals. However, many interventions with which nurses are concerned are not straightforward. Many interventions are 'complex' in that they comprise a number of components that act both independently and interdependently. Typically, these interventions are:

- hard to define or control;
- not received passively, but are modified by the people they impact on;
- powerfully affected by structural and cultural contexts and by interpersonal influence;
- constantly under negotiation, with respect to their goals, means and objectives, and are not stable over time;
- conducted in the midst of and influenced by other programmes (past and present);
- subject to constant self-scrutiny and feedback (including that from any formal evaluation) and this itself transforms the intervention;

never alike in different incarnations, although a limited repertoire of comparable mechanisms for change are generally identifiable.

As noted by evaluators of Health Action Zones (Judge & Bauld 2001), such characteristics pose a number of challenges for evaluators. For example:

- It is difficult (perhaps impossible) to measure/ monitor all the factors and contingencies that may influence the conduct and outcome of evaluation.
- It is difficult to identify, separate and compare treatment and control sites or settings.
- It is difficult to ascribe cause and effect, to identify core mechanisms or to say what would have happened in the absence of the intervention.

Examples of complex interventions include: interventions at level of individual patients, such as cognitive behaviour therapy delivered by nurse therapists, in which not only the treatment techniques but the personality and approach of the individual therapist are important; organisational or service improvements, such as the introduction of an incontinence nurse specialist into a hospital; interventions designed to improve the competence and performance of individual nurses, such as education programmes; and interventions designed to improve the health of populations, such as no smoking and other health promotion campaigns.

Opening the black box

Complex interventions raise the question of what mechanisms within the intervention create its effect. This is not a problem for classical experimental evaluators with respect to simple interventions. If it is clear to those who read the evaluator's report how the intervention can be transported and put into place in other contexts, then it might be argued, quite reasonably, that it is not essential to discover the precise mechanisms of action. In the case of complex evaluations, it is rarely possible to recreate the conditions under which the intervention was first implemented and essential mechanisms may inadvertently be lost.

There seems to be reasonable consensus between evaluators that, in the case of complex interventions,

it is important to establish by what specific ingredients a complex intervention is effective. However, evaluators vary in how these ingredients are discovered. Below we compare the very different approach to the problem of complex interventions from within and outwith the classical experimental evaluation tradition.

The classical tradition

The Medical Research Council (2000) propose a well-developed approach to evaluating complex interventions, from within the experimental evaluation tradition. This involves a framework comprising a sequential series of phases of investigation, together with the objectives to be met at each phase. The phases, summarised in Figure 6.1, are described below.

(1) 'Pre-clinical' or theoretical phase. This phase involves identification of mechanisms of action that explain how the intervention being evaluated should have the effect(s) expected. Researchers may draw upon formal theory of, for example, individual or organisational behaviour or may need to rely upon informal evidence which helps to promote or inhibit change in the behaviour of health care professionals or patients; for example what is known about organisational constraints or patients' or health professionals' beliefs. Insights about the theoretical basis for an intervention can inform the kind of intervention needed and aspects of the evaluation design. This phase is particularly important with respect to interventions that are novel, or not in widespread use, and for which mechanisms of action are little understood.

(2) Phase I or 'modelling'. The second phase builds on the first by modelling the essential components of an intervention, their interrelationships and how the proposed mechanisms of action relate to these components and to either surrogate or final outcomes. Thus, the aim is to predict how these components and mechanisms work together. Modelling may involve diagrammatic representation of the intervention, computer simulation or economic modelling. It might also involve testing through

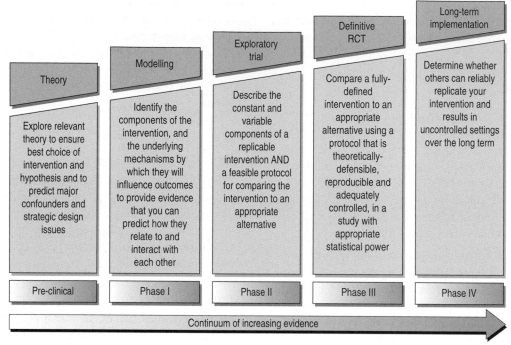

Figure 6.1 – *Framework for the development and evaluation of RCTs for complex interventions. (From MRC 2000, with permission.)*

preliminary surveys, small observational studies or focus groups.

(3) Phase II or exploratory trial. This third phase involves testing all the evidence collected, and is essential prior to the main RCT. The evaluator may vary the different components of the intervention and monitor changes in its effects; for example, changes in the form (dose) of the intervention. Insights are gained also into the likely challenges presented by a main trial and how these might be overcome: for example, how adaptive the intervention is within a particular context and so how much control is possible; what control group might be most appropriate and how they might be recruited; which outcome measures are most sensitive to the intervention; what evidence is there that expected mechanisms of action are producing effects; and what changes need to be made to the study design and strategy for analysis.

(4) Phase III or main trial. The fourth step is the main randomised controlled trial, which requires

attention to the standard features of well-designed trials including adequate power, randomisation and blinding (where feasible), appropriate outcome measures and informed consent of participants.

(5) Phase IV or long-term surveillance. A final, and often neglected part of a comprehensive evaluation of a complex intervention is a separate observational study to establish the long-term and real-life effectiveness and sustainability of the intervention and identify of long-term adverse events.

Critique

In our experience, the MRC guidelines are widely accepted, particularly amongst medical scientists. They see them as providing an approach to evaluation which accommodates the features of complex interventions, but, at the same time, retains the rigour of the traditional randomised controlled trial, which is widely regarded as the gold-standard research design for studying the effectiveness of health care interventions. However, even within the ranks of med icine, there is a minority view that the MRC's refinement of the randomised controlled trial is inadequate as a research design for evaluations of complex interventions. A letter published in the *BMJ* by Kernick (2000), a general practitioner, criticises the MRC group for getting the 'wrong end of the stick' entirely, and missing an important opportunity to develop an adequate methodology for evaluating complex interventions.

Kernick's main argument is that the MRC group is trapped within a postpositivist framework, which results in them misunderstanding what complex interventions really are. In particular, they confuse complicated (that is linear, predictable, understandable by a breakdown into component parts) with complex. Complexity, Kernick says, is the result of a rich interaction of simple elements that only respond to the limited intervention each of them is presented with. Complex systems are not linear, cannot be disaggregated into component parts and are unpredictable. These remarks in the *BMJ* reflect more fundamental criticisms of classic evaluation research, to which we now turn, drawing particularly on the realist critique of experimental evaluation developed by Pawson and Tilley (1997), in *Realistic Evaluation*.

Like Kernick, Pawson and Tilley are highly sceptical of experimental evaluation in the classic tradition and are doubtful of its value as a method of finding out which programmes do and which do not produce intended and unintended consequences. Nor do they believe it to be a sound way of deriving sensible lessons for policy and practice. Tilley (2000) illustrates their critique of classic evaluation with reference to mandatory arrest for domestic violence. This intervention, which aims to reduce rates of repeated assault, is one of the most widely evaluated interventions in the criminal justice system. The first evaluation of this intervention was in Minneapolis where police officers were randomly allocated three alternative responses in response to incidents of domestic violence in which there was no serious injury. These were to:

- arrest the assailant, although not necessarily charge them (the intervention condition);
- provide advice; or
- send the assailant away.

According to Tilley (2000), the mandatory arrest policy was found to be significantly more successful than the other two responses in reducing the risk of repeated calls for domestic violence; there was only 10% of repeat incidents in the mandatory arrest group, compared with 19% for those given advice and 24% for those sent away. On the basis of this finding, many other cities in the USA adopted a mandatory arrest policy in relation to domestic violence as a means of reducing repeat assaults, rising from only 10% of US cities with a population of over 100 000 in 1984 to 43% in 1986 and 90% by 1988.

However, the results of six follow-up studies to the original experiment in Minneapolis found mixed results. Three studies found a higher rate of repeated incidents of domestic violence and the other three a lower rate for the mandatory arrest group compared with the other two responses. As Tilley points out, in some cases adoption of a mandatory arrest policy actually increases the risk of repeated domestic violence – but why?

Tilley cites Sherman (1992) whose explanation points to the influence of the very variable communities, employment and family structures in the different cities. He suggests that, in cities with high levels of employment and stable family structures, arrest generates feelings of shame for the assailant, who is then less likely to reoffend. However, in communities characterised by high rates of unemployment, arrest triggers not shame but anger in the assailant, who in turn is likely to behave in a more violent fashion. Thus, the context within which the new policing response is introduced is crucial to its success or otherwise in reducing future episodes of domestic violence. Context influences the way in which the same intervention is experienced and so responded to by those towards whom it is targeted. Tilley argues that the classic evaluation studies of the mandatory arrest policy are typical of classical evaluations of other complex interventions, where typically a series of evaluations produce mixed results – an outcome that is unhelpful for policy makers.

Realistic evaluation

Pawson and Tilley's (1997) starting point in addressing the problem of evaluating complex interventions is to revise the key research question. Whereas the classical evaluator asks: 'Does it work'? or 'What works?' the key question asked by realistic evaluators is 'What works, for whom in what circumstances?' Their expectation is that the effects of an intervention or programme will vary according to the context in which it is introduced. The task for evaluators is to discover how and under what circumstances it will produce positive (and negative) effects, so providing a sound knowledge base for policy makers and practitioners.

Realistic evaluation is based upon a different view of causality than that which underpins classical experimental evaluation. The assumption of traditional experimental evaluation is that one event will be succeeded by another, so-called 'successive causality' (Pawson & Tilley 1997). In contrast, the realist evaluator understands causality in terms of underlying mechanisms generating observed patterns, so-called 'generative causality'. The natural world has many examples of such mechanisms at work, many of which cannot be observed directly; for example, the mechanism of gravity in making things fall to the earth. Scientific experimentation, according to realist evaluators, involves the creation of conditions under which mechanisms will be activated and discovered. From such experiments, scientists infer that such mechanisms, which they conjecture to exist, will also operate in the natural world. Tilley gives the example of gunpowder (mechanism), which will only operate (explode) within a particular set of conditions (context) – enough of it, dry, closely packed and so forth. For Tilley (2000), realistic evaluation is simply the application of these insights to the evaluation of social programmes or other complex interventions.

Thus, realistic evaluation is concerned with the following elements:

- Mechanisms (M) for change triggered by the complex intervention; that is, what it is about the intervention that might lead to a particular outcome in a given context.
- Contextual (C) conditions necessary for the change mechanisms to operate, and so to produce particular outcomes.
- Outcomes (O) that result from the intervention; that is the effects of a particular mechanism being triggered in a given context.

Realist evaluation studies draw upon these elements to produce 'context–mechanism–outcome pattern configurations' (Pawson & Tilley 1997, p. 77), which links together the context, mechanisms and outcomes. The task for evaluators is to identify, articulate, test and refine conjectured context–mechanism–outcome (CMO) configurations.

A frequently cited simple example, originally from Tilley (1993) and detailed in Pawson and Tilley (1997) to illustrate realistic evaluation, is of the deployment of closed-circuit television (CCTV) in car parks to reduce car crime. This intervention does not meet the criteria of a complex intervention. Indeed it seems very simple and so a good candidate, one might think, for a randomised controlled trial in which car parks are allocated randomly to an intervention (CCTV) or a control group (no CCTV) and the primary outcome (incidents of car crime) is compared across the groups. However, as realistic evaluation suggests, even apparently simple interventions are less simple than they appear.

The first step in a realistic evaluation of CCTV in car parks would be identification of potential mechanisms. Here are four examples of possible mechanisms that Pawson and Tilley (1997) come up with:

Ma) The 'caught in the act' mechanism. CCTV might reduce car crime by increasing the chances of offenders being videotaped committing their crimes, so leading to their arrest, conviction and so being deterred from future offences.
Mb) The 'you've been framed' mechanism. CCTV might reduce car crime because potential offenders are deterred by the risk they perceive of being

caught and convicted because of the evidence on videotape.

Mc) The 'effective deployment' mechanism. CCTV might reduce car crime through enabling security guards to be deployed more quickly if suspicious behaviour is detected by CCTV monitors. This deters potential offenders because of the guards' high visibility.

Md) The 'memory jogging' mechanism. CCTV cameras and notices act as a reminder to drivers of the possibility of car crime and so to lock their vehicles and place valuables out of sight.

The next element is 'context'. Are all car parks and all car park crime problems the same? The realistic evaluator would suggest not. Here are some contextual variations that Tilley (1993) identifies:

- The 'criminal clustering' context. The rate of car crime may arise from the activity of a large number of occasional offenders or a few very active offenders. Given this, the 'caught in the act' mechanism (Ma) will deliver good outcomes, in relation to the offender/offence ratio – being more effective if there are fewer offenders.
- The 'lie of the land' context. The vulnerability of cars parked in CCTV blind spots will be higher if the 'you've been framed' mechanism (Mb) operates, since this relies on increased chances of being caught through videotaped evidence of the offence. However, the risk to cars in CCTV blind spots is not increased if the operating mechanism is the changed security behaviour of drivers, as in the 'memory jogging' mechanism (Md).
- The 'alternative targets' context. Ready availability or relative absence of substitute targets of crime, together with the particular preference of offenders, provides the context for potential displacement of criminal activity away from car parks. In contexts where there are alternative targets, the 'you've been framed' mechanism (Mb) is likely to deliver better outcomes than in contexts where other suitable targets for crime are scarce.

What this example highlights is that, even in relation to a relatively simple intervention in a relatively simple setting, it is unlikely that the same intervention will have the same effect in all cases. The range of possible mechanisms and contexts at work are too varied.

Conclusion

This chapter has provided an overview of evaluation research and has presented two contrasting approaches to evaluating complex interventions. Which approach might be preferred? Our own view is that the UK MRC guidelines provide excellent advice on how to do cluster-based randomised controlled trials. But they do not acknowledge the value of having a variety of approaches to call upon to evaluate complex interventions. Realistic evaluation is an attractive alternative approach, which has yet to be adequately tested in the health care field. However, we have gained some insights into its use from an evaluation of Mental Health Link, a facilitated programme which aimed to develop systems within primary care and links with specialists to improve care for patients with long-term mental illness (Byng et al 2005). This is the first known evaluation to use realistic evaluation (RE) to complement a cluster randomised controlled trial, and demonstrated the potential complexity of using RE in practice. In summary, Byng et al's (2005) experience of using RE in a health care context suggests that Pawson and Tilley's (1997) emphasis on single mechanisms and search for contingent contexts does not adequately represent the reality of health care interventions. Complex interventions, such as Mental Health Link, may involve multiple mechanisms which may be active and sometimes countervailing. Nevertheless, so long as the CMO notation is regarded as a methodological technique, with the split between mechanisms and context being pragmatic rather than theoretical, the search for CMO configurations can enhance our understanding of complex interventions and how they produce their effects.

EXERCISES

1. Debate the pros and cons of a realistic versus experimental approach to evaluating a nurse-led unit for older people with chronic health problems.
2. Read the following paper: Holm L, Smidt S 1997 Uncovering social structures and status differences in health systems. *European Journal of Public Health* 7: 373–378. Consider the value of combining quantitative and qualitative data research methods to inform and evaluate service improvement.

References

Byng R, Norman I J, Redfern S J 2005 Using realistic evaluation to evaluate a practice-level intervention to improve primary healthcare for patients with long-term mental illness. Evaluation 11: 69–93

Campbell D 1969 Reforms as experiments. American Psychologist 24: 409–429

Judge K, Bauld L 2001 Strong theory, flexible methods: evaluating complex community-based initiatives. Critical Public Health 11: 19–38

Kernick D 2000 Focusing on being precisely wrong rather than vaguely right. Rapid Response to Campbell M, Fitzpatrick R, Haines A et al Framework for design and evaluation of complex interventions to improve health. British Medical Journal 321: 694–696

Langley C, Nolan K, Nolan T et al 1996 The Improvement Guide: A Practical Approach to Improving Organisational Performance. Jossey-Bass, San Francisco

Medical Research Council (MRC) Health Services and Public Health Research Board 2000 A framework for development and evaluation of RCTs for complex interventions to improve health. MRC, London

Pawson R, Tilley N 1997 Realistic Evaluation. Sage, London

Popper K 1945 The Open Society and its Enemies, Volume 2: Hegel and Marx. Routledge, London

Portney L G, Watkins M P 1993 Foundations of Clinical Research. Applications To Practice. Appleton & Lange, Norwalk

Sherman L 1992 Policing Domestic Violence. Free Press, New York

Tilley N 1993 Understanding car parks, crime and CCTV: evaluation lessons from safer cities. Crime Prevention Unit Series paper 42. Home Office, London

Tilley N 2000 Realistic evaluation: an overview. Paper presented at the Founding Conference of the Danish Evaluation Society, September 2000

Section 2

The Process of Research

Chapter 7

Asking Research Questions

Ian Atkinson

Introduction

Deciding upon a suitable research question often poses a formidable obstacle for students engaged in their first encounters with research. However, once a well-thought-out question is finalised then invariably the research goes ahead and answers are found with relatively few problems. In this chapter we consider the role of the research question to be absolutely central to the development of successful research. As a preliminary step to formulating a research question it is important first to select and analyse a topic for investigation. A method for doing this is introduced. Research questions can be framed in different ways, from the interrogative question to the precise research hypothesis. These are discussed in some length and guidelines are presented to assist in assessing their viability.

Developing a research question

Developing a clear research question is key to the development of any research investigation and is needed for a variety of other reasons. It is unlikely that providers of research funds would wish to spend substantial sums of money on projects which set out to conduct some vague and unspecified exploration. We need to know from the beginning what we want to find out even though in some studies this may evolve in the course of the investigation.

Once a research question is clarified then a study design and methods will evolve from it. In other words, once the research question is fixed then so are the choices of design and methods which can be employed to obtain the data to answer the question.

If this is accepted then we must also accept that arguments over which research approach is the better, i.e. quantitative or qualitative, are of little value. If we ask a qualitative research question then we are left with little alternative but to employ qualitative methods. If we ask a quantitative research question then equally we must employ quantitative research methods (Sackett and Wennberg 1997). Although this should not be taken to mean that both types of question and both types of methods could not be part of the same piece of research.

There is little doubt that nursing and health care in general provide an extraordinary source of the most interesting questions for research. No matter what background a researcher may have, be it from management science to geography or from chemistry to social anthropology, nursing and health care will be able to pose valuable questions which require such a range of disciplines to provide answers.

In the selection of subjects for research we follow a process of narrowing an initial broad area to a refined topic, followed by a specific research question and finally deciding upon precisely what information we need in order to answer that question. Selecting a broad area in which to conduct research will rarely pose any great difficulty and may be determined simply by personal knowledge, experiences and interests, or indeed those of colleagues and other associates. The availability of research funding obviously plays a key role in determining research areas but the requirements of funding bodies rarely play a significant role in undergraduate and Masters level research projects. Research areas are by definition very broad, for example a diagnosis such as stroke, or a particular aspect of care such as nurse patient communication. In themselves these present such wide areas that they must be first narrowed down to a specific topic before we can begin to start developing a research question.

Choosing a topic

A narrow topic for research will generally be derived from a number of considerations. A range of different factors are likely to influence and direct the choice of topic. An awareness of material already published in the area is going to be of key importance. The types of publication which should be of interest will include not only academic papers but outputs from government, the mass media, and the internal publications of various public and private organisations. Discussion among colleagues with interests and experience in the area can be invaluable. Conferences and study days provide ideal opportunities to meet and discuss ideas. In the case of student research, supervisors are generally consulted at an early stage of topic selection and often take a major role in narrowing the research topic.

At this stage the topic may still be too broad for a focused research question to have emerged. A variety of methods are available for analysing a broad topic which may help to identify a specific topic for research. One of these is the construction of relevance trees and this can be usefully applied here (Futures Group 1994). The approach is simple in principle and is likely to lead to new insights and a clear understanding of a topic. However, it does entail a good deal of effort and concentration by the user!

Construction of the relevance tree involves writing the topic at the head of a sheet of paper then breaking it down into components. Figure 7.1 gives an illustration using 'blood glucose monitoring' as an example topic. The root is labelled 'Use of glucose self monitoring' and this is broken down into three components. These are 'patient experiences', 'accuracy of assessment' and 'glycaemic control'. Each of these components is further broken down into sub-components and so the process continues. This continual breaking down could continue ad infinitum and has to be limited in some way. Certain parts of the branching would soon become less interesting and those with more appealing topics would become the focus of attention. The tree in Figure 7.1 is quite limited in its breakdown of the topic but its purpose is only to illustrate the approach. The intricacies of the method are fully discussed in the Futures Group paper (1994). Connections and overlaps between the different branches soon become apparent and these can be developed. In the example, issues of patient empowerment could be easily linked to the prevention of

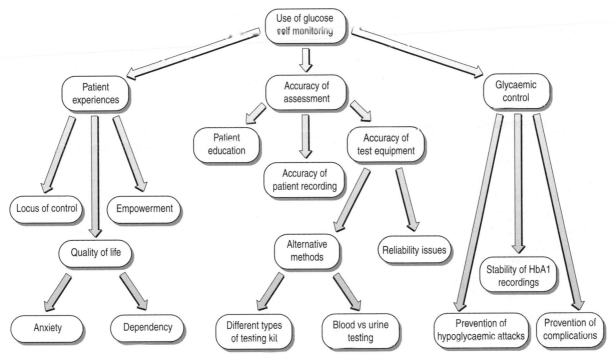

Figure 7.1 – *Example of a relevance tree for identifying the components of a research topic.*

hypoglycaemic attacks. Extensive development of such a tree may eventually lead the user to ideas which otherwise would not have been identified. The method has to be used creatively to be of most value.

Formulating the research question

Now the research question should be in sight and can be formulated either as an interrogative question or as an hypothesis. Often confusion arises as to whether a study should use a research question or a hypothesis. As a general rule it is the more structured studies, for example experiments, which tend to use hypotheses while the less structured surveys and qualitative studies use interrogative questions (Punch 2005). Whether we choose to use either a question or a hypothesis it will not affect the type of data required and the logic of the design needed to provide an answer.

The interrogative research question just states what the research is trying to find out and is written as a question. For example, 1: 'Does self monitoring of blood glucose lead to a change in the number of hypoglycaemic attacks experienced?' Sometimes research questions are not quite so precisely stated but nevertheless still serve their purpose quite adequately. For example, 2: 'What are the perceived benefits of self-monitoring of blood glucose among insulin-dependent patients?'

Question 1 could be reformatted as a study hypothesis as an alternative to the question format. An hypothesis is a statement which identifies at least two variables and makes an assertion about their relationship to each other. By implication the research hypothesis can be tested empirically (see Graziano & Raulin 2000). It is usual to formulate an hypothesis as two statements, one predicting no relationship exists between the variables and a second predicting a relationship does exist.

The following two statements are the equivalent of question 1 only this time formatted as hypotheses:

1. Glycaemic self-monitoring will not lead to a reduction in the number of hypoglycaemic attacks experienced.
2. Glycaemic self-monitoring will lead to a change in the number of hypoglycaemic attacks experienced.

The first of these statements predicts that self-monitoring will make no difference to the number of attacks and is often called the 'null' hypothesis or the hypothesis of 'no difference'. The second statement is predicting that self-monitoring will actually change the number of attacks and is often referred to as the 'alternative' hypothesis or the hypothesis of 'difference'. It should be noted that the second or alternative hypothesis in this example does not state the direction of the relationship between self-monitoring and the number of attacks. Our hypothesis of difference only states that the number of attacks will change with self-monitoring; therefore it is 'non-directional'. It is possible that for a variety of reasons we would actually expect the number of attacks to go down as a consequence of self-monitoring and in this case we would be justified in using what is called a 'directional hypothesis'. That is, we would specifically state in the hypothesis of difference that the number of attacks will go down. The second hypothesis therefore would be:

2. Glycaemic self-monitoring will lead to a reduction in the number of hypoglycaemic attacks experienced.

To justify the use of a directional hypothesis we must have a prior knowledge of what the effect of one variable is likely to be on the other. This could be based upon knowledge derived from previously completed research or upon theoretical prediction.

Having formulated the hypothesis, all that is required are data to confirm the truth of one or the other of the two hypothetical statements. This way to acquiring knowledge is in the tradition of the hypothetico-deductive approach to scientific enquiry. Science moves forward by developing hypotheses on the basis of theory and testing them using empirical evidence. For the above example the evidence required to confirm the truth or falsity of the hypotheses is exactly the same as that needed to answer the problem when stated as a question. The way in which the problem is written, either as a question or a hypothesis, makes no difference to the evidence we have to obtain to find an answer.

There is little doubt that a good research question is one for which there is an answer and the above questions suggest ways in which they could be answered. It is fairly obvious that the answer to question 1 is going to be expressed numerically. The data required is a count of the number of hypoglycaemic attacks and we could obtain this by asking patients themselves. The question is quantitative in nature and requires a quantitative answer. Question 2, on the other hand, is rather different. There are no obvious numerical values which we could collect to provide an answer. The question addresses subjective human experience and is by nature a qualitative question requiring a qualitative answer. The data we require here are subjective expressions or verbal accounts of the experiences people have had in relation to self-monitoring blood glucose. These could be collected by in-depth interviews with patients.

Both of our example research questions have implications for study design. For readers who are not entirely certain of the terms research methods and research design it may be helpful to define these terms again. Research methods are the processes and procedures we carry out during a study; for example, the ways of collecting data, such as questionnaires, interviews, observation etc., are all research methods. Research design, on the other hand, is a rather more abstract concept; it is the logic of a study or the overall plan which bonds the methods together. For example, if we want to see how effective a new medication is for reducing blood pressure then we could observe patients' blood pressures using the relevant equipment after taking the medicine. But such a set of data would not allow us to draw conclusions which would answer the question. It could be that the blood pressures have hardly changed but we do not know this with the data at hand. What is needed to answer this study question are two measurements of blood pressure, one taken before the medication and one taken afterwards. In terms of design what is needed to answer the question is a type of before and after design. It is the logic or design of the study which enables us to answer the research question (Ploeg 1999, Roberts & DiCenso 1999).

As in the above problem, a complete answer to example research question 1 requires that a comparison be made. That is, there will be '. . .a reduction in the number of hypoglycaemic attacks'. The implications of this are that not only do we need to count the number of attacks but counts have to be made before patients use self-monitoring and then afterwards once self-monitoring is in progress. Only then can we tell if there has been a reduction. With this logic, which is afforded by the design, we are able to answer the question properly. Questions such as this which require before and after studies often require full experimental designs to be applied to rule out alternative explanations for the changes which may be observed. These designs are considered in Chapter 18 of this book.

The second example question about the experiences of people using self-monitoring equipment also has specific design requirements. The answer makes no demands for comparison, consequently a single data collection exercise with one group of patients would be appropriate. The question also requires an answer derived from a flexible exploration of unknown human experiences, so clearly a qualitative approach to this problem would be the research design to employ.

Once having arrived at our research questions, there are several things that we should ask of the question itself to ensure it will be suitable to pursue with a research enquiry. A novel question is always desirable and will catch the attention of others, although apparently mundane questions will often yield findings of equal importance. Neither need the question be original, but this might be a requirement if it is to be submitted for a research degree.

A first and rather obvious question to ask is, are we going to be able to answer this research question

and are the implications for research design and methods practicable? This involves a wide assessment of what the problem is going to involve. The research question itself must suggest the types of information needed and the design logic for its collection.

Sometimes assumptions about the existence of data could be made when in truth it does not exist or it is held in a format rendering it unusable for research purposes. Information may exist but permission to access it may be denied. Will the data required take an excessive length of time or be difficult to obtain? In studies which depend upon recruiting patients, no matter how carefully recruitment rates are predicted once the study begins then the supply of suitable patients invariably falls away. Some researchers have referred to this as the 'law of the disappearing patient'! This affects the time it will take to answer the question and may have important implications for resources.

The above points lead us to the need to assess the risk of not being able to complete the study. Many things could occur in the course of a research project resulting in non-completion and often these are quite unpredictable. Some predictors of such catastrophes can be noted at an early stage and should be carefully assessed. For example, the greater complexity of questions and the designs they require may lead to escalating problems. Often such studies depend on the collaboration of many organisations and inevitably some will either refuse or not give the extent of cooperation needed. Longitudinal studies planned to take place over several years, or even decades, may run into problems when staff change or respondents cannot be traced for follow-up.

The availability of resources can accentuate the above if the work is being carried out on limited funds. Resources also include the abilities and skills of those who will be conducting the work. Many, if not all research projects will involve the investigator learning some new skills and this takes up time. It is quite acceptable to learn how to run a new database or a statistical software package as the work goes on. On the other hand, if such training is going to involve very extensive periods of study, then such knowledge should be attained before the research is proposed.

A very important exercise, especially for student researchers, is to look at what possible answers to our questions might reveal. It is desirable, especially for novice researchers, to ensure that no matter what the outcome, the research findings will be valuable and preferably have implications for increasing knowledge and/or improving clinical practice. This characteristic of a research study could be termed equilibrium or equipoise. An example of a study question where the possible findings would be out of equilibrium is one that sets out to develop a new method of assessing risk of relapse among patients with chronic illness. There are two possible outcomes here. The first would be a fully validated method which would justifiably receive great acclaim from colleagues. On the other hand, if the model produced was completely invalid then the project has failed. Very little credit would be given to the investigator and very few people would be interested. Inevitably for a new researcher such an outcome would be extremely disappointing. This is not to say that unbalanced studies are not worth conducting. Indeed the opposite is the case as no study could be more out of equilibrium than the randomised controlled trial of a new treatment – a type of study held to produce evidence of the highest quality.

Finally we must look at the value that our study question and the findings may have. This is often not easy to see through an objective eye and is possibly something left to the judgement of others. The response of colleagues to your ideas might be one of the best sources of help here before a proposal is produced and put before the ultimate arbiter on value, i.e. a research funding panel!

Conclusion

In conclusion we have seen that research topics need to be refined prior to devising research questions. There are a number of systematic ways of doing this but it is recommended that relevance trees are used, at least at first given their simplicity. The research questions which follow can be posed as interrogative questions or more formally stated as research hypotheses. Most importantly, because research design evolves directly from the question, it is crucial that research questions are developed with the utmost clarity. Once this is done, the nature of data needed and the logic of research design required to answer the question will become obvious. The feasibility of being able to answer the question must be established before embarking on a study and a number of qualities to help assess this have been presented.

EXERCISES

1. Take a subject area or broad topic in which you have a particular interest and analyse it by constructing a relevance tree. Once you have constructed the relevance tree, examine the contents of the tree to identify a subject you might be interested in following and develop some possible research questions.
2. Suppose you wish to establish the extent of community nursing support provided to frail older people and their informal carers living at home. Your intention is to recruit a sample of older people from day centres and ask them about the services they receive.

   a. Develop an appropriate research question for this study.
   b. Evaluate the quality of your research question by applying the qualities which it is desirable for a research question to have, as discussed in this chapter.
   c. During the exploratory work, you begin to suspect that frail older people with female carers are less likely to receive community nursing support than those with male carers. Formulate a study hypothesis which you could use to test this proposition.

References

Futures Group 1994 Relevance trees and morphological analysis. Online. Available: http://www.futurovenezuela.org/_curso/12-tree. pdf June 2006

Graziano A M, Raulin M L 2000 Research Methods, 4th edn. Allyn & Bacon, Boston

Ploeg J 1999 EBN notebook. Identifying the best research design to fit the question. Part 2: qualitative designs. Evidence-Based Nursing 2(2): 36–37

Punch K F 2005 Introduction to Social Research. Quantitative and Qualitative Approaches. Sage, London

Roberts J, DiCenso A 1999 EBN notebook. Identifying the best research design to fit the question. Part 1: quantitative designs. Evidence-Based Nursing 2(1): 4–6

Sackett D L, Wennberg J E 1997 Editorial, Choosing the best research design for each question. British Medical Journal 315: 1636

Chapter 8

Accessing the Nursing Research Literature

Paul Murphy and Seamus Cowman

Introduction

With a continuing increase in the volume of nursing information being published, there is a growing need to make that information accessible. One current directory of periodicals lists over 700 nursing journals and many more health care journals are potentially relevant (Ulrichs 2006). As we cannot read everything, we need to develop the information skills to identify and locate relevant documents when needed. There are some core information skills which can be applied across a range of publication formats and media.

Choosing the best sources is a skill acquired through familiarity with a range of nursing publications. For example, a pharmacopoeia might give sufficient information on a medication query; a review article summarising recent evidence-based research may be the solution to a clinical problem; guidelines for practice might be available on a reputable website. In other clinical and research contexts, there may be more complex problems to be solved and a more systematic search for information is needed. A literature review is conducted to create a picture of what is currently known about a problem situation and to identify what knowledge gaps may exist. Identifying pertinent studies, reviewing them and then clarifying the areas of further investigation all contribute to the development of research (Younger 2004).

Nursing information may be categorised according to the degree to which it is based upon empirical evidence from research or practice. Primary, research information derives mainly from original data collected and analysed in methodologically rigorous studies. Secondary information derives from authors presenting and discussing the work of others. Theoretical works contribute to other levels of knowledge building. Descriptive accounts and case reports may be valuable in presenting information on areas where there has been little or no formal research.

The impact of evidence-based medicine on nursing literature was noted by Morrisey and DeBourgh (2001), as was the subsequent drive to develop access to the literature among nurses. The growth of evidence-based practice has led to a clearer focus upon identifying specific types of scientifically sound studies in the literature. The study types concerned range from systematic reviews and randomised controlled trials to cohort and case studies. The Centre for Evidence Based Medicine at Oxford has a useful guide to the various levels of evidence in published research (Centre for Reviews and Dissemination 2005a) (Table 8.1).

Journals are now commonly published on the web, but searchers cannot rely on general web search engines to discover articles. Web search engines work well for general information but specialist bibliographic databases such as CINAHL (Cumulative Index to Nursing and Allied Health) and MEDLINE have been developed specifically to index journal articles. Human indexers evaluate the articles and add abstracts and subject information to aid the searcher in assessing the work described. Bibliographic databases are professional finding tools; however, they do not always include the complete full text of all articles indexed. Accessing the full text of articles is often another stage in the search process. Much will depend for instance upon whether an institution or a library has a subscription to a journal.

Choosing a database

There are a significant number of nursing databases, each with a different coverage of nursing sources (Table 8.2). The journals included for indexing are

selected by the database publishers; not all journals relevant to a particular sub-specialty or geographic area may be included in any one database. Morrisey and DeBourgh (2001) discuss the spread of nursing literature across medical, nursing and social science sources and they suggest that nurses must refine their literature search skills to improve effectiveness. Hek et al (2000) identified over 20 databases being used in some systematic reviews.

There is potential for some overlap between databases, but there may also be gaps; some databases will not index reports, books or theses. Newly published journals may publish on emerging issues but it may be some time before databases start indexing them. There are also access and subscription issues; many of the most important databases are offered by different vendors with various search interfaces and features. CINAHL for instance is available from publishers such as OVID, DIALOG and EBSCO.

Other sources of information

The UK's national gateway for nursing information, NMAP – Nursing, Midwifery and the Allied Health Professions (http://nmap.ac.uk), is a good source of information on health care resources.

Nursing dissertations are included in ProQuest's Dissertations & Theses Database (http://www.proquest.com) and the Index to Theses (http://www.theses.com).

Search process

Searching is often an intuitive, iterative process with the results retrieved at each stage informing the steps used to proceed further. Searches on most systems can range from basic searches using a few keywords to more complex searches which use the many advanced search features. In the simplified record from CINAHL on the OVID system presented in Table 8.3 the words and phrases in the title, abstract and subject headings fields are the basis for successful search matches. If the system matches the search words with terms in article records, then these articles will be deemed to be relevant and will be presented in the results.

Table 8.1 – *Publication formats and access tools*

Study or document type	Publication format (printed or electronic)	Access tool
Systematic reviews Meta-analysis Randomised controlled trials Clinical trials Cohort studies Case-based studies Reviews	Journal article Cochrane Review	Journal index databases and evidence-based databases: CINAHL MEDLINE Cochrane Library Other bibliographic databases
Opinion, editorial, letters Textbooks, monographs	Journal Book	Journal index databases Local and national library catalogues Online book services Web search engines CINAHL
Conference proceedings	Published proceedings	CINAHL Health care web portals Web search engines
Reports	Report	Library catalogues Health care web portals Web search engines Official agencies
Clinical guidelines	Guideline	CINAHL Health care web portals Web search engines Health care agencies
Theses	Thesis	Dissertation abstracts Index to theses CINAHL
Reference data, drug information	Reference book	Manual Pharmacopoeia Formulary website
News and general information	Journal Magazine Website	Keyword search engines Health care web portals Practitioner journals

Table 8.2 – *Key bibliographic databases in nursing*

Database	Type	Features
CINAHL – Cumulative Index to Nursing and Allied Health	CINAHL has indexed over 3000 nursing and allied health journals online from 1982. CINAHL covers nursing, biomedicine, complementary medicine, consumer health and many allied health disciplines. Selectively indexes health care books, dissertations, conference proceedings, standards of practice, educational software and book chapters	www.cinahl.com Commercial, subscription database available on a number of search systems and interfaces Indexes over 1000 journals Full text option with over 300 journals
MEDLINE	The US National Library of Medicine's bibliographic database covering the fields of medicine, nursing, the health care system, and the pre-clinical sciences worldwide. MEDLINE contains bibliographic citations and author abstracts from more than 4800 biomedical journals	Available on a number of search services Free version (PubMed www.pubmed.gov) 12 million + citations from mid 1960s with some older material
The Cochrane Library	The Cochrane Library consists of a regularly updated collection of evidence-based medicine databases including the unique Cochrane Reviews (over 4000) produced by the global Cochrane Collaboration. Cochrane Reviews are systematic reviews of the most reliable information on the effects of interventions in health care. The Library as a whole is a mix of fulltext reviews, references to articles and reports and registries of trials with over 500 000 items in all	www.cochrane.org Cochrane Database of Systematic Reviews Database of Abstracts of Reviews of Effects (DARE) Central Register of Controlled Trials Database of Methodology Reviews Methodology Register Health Technology Assessment database NHS Economic Evaluation Database
Web of Science	Includes the Social Sciences Citation Index, a multidisciplinary index to over 1725 journals across 50 social sciences disciplines and indexed overall from 1956 forward; included are Nursing, Public Health, Social Issues, Law, Sociology, Psychology and Psychiatry	scientific.thomson.com Citation indexes enable tracking all of whom reference an author or work
PsycINFO	PsycINFO covers behavioural sciences and mental health. Indexes journals in psychology and related fields such as psychiatry, management, business, education, social science, law, medicine, and social work	www.apa.org/psycinfo/ over 2 350 000 records Nearly 2000 journals Selected book indexing Dissertations Historic records

Table 8.2 – *Key bibliographic databases in nursing—Cont'd*

Database	Type	Features
British Nursing Index	*BNI* is a nursing and midwifery database, covering over 200 UK journals and other English language titles. A collaborative production involving UK nursing libraries, it is available from a number of vendors	www.bniplus.co.uk
MIDIRS (Midwives Information and Resource Service)	MIDIRS contains over 100 000 references to articles, book chapters, reports relating to midwifery, pregnancy, childbirth and infant care	www.midirs.org Specialist database now available through OVID
AMED – Allied and Complementary Medicine Database	AMED is produced by the Health Care Information Service of the British Library. It covers selected journals in professions allied to medicine (physiotherapy, occupational therapy, speech therapy), in complementary medicine and in palliative care	www.bl.uk/collections/health/amed.html Specialist database
ASSIA: Applied Social Sciences Index and Abstracts	ASSIA indexes health, social services, psychology, sociology, economics, politics, and education journals. Covers anxiety disorders, ethnic studies, family, geriatrics, nursing, immigration, child abuse, psychology and social issues	www.csa.com US-based publisher Coverage from 1987 500 journals from 16 countries

Search strategy

There are a number of factors to be considered in choosing the best terms. Simple spelling variations can affect retrieval in database systems: *pediatric nursing* or *paediatric nursing*; *anesthesia* or *anaesthesia* produce quite different results in textword searches. Databases do not always translate synonyms; all alternative terminology must be considered separately:

- nurses' aides OR health care assistants;
- pressure ulcer OR pressure sores OR bed sores OR decubitus ulcers.

In addition to thinking of all possible variants, there is some control possible by truncating words; 'therap*' (with an asterisk), for example, will find the terms 'therapy', 'therapist' and 'therapeutic' in most databases.

Relationships between different variables may also have to be considered. Suppose you are interested in investigating the relationship between stress, health beliefs and chronic fatigue syndrome. A search on the general aspects of stress and beliefs is one component. You may need to discover more about chronic fatigue syndrome and related conditions separately. You then need to bring all elements together to discover if any research links both. In CINAHL terms, the search elements might be grouped like this:

- stress OR stress, psychological;
- health beliefs OR attitude to health;
- chronic fatigue syndrome OR myalgic encephalomyelitis OR post viral fatigue syndrome.

Table 8.3 – *Simplified database record (from CINAHL)*

Title	Post-operative pain management in day surgery
Author	Skilton, M.
Source	Nursing Standard 2003 Jun 4–10; 17(38): 39–44. (17 ref)
Abstract	The author carried out a literature review of post-operative pain management in day surgery units...
Journal subset	Double Blind Peer Reviewed. Expert Peer Reviewed. Nursing Journals. Peer Reviewed Journals
CINAHL subject headings	Ambulatory Care Nursing Ambulatory Surgery/ae [Adverse Effects] Narcotics/tu [Therapeutic use] Pain/pa [Pathology] Postoperative Pain/dt [Drug Therapy] Postoperative Pain/ep [Epidemiology] Postoperative Pain/nu [Nursing] Postoperative Pain/pf [Psychosocial Factors] *Postoperative Pain Reflection
Publication type	Journal Article, Review, Tables/Charts

Table 8.4 – *CINAHL search, postoperative pain and hip replacement*

Search type	Search term	Articles
Keyword	Postoperative pain	2894
Keyword mapped to subject heading	*Postoperative Pain/	1753
Subject heading with therapy subheadings	*Postoperative Pain/dh, dt, th	1035
Subject heading	Arthroplasty, Replacement, Hip/	947
Combine with AND	*Postoperative Pain/dh, dt, th AND Arthroplasty, Replacement, Hip/	9
Limit to Research articles only		6

The / symbol denotes a subject heading.
The * symbol denotes a major subject heading.
Subheadings are coded (th for therapy, dt for drug therapy, dh for diet therapy).

By entering 'postoperative pain' into the main search box, the terms are immediately 'mapped' or translated to the nearest matching term in the CINAHL Subject Headings. The 'mapping' function has been developed to translate keywords into the preferred language of the database and thereby give better matches.

Records are enhanced with a range of subheadings which categorise general aspects of many clinical topics, for example epidemiology, pathology or therapy. As the interest here is in treatment options, three applicable subheadings ('diet therapy'; 'drug therapy'; 'therapy') are chosen to focus results further.

Subject headings

The thesaurus of CINAHL Subject Headings has a hierarchical tree or branch structure, with broader

Subject headings, Boolean and related features

Assume a searcher wants to find references relating to treatment options for *postoperative pain after hip replacement*. The search can be built up in various ways in a number of steps using three essential search techniques: subject headings, Boolean logic and limits. The search shown in Table 8.4 is based upon CINAHL on the OVID platform but the principles apply equally to other systems.

Table 8.5 – *CINAHL subject headings*

Narrower subject headings for 'Pain'	Selected subheadings
Back pain	Complications
Facial pain	Diagnosis
Headache	Drug effects
Muscle pain	Drug therapy
Neck pain	Metabolism
Neuralgia	Nursing
Phantom pain	Pathology
	Physiology
	Prevention and control
	Prognosis
	Psychosocial factors
	Symptoms
	Therapy

and narrower terms adjacent to the first entry term (Table 8.5). The tree presents a searcher with the context of a term and allows the selection of a broader or narrower emphasis. The subject headings can be used individually as precise search terms but may also be combined with any number of keyword or free text terms.

Subject heading terms usually include a means of emphasising how specific a term should be. Having selected a subject term, CINAHL offers another step guiding a searcher to *focus* the term or to *explode* the term. 'Focus' retrieves only those results in which that term represents the central concept of the records. With 'explode', a search for the selected term combines it with all of its conceptually narrower terms from the subject heading display. Exploding 'Pain' will also include articles on 'Back Pain', 'Facial Pain', 'Headache' and all other narrower terms.

A number of important aspects of articles are defined from the main subject heading by choosing from a range of standard *subheadings* such as 'therapy' or 'diagnosis'. This enables the searcher to specify that articles must emphasise the selected aspect. There are 44 subheadings representing

various health care aspects associated with the term 'pain' in CINAHL (Table 8.5). Multiple subheadings may be selected to include other aspects of interest.

Boolean

The use of the Boolean operators 'AND' and 'OR' is one method used to control relationships between search concepts. In our hip replacement example, the 'AND' operator is used to link the main concepts *postoperative pain 'AND' hip replacement*. All articles retrieved will now discuss both concepts together. 'AND' is usually the default combination in database search engines.

The 'OR' operation broadens the scope of searches and specifies that either one or the other or both terms appear in each of the articles retrieved. The search statement *hip replacement 'OR' arthroplasty replacement* serves to broaden this search considerably.

The 'NOT' operator is sometimes available but it is rarely used. The NOT operator excludes any record where the term appears in the record. For example, the search statement *terminal care 'NOT' cancer* will exclude all records where the term cancer appears.

Limits and related features

Limits can be used to focus further and refine that set. Standard limits are available in both MEDLINE and CINAHL.

CINAHL has an extensive set of limits that includes document formats such as books, dissertations and conference proceedings. There is also a set of 'Special Interest' categories from *critical care* to *wound care* indicating that articles will be of particular interest to practitioners in these areas.

Evaluation of search strategy

As a search strategy is elaborated and refined on the basis of the references retrieved, an ongoing process of evaluation, combining formal and intuitive elements, is involved. Articles judged important are worth acquiring and reading in full. This may be as simple as clicking for the full text on-screen to see if it is available on the local system.

In addition there are other measures of success of a search strategy, usually expressed in the form of degrees of *sensitivity* and *specificity* (Eysenbach & Diepgen 1998). Sensitivity is the likelihood of retrieving all relevant items from a given set of documents and is an indication of extent of the scope of the search. The higher the sensitivity, the more articles retrieved, even though some may not be relevant. In practical terms, if the results you retrieve are too narrow, increase the sensitivity of the search by using these broadening techniques:

- choose to combine more terms with OR;
- explode the term and include all subheadings;
- do not use any limits;
- search on other databases.

Specificity is the likelihood of finding only the most relevant items and excluding irrelevant articles. In practical terms if the results you retrieve are too broad, increase the specificity of the search by using these narrowing techniques:

- use the most specific term or subject heading;
- specify that the subject heading must be a major subject of the article;
- use an appropriate subheading;
- use the focus feature; do not explode;
- limit by population, clinical study type, language, type of journal.

Identifying evidence-based studies

Finding evidence-based studies begins at the source selection stage; choosing to search the Cochrane Library will, by the nature of the Library's content, ensure that the initial extent of evidence on the topic will be discovered. *Clinical Queries* are a series of preset filters and they specify the search terms and limits used in search strategies for MEDLINE, CINAHL, PsychINFO and other databases (Health Information Research Unit 2005). The UK's Centre for Reviews and Dissemination has also developed search strategies for reviews and meta-analysis (Centre for Reviews and Dissemination 2005b).

Table 8.6 – *Clinical Query search, CINAHL*

Set number	Search history	Results
1	Pain	8287
2	Osteoarthritis	1889
3	1 and 2	152
4	Limit 3 to Clinical Query 'treatment (high specificity)'	17
5	Limit 3 to Clinical Query 'reviews (high specificity)'	4

The 'Clinical Queries' features in MEDLINE and CINAHL each have a clinical category element (which includes diagnosis, therapy, prognosis) and scope elements (sensitivity, specificity). The scope element defines how broad or how narrow the results will be.

Table 8.6 outlines the results of a search for evidence-based studies using a narrow strategy with focused searches of the subject headings *pain AND osteoarthritis*. The result is limited to the Clinical Query 'treatment (high specificity)'. The search has retrieved a high proportion of randomised controlled trials. Using a different Clinical Query filter on the main topic, 'reviews (high specificity)' finds four systematic reviews and meta-analyses. Identifying evidence-based studies is a combination of clinical query searching and document type limits in both MEDLINE and CINAHL. The main options both in MEDLINE and in CINAHL as presented in Table 8.7 are derived from the Centre for Reviews and Dissemination's documentation (Centre for Reviews and Dissemination 2005b).

Additional evidence-based health care resources

While searches of the Cochrane Library, CINAHL and MEDLINE cover the main categories of evidence we have discussed, there are some other additional sources which might be included in more comprehensive searches and these sources are presented in Table 8.8.

Table 8.7 – *Evidence-based filters in MEDLINE and CINAHL*

Query/Study type	MEDLINE		CINAHL	
	Publication type limit	*Clinical query*	*Publication type limit*	*Clinical Queries limit*
Diagnosis		Yes		
Aetiology		Yes		Yes
Prognosis		Yes		Yes
Therapy		Yes		Yes
Randomised controlled trial	Yes	Yes		
Clinical trial	Yes		Yes	
Meta-analysis	Yes			
Systematic review		Yes	Yes	
Review	Yes		Yes	Yes
Guideline	Yes		Yes	
Protocol			Yes	
Practice guideline	Yes		Yes	
Case study			Yes	
Clinical prediction quides		Yes		

Searching the open web

The unregulated internet enables anybody to present any information to a global readership. Information may be incorrect or misleading. Material may be out of date and may never have been revised. The responsibility for evaluating information has now more than ever shifted to the reader at the point of use.

Due to the scale of the internet, effective information retrieval is more difficult as clinical research information is a very small proportion of the public web. Websites and web documents become visible to web search engines only when opened to the automatic software agents which 'spider' the web, collecting data to index. Search engines typically index only a portion of the text on a website when they visit. The 'invisible' web comprises an enormous amount of data that is either not indexed by web search engines or, if indexed, is otherwise inaccessible for a variety of reasons (University of California Berkeley 2005). Institutional websites may block search engines; other sites may require a payment to view material, as with journals. Therefore, while web searches often produce large numbers of documents, a significant proportion of the most relevant information may be hidden or the final document may be inaccessible.

Discovery and web search techniques

One common feature of the general search engines is that they use some variation of the 'popularity' of a site; search engines are all-purpose tools unsuited to some purposes. Some search engines have been developed to focus upon scientific and research information and they filter out much of the lower grade information. Scirus (www.scirus.com) is one such engine which emphasises results from educational and research organisations and it produces excellent results on most nursing topics. It is useful to consult a current guide. SearchEngineWatch (http://searchenginewatch.com) is a source which reviews search services and which offers a guide to web search techniques.

Table 8.8 – *Additional evidence-based resources*

Resource	Type	Source
Joanna Briggs Institute	The Institute coordinates centres worldwide to disseminate 'best evidence' and it produces a range of resources from 'Best Practice Clinical Reviews', a database of systematic reviews, evidence-based support material and consumer summaries	Australian research body http://www.joannabriggs.edu.au
NHS Centre for Reviews and Dissemination	The Centre for Reviews and Dissemination (CRD) produces: systematic reviews of research, scoping reviews mapping research, the Database of Abstracts of Reviews of Effectiveness (DARE), NHS EED and the HTA database CRD Reports, Effective Health Care, and Effectiveness Matters	UK University of York http://www.york.ac.uk/inst/crd/
National Guideline Clearinghouse	The Agency for Healthcare Research and Quality established the Clearinghouse as a freely available database of evidence-based clinical practice guidelines and documents including structured abstracts and bibliographies on guideline development	US official agency http://www.guideline.gov/
Royal College of Nursing	The RCN College of Nursing produces a major series of clinical practice guidelines for nursing and a range of supporting documents and databases	UK professional body http://www.rcn.org.uk
National Institute for Health and Clinical Excellence (NICE)	NICE provides national guidance on the promotion of good health in the UK including technology appraisals, guidance on medicines, clinical guidelines and interventional procedures	National UK body http://www.nice.org.uk/
Evidence-Based Nursing (BMJ)	*Evidence-Based Nursing* (BMJ) surveys a wide range of international journals and is designed to alert practising nurses to clinical advances	Journal http://ebn.bmjjournals.com/

The same general retrieval principles and methods apply to using keyword search engines as apply to bibliographic databases. Problem definition, keyword choice and spelling have to be considered. Explore the 'advanced search' mode features of a search engine; advanced techniques will significantly increase your control over the results and improve the relevance of searches (Table 8.9).

Web searches are especially important to source document types not covered in bibliographic databases. Many reports of local health care agencies, private institutions, governments, non-governmental agencies and international bodies can be identified by keyword web searches. The catalogues of virtually all major publishers and libraries are also accessible. Resources in visual and sound media can also be discovered; educational materials, video, presentations,

Table 8.9 – *Search results Google search engine (Jun 2006)*

Search statement	Sites retrieved
Pain control chest tube removal	1 430 00
'pain control' 'chest tube' removal	929
'pain control' 'chest tube' removal Limited to English sites in the educational domain .edu updated within the past year	126

sounds and images can usually be specified in most search engines.

Directories, gateways and portals

The limitations of keyword searching led to the development of directory sites which list resources and organisations in an organised structure by category. Subject-specific *gateways* to medical and nursing resources were created to direct users to the best websites. The advantage of gateway services is that the websites in the directories have been evaluated by health care professionals and that the content meets quality standards.

The UK's BIOME (http://biome.ac.uk) collection of subject gateways in biomedical subjects includes the OMNI – Organising Medical Networked Information gateway (http://omni.ac.uk) and the NMAP (Nursing, Midwifery and Allied Health Professions) gateway. NMAP (http://nmap.ac.uk) is a database of web-based nursing resources selected in consultation with the key providers.

Research agencies and universities pioneered the development of guided gateways as in these services:

- Hardin MD, University of Iowa (http://www.lib.uiowa.edu/hardin/md/nurs.html).
- HealthWeb (http://www.healthweb.org/nursing/).
- Health on the Net Foundation (http://www.hon.ch/).

Portals have been established as gateways to information for entire health systems on a national

basis. A well-developed example is the UK National Health Service's NeLH – National electronic Library for Health (www.nelh.nhs.uk). In addition to structuring access to free internet services, NeLH has subscribed services including CINAHL, MEDLINE, BMJ's Clinical Evidence, and the Cochrane Library.

Quality control on the web

A number of criteria which may be used in determining the quality of a website are offered in Table 8.10, which is based upon a number of sources including these:

Table 8.10 – *Quality criteria*

Ownership and influence	Who runs the site? Is the funding support apparent? Are there commercial or political influences evident?
Purpose and audience	What is the purpose of the site? Who is it intended to serve? Is it targeted at researchers and practitioners?
Authorship and authority	Who wrote the information? Do the authors have clinical credibility? Is there an editor(s) and can they be contacted?
Content and evidence	Are sources of data referenced? How verifiable is the information presented? Are links relevant and appropriate?
Currency	Is the information up-to-date? Is material dated? Are there statements of editing and revision?
User factors	How easy is it to use? Is it well structured, clear and logical? Does the content require browser enhancements? Would you recommend it?

- US National Library of Medicine's MEDLINEPlus *Evaluating Health Information* (http://www.nlm.nih.gov/medlineplus/evaluatinghealthinformation.html).
- The Health on the Net Foundation has produced a *Code of Conduct* aimed at website producers. Eight clear principles are articulated, including transparency and honesty, and the code forms a basis for rating sites (http://www.hon.ch/HONcode/Conduct.html).

The criteria in Table 8.10 are general criteria which might be applied by any critical reader. It was also recognised by Murray that the new mixture on websites, with additional media such as video and presentations, might pose the greater challenge (Murray & Rizzolo 1997). Building upon the studies identifying the role of intuition in clinical decision making, some (Cader et al 2003) highlight the value experienced nurses place upon intuition in their assessment of practice-based information appearing on the web. Their conclusions emphasise that nurses themselves are likely to favour a range of general criteria and their own assessment of how information is likely to be care related and practice enhancing.

Conclusion

Key databases for accessing the nursing literature include CINAHL, MEDLINE and the Cochrane Library. Understanding these databases in terms of what they include establishes the scope of the search across the range of resources and formats. Databases are offered in a variety of search interfaces and they often change in appearance and functionality. The searcher is sometimes challenged to discover the common pattern of search procedure which underlies the systems. Adopting a systematic approach to search strategy and taking the time to learn from the many guides and search aids available will enhance a searcher's information skills. The formulation of flexible search strategies using the many retrieval features of the databases is the core search skill. Being able to broaden and narrow and being able to specify the level of evidence or discussion is the essence of successful searching.

While the professional tools gather research evidence and channel it to practitioners, the open web has made much valuable health care information in many hitherto inaccessible formats available to nurses and patients worldwide. Whether accessed through a search engine or an advanced gateway, the nature of published information on the web challenges every reader to adopt a critical and sceptical point of view.

EXERCISE

Identify major research on the effectiveness of therapies for anorexia nervosa.

Search terms, subject headings and related terms might include: anorexia, eating disorders, bulimia, body image, eating behaviour, appetite.

- Search MEDLINE/Pubmed using keyword terms and Medical Subject Headings.
- Search CINAHL using keyword search and map to subject headings.
- Compare results from MEDLINE and CINAHL.
- Find systematic reviews in the Cochrane Library for anorexia nervosa.
- Use the NMAP gateway (http://nmap.ac.uk) to find authoritative patient information resources on anorexia nervosa.
- Search the phrase 'eating disorders' in both the search engines Google (http://www.google.com) and Scirus (http://www.scirus.com) and compare the first 30 results.

References

Cader R, Campbell S, Watson D 2003 Criteria used by nurses to evaluate practice-related information on the world wide web. CIN: Computers, Informatics. Nursing 21: 97–102

Centre for Reviews and Dissemination. 2005a Finding studies for systematic reviews: a checklist for researchers. University of York. Online. Available: http://www.york.ac.uk/inst/crd/revs.htm 23 Jan 2006

Centre for Reviews and Dissemination. 2005b Search strategies to identify reviews and meta analyses in MEDLINE and CINAHL. University of York. Online. Available: http://www.york.ac.uk/inst/crd/search.htm 23 Jan 2006

Eysenbach G, Diepgen T 1998 Towards quality management of medical information on the internet: evaluation, labelling, and filtering of information. BMJ 317: 1496–1500

Health Information Research Unit 2005 Search Strategies for MEDLINE in Ovid Syntax and the PubMed translation. Online. Available: http://hiru.mcmaster.ca/hedges/30 Jan 2006

Hek G, Langton H, Blunden G 2000 Systematically searching and reviewing literature. Nurse Researcher 7: 40–57

Murray P J, Rizzolo M A 1997 Web site reviews and evaluations. Nursing Standard. 11(45): 1–8. Online. Available: http://www.nursing-standard.co.uk/archive 7 Feb 2006

Morrisey L J, DeBourgh G A 2001 Finding evidence: refining literature searching skills for the advanced nurse practice nurse. AACN Clinical Issues 12: 560–577

Ulrich's Periodicals Directory Online Database. Available: http://www.ulrichsweb.com/ulrichsweb/30 Jan 2006

University of California Berkeley 2005 Invisible web: what it is, why it exists, how to find it, and its inherent ambiguity. UC Berkeley – Teaching Library Internet Workshops. Online. Available: http://www.lib.berkeley.edu/TeachingLib/Guides/Internet/InvisibleWeb.html 7 Feb 2006

Younger P 2004 Using the Internet to conduct a literature search. Nursing Standard 19: 45–51

Chapter 9

Synthesising Qualitative and Quantitative Evidence within a Systematic Review

Mary Dixon-Woods, Shona Agarwal, David R. Jones, Bridget Young, Alex J. Sutton and Jane Noyes

- Introduction
- Systematic reviews
- Methods for synthesis
- Issues in synthesis
- Conclusion

Introduction

In this chapter we briefly describe systematic review methodology, signpost examples of guidance, and present a brief overview and critique of a selection of approaches for synthesising qualitative and quantitative forms of evidence, illustrated with examples. The challenge for nurses is to synthesise evidence from studies in a rigorous and meaningful way (Oliver et al 2005). Along with others (e.g. Dixon-Woods & Fitzpatrick 2001, Dixon-Woods et al 2005), nurse researchers (e.g. Morse 2006, Pearson et al 2005, Sandelowski et al 1997) have been at the forefront of developing methods for review and synthesis. Likewise, nurse researchers have been prominent in publishing their experiences of synthesising studies in nursing journals (e.g. Henderson 2005, Whittemore & Knafl 2005).

Systematic reviews

Several resources exist to guide nurse researchers on methods of systematic review. These vary in complexity, and include the University of Plymouth's webguide (Barbour 2004), which is a comprehensive but basic resource for novice nurse researchers. Other sources of guidance include the *Cochrane Reviewers' Handbook* (Alderson et al 2004), the

Centre for Reviews and Dissemination guidance (CRD 2001), and publications of the Evidence for Policy and Practice Information and Co-ordinating Centre (EPPI-Centre) (e.g. Rees et al 2001). The search strategy is usually developed in association with an information specialist to minimise bias and searcher oversight. A variety of sources should be searched to minimise a range of biases. The types of studies to be sought depend on the nature of the review (Glanville 1999, Dixon-Woods et al 2004).

Systematic review methodology has traditionally tended to favour quantitative forms of evidence – particularly from randomised controlled trials (RCTs). However, nurses are increasingly aware of the limitations regarding RCTs as the sole source of 'evidence'. This has resulted in growing calls for more inclusive forms of review, so that better use may be made of primary data, including qualitative research (Davies & Boruch 2001, Kelly et al 2002, Pound et al 2005, Speller et al 1997, Thorne 1994). Using multiple forms of evidence allows maximum value to be gained from studies that have overcome problems with access to sensitive or hard-to-reach settings; contradictions in the evidence base can be identified and examined; and theory development or specification of operational models can be optimised. Excluding any type of evidence on grounds of its methodology could have potentially important consequences.

In characterising the different approaches to synthesis, Noblit and Hare (1988) introduce a useful distinction between *integrative (or what we term aggregative)* and *interpretive* reviews. Aggregative synthesis involves techniques, such as meta-analysis, that are concerned with assembling and pooling data, and require a basic comparability between phenomena studied so that the data can be aggregated for analysis. Interpretive reviews, by contrast, see the essential tasks of synthesis as involving both induction and interpretation. Interpretive reviews achieve synthesis through subsuming the concepts identified in the primary studies into a higher-order theoretical structure.

We suggest that *aggregative* syntheses of the type most commonly found in systematic reviews are those where the focus is on *summarising data*, and where the concepts (or variables) under which data are to be summarised are assumed to be largely secure and well specified. For example, in an aggregative synthesis of the impact of educational interventions on uptake of influenza immunisation in older people, the key concepts (educational intervention, uptake, older people) would be defined at an early stage in the synthesis and would effectively form the categories under which the data extracted from any empirical studies are to be summarised. This summary may be achieved through pooling of the data, perhaps through meta-analysis, or less formally, perhaps by providing a descriptive account of the data. It is important not to exaggerate how secure such categories are (for example, how to define 'older people' might be debated), nor is it impossible for an aggregative synthesis to fulfil theoretical functions (though these are most likely to be theories of causation).

The defining characteristic of an *interpretive* synthesis is its concern with the development of concepts, and with the development and specification of theories that integrate those concepts. An interpretive synthesis will therefore avoid specifying concepts in advance of the synthesis. It will not be concerned to fix the meaning of those concepts at an early stage to facilitate the summary of empirical data relating to those concepts. The interpretive analysis that yields the synthesis is conceptual in process and output, and the main product is not aggregations of data, but theory. Again it is important not to caricature an interpretive synthesis as therefore floating free of any empirical anchor: an interpretive synthesis of primary studies must be grounded in the data reported in those studies. An interpretive synthesis may be able to address questions that are difficult to address through aggregative syntheses, and be concerned with the generation of middle-range theories – explanations which apply in a specified domain, such as seeking to explain why people defer help-seeking for some types of symptoms. *Interpretive* syntheses, therefore, can be carried out on all types of evidence, both qualitative and quantitative.

There is considerable overlap between interpretive and aggregative forms of synthesis. Whilst most forms of synthesis can be characterised as being either primarily interpretive or primarily aggregative in form and process, every aggregative synthesis will include elements of interpretation, and every interpretive synthesis will include elements of aggregation of data.

Methods for synthesis

The different methods can be broadly grouped in terms of their epistemological and ontological foundations and whether the aim of synthesis is primarily interpretive or primarily aggregative. Clustering towards the interpretive end of the spectrum are the methods of narrative summary, grounded theory, meta-ethnography, meta-synthesis, meta-study, realist synthesis and Miles and Huberman's (1994) data analysis techniques, while lying at the more aggregative end of the spectrum are content analysis, case survey, qualitative comparative analysis and Bayesian meta-analysis. Within these clusters or groups, elements of the methods show considerable overlap.

Narrative summary

Narrative summary typically involves the selection, chronicling and ordering of evidence to produce an account of the evidence. Its form may vary from the simple recounting and description of findings through to more interpretive and explicitly reflexive accounts that include commentary and higher levels of abstraction. Narratives of the latter type can account for complex dynamic processes, offering explanations that emphasise the sequential and contingent character of phenomena (Abbot 1990). Narrative summary is often used in systematic reviews alongside systematic searching and appraisal techniques, as exemplified by Fairbank et al (2000). It can 'integrate' qualitative and quantitative evidence through narrative juxtaposition. Under the UK ESRC Methods Programme, methodological guidance on the conduct of narrative summaries has been developed, which informs good practice in this area (Popay et al 2006).

Thematic analysis

Thematic analysis, clearly sharing some overlaps with narrative summary and content analysis, involves the identification of prominent or recurrent themes in the literature, and summarising the findings of different studies under thematic headings. Summary tables, providing descriptions of the key points, can then be produced (Mays et al 2001). Several recent attempts at providing structured or systematic overviews of diverse areas of evidence have adopted this kind of approach (e.g. Garcia et al 2002).

Thematic analysis allows clear identification of prominent themes. It is flexible, allowing considerable latitude to reviewers and a means of integrating qualitative and quantitative evidence. It can be either data driven – driven by the themes identified in the literature itself – or theory driven – oriented to evaluation of particular themes through interrogation of the literature. However, there is frequently a lack of explicitness about procedures and aims in this area, including failure to specify the extent to which thematic analyses are descriptive or interpretive. Questions remain about whether the structure of the analysis should reflect the frequency with which particular themes are reported, or should be weighted towards themes that appear to have a high level of explanatory value. If thematic analysis is limited to summarising themes reported in primary studies, it offers little by way of theoretical structure within which to develop higher-order thematic categories beyond those identified from the literature.

Grounded theory

Grounded theory, originally formulated by Glaser and Strauss (1967), describes methods for qualitative sampling, data collection and data analysis. It sees the overriding concern of qualitative research as the generation of theory (generalisable explanations for social phenomena). The constant comparative method, the most widely used element of grounded theory, has the most obvious potential for application for systematic review in part (especially in later formulations) because it offers a set of procedures by which data may be analysed (see Strauss & Corbin 1998).

One of the most robust and theoretically sophisticated examples of the use of grounded theory for synthesis is Kearney's (2001) grounded theory analysis of 15 qualitative papers on women's experience of domestic violence. This study shows how grounded theory can deal with sampling issues and allow a synthesis of studies by treating study reports as a form of data on which analysis can be conducted using the constant comparative method. The generation of higher-order themes as a means of synthesis encourages reflexivity on the part of the reviewer while preserving the interpretive properties of the underlying data. Grounded theory, in the notions of theoretical saturation and theoretical sampling, also offers a means of limiting the number of papers that need be reviewed, especially where the emphasis is on conceptual robustness rather than on completeness of data.

Grounded theory does, however, have several disadvantages as a method for review. Even in its more proceduralised forms, it inherently lacks full transparency because it is an interpretive method. It also offers no advice on how to appraise studies for inclusion in a review. There are several important epistemological issues to be resolved, including the status of the accounts offered in the studies and how to deal with the varying credibility of these accounts. Moreover, the methodological anarchy that characterises the area, with 'grounded theory' being used to label many different types of analysis, should not be underestimated as a barrier to the development of this approach as a means of synthesising primary studies (Dixon-Woods et al 2004).

Meta-ethnography

Meta-ethnography is a set of techniques specifically developed for synthesising qualitative studies. First proposed by Noblit and Hare (1988), it involves three major strategies:

1. Reciprocal translational analysis (RTA). The key metaphors, themes, or concepts in each study are identified. An attempt is then made to translate these into each other. Some analogies can be drawn between RTA and content analysis.

2. Refutational synthesis. Key metaphors, themes or concepts in each study are identified, and contradictions between the reports are characterised. Possible 'refutations' are examined and an attempt made to explain them.

3. Lines of argument synthesis (LOA). This involves building a general interpretation grounded in the findings of the separate studies. Some analogies can be drawn between LOA and the constant comparative method.

Britten et al (2002) offer a well-documented demonstration meta-ethnography to synthesise four papers on the meanings of medicines, drawing on Schutz's (1962) notion of first and second order constructs. 'First order constructs' refer to the everyday understandings of ordinary people, whereas 'second order constructs' refer to the constructs of the social sciences. Britten and colleagues built on the second order constructs reported in the studies they reviewed to develop what they call 'third order interpretations', which were consistent with the original results but extended beyond them.

Meta-ethnography represents one of the few areas in which there is an active programme of funded methodological research for qualitative synthesis. It offers several advantages, including its systematic approach combined with the potential for preserving the interpretive properties of the primary data. Like grounded theory, it can potentially deal with quantitative data.

Several issues need to be resolved if meta-ethnography is to develop in ways that are helpful and useful to reviewers. Meta-ethnography, at least in its original form, offers no guidance on sampling or appraisal, and is solely a means of synthesis. It is demanding and laborious, and might benefit from the development of suitable software. Like most interpretive methodologies, the process of qualitative synthesis cannot be reduced to a set of mechanistic tasks, and meta-ethnography thus runs into the usual problems of transparency. Campbell et al (2003), for example, point to the problem of determining in which order the papers should be synthesised for reciprocal translational analysis. Other difficulties arise when a large number of reports need to be synthesised, because RTA appears to be most suitable for small stable sets of papers. Finally, RTA provides summaries in terms that have already been used in the literature, and there is therefore a danger that it will tend towards conservatism.

Meta-study and meta-synthesis

Paterson et al (1998a, 1998b) use the term 'meta-study' to encompass the overview of theory, method and data. They distinguish between meta-data synthesis, meta-method synthesis and meta-theory synthesis. Meta-data synthesis refers to the synthesis of data presented in reports; they suggest that the choice of analytic approach is up to the reviewers, with possible choices including grounded theory, meta-ethnography, thematic analysis and interpretive descriptive analysis (by which they seem to mean a narrative critical review).

Paterson et al propose that the key concern in meta-method is with identifying how the methods applied to an area of study shape understandings of it (e.g. interview-based studies compared with ethnographics). Meta-theory, on the other hand, involves a critical exploration of the theoretical frameworks that have provided direction to research (e.g. psychological and sociological approaches to understanding people's experiences of chronic illness). They use the term 'meta-synthesis' to describe bringing together the ideas that have been deconstructed in the three meta-study processes. The primary goal of such an analysis is to develop mid-range theory (i.e. theories that are moderately abstract and have direct applications for particular defined areas of practice). However, the term 'meta-synthesis' is often deployed as a way of distinguishing reviews of qualitative studies from systematic reviews or meta-analyses (Walsh & Downe 2005). In this latter sense, 'meta-synthesis' has become widely used to describe an approach to synthesising qualitative research that draws broadly on the meta-ethnography tradition, and does not necessarily involve the strategies specified by Paterson et al. Though meta-study provides

a very useful framework it also suffers from the limitations that it does not explicitly cope with quantitative evidence, and its processes are laborious and time-consuming.

Realist synthesis

Realist synthesis is an explicitly theory-driven approach to the synthesis of evidence (Pawson 2002a). Beginning with the theory that (apparently) underlies a particular programme or intervention, it seeks evidence in many forms, including formal study reports (both qualitative and quantitative) as well as case studies, media reports, and other diverse sources, and integrates them by using them as forms of proof or refutation of theory.

Examples of the approach have been provided in relation to the provision of smoke alarms as a means of improving safety, and public disclosure (Pawson 2002b). Key problems include the tendency to treat all forms of evidence as equally authoritative, the contingency of the chains of evidence, the vulnerability to the robustness of the theory being evaluated rather than the evidence being offered, and the lack of explicit guidance on how to deal with contradictory evidence.

Cross-case techniques

Miles and Huberman's cross-case techniques (1994) offer a number of strategies for conducting cross-case analyses, which might also be suitable for synthesising across different studies. These include meta-matrices for partitioning and clustering data in various ways, sometimes involving summary tables based on content analysis, case-ordered displays, or time-ordered displays. Though Miles and Huberman appear to be discussing the analysis of primary data, their techniques are readily transferable to the synthesis of study reports. McNaughton (2000) describes using these techniques to conduct a synthesis of 14 qualitative reports of home visiting research.

Miles and Huberman's approaches are highly systematic. The emphasis on data display assists in ensuring transparency, and the results of the synthesis are likely to be capable of being readily converted to quantitative variables. Software is available that can cope with this approach. However, Miles and Huberman's emphasis on highly disciplined procedures is seen by some as unnecessarily and inappropriately stifling. Miles and Huberman offer no advice on sampling or appraisal of the primary papers.

Content analysis

Content analysis is a technique for categorising data and determining the frequencies of these categories (Bryman 2001). It differs from more 'qualitative' qualitative methods in several ways. First, content analysis requires that the specifications for the categories be sufficiently precise to allow multiple coders to achieve the same results. Second, it relies on the systematic application of rules. Third, it tends to draw on the concepts of validity and reliability more usually found in the positivist sciences (Silverman 2001). Content analysis offers a means of synthesising study reports by allowing a systematic way of categorising and counting themes. Evans and Fitzgerald (2002) describe using content analysis in a systematic review of reasons for physically restraining patients and residents. They identify 'safety' as one of the categories, and show that this is cited in 92% of reports as a reason for using physical restraint.

Content analysis is well developed and widely used in the social sciences. It is (largely) transparent in its processes and easily auditable. Software packages are available. The data resulting from content analysis lend themselves to tabulation. Content analysis converts qualitative data into quantitative form, making it easier to manipulate within quantitative frameworks should this be appropriate.

The disadvantages of content analysis include the fact that it is inherently reductive, and tends to diminish complexity and context. It may be unlikely to preserve the interpretive properties of underlying qualitative evidence. Frequency-counting may lead to failure of the results to reflect the structure or importance of the underlying phenomenon. A related problem is the danger that absence of evidence (non-reporting) could be treated as evidence of absence (not important).

Case survey

The case survey method proposed by Yin and Heald (1975) is a formal process for systematically coding relevant data from a large number of qualitative cases for quantitative analysis. A set of highly structured closed questions is used to extract data from individual case studies. These data are converted to quantitative form subsequently used for statistical analysis. Developments of the approach use multiple coders to score the cases (Larsson 1993) and meta-analytic schedules (Jensen & Rodgers 2001).

The case survey method's ability to synthesise both qualitative and quantitative evidence is a strength. It converts qualitative evidence into a quantitative form, making it easy to manipulate within quantitative frameworks. The approach may make it possible to synthesise case studies from areas outside health care in addressing questions relating to organisation or policy.

The approach also has a number of important limitations. It relies on having a sufficient number of cases to make quantitative analysis worthwhile. Many qualitative researchers would probably reject the description of their studies as 'cases'. The approach might have difficulty in coping with the interpretive properties of qualitative data; contextual factors that might be important in explaining the features of particular cases may be 'stripped out' as the data are reduced to quantitative form; and it may be more suited to studies of outcomes than processes.

Qualitative comparative analysis (QCQ) Method

The qualitative comparative method, originally proposed by Ragin (1987), was based on the view that the same outcome may be achieved in different combinations of conditions, and that causation must be understood in terms of necessary and sufficient conditions. Complex causal connections are analysed using Boolean logic to explain pathways to a particular outcome. Cress and Snow's (2000) review used QCA to look at outcomes of mobilisation by the homeless.

QCA requires the construction of a 'truth table', showing all logically possible combinations of the presence and absence of independent variables and the corresponding outcome variable. Actual cases in the data that match each possible combination of independent variables and the outcome are sought. A Boolean minimisation process then eliminates all logically inconsistent variables. From many potential explanations, only a small number of combinations of variables to account for particular outcomes is left. This yields a parsimonious and logically consistent model of the combination of variables associated with the outcome under study (Haggerty 1992). Recent refinements of the method have included the introduction of 'fuzzy' logic, so that it is not necessary to dichotomise variables so precisely (Ragin 2000).

Qualitative comparative analysis has the advantage that it may not require as many cases as the case survey method. It can be used with previously conducted studies as well as with new studies, and thus encourages an evolutionary and integrative approach to knowledge creation. It allows easy integration of both qualitative and quantitative forms of evidence, and is (largely) transparent and systematic. Complex and multiple patterns of causation may be explored.

However, as with any approach that relies on converting qualitative evidence into quantitative form, qualitative researchers are likely to argue about the ontological and epistemological assumptions of QCA. QCA is mainly appropriate when a causal pathway is sought, and may be ill-suited to the more usual concerns of qualitative research, including the meanings that people give to their experiences. QCA appears to be designed primarily to deal with case studies, and may not cope well with the more usual form of qualitative study reports.

Bayesian meta analysis

Meta-analysis is the quantitative synthesis of data, in which evidence is pooled using statistical techniques. Bayesian forms of meta-analysis offer flexibility in handling data from diverse study types. It begins with beliefs that are temporally or logically prior to the main data, formally expressed as a probability distribution, and updates these beliefs using the study data to produce an assessment of current evidence.

It allows the integration of qualitative and quantitative forms of evidence, and explicitly allows qualitative evidence to contribute to meta-analysis by identifying variables to be included and providing evidence about effect sizes. It therefore reflects important precedents from primary research, where qualitative research is often used to identify the variables of interest before conducting a quantitative study.

The method proposed by Roberts et al (2002) used the qualitative studies about childhood immunisation as a source of external evidence to identify the relevant variables to include in the synthesis and to contribute to informing initial judgements about the likely effects of these variables. These were then synthesised with quantitative studies. The synthesis showed that exclusion of either the quantitative or the qualitative studies from the meta-analysis would have resulted in only a partial synthesis of the available evidence.

However, Bayesian meta-analysis, though conceptually straightforward, is not necessarily easy to implement and may lack appeal to some sections of the qualitative community. The techniques for achieving this form of analysis are still under development, and many methodological issues remain to be resolved, including those relating to elicitation of the priors and the impact of different methods of qualitative synthesis.

Issues in synthesis

Questions can be asked about whether apparent differences between the strategies reflect superficial differences in terminology and the degree to which methods have been specified. Work that compares the results of applying the different methods of synthesis will be useful in distinguishing trivial from non-trivial divergences between the methods. In the longer term, methods that incorporate the most useful elements of these approaches may be developed; it is important that future work builds on the existing approaches.

Is it acceptable to synthesise studies?

There are arguments about whether it is feasible or acceptable to conduct syntheses of qualitative evidence at all (Sandelowski et al 1997), and whether it is acceptable to synthesise qualitative studies derived from different traditions. The distinctions, tensions and conflicts between these have been vividly described (Barbour 1998). Some have argued (Estabrooks et al 1994, Jensen & Allen 1996) that studies to be synthesised should share a similar methodology. They suggest that even when similar themes can be identified across all studies, the mixing of methods leads to difficulties in developing theory because of differences in their epistemological foundations. Others have taken a more pragmatic approach (Paterson et al 1998b).

Perhaps even more likely to generate controversy are attempts to synthesise qualitative and quantitative evidence. It is evident from the discussion above that synthesis of diverse forms of evidence will generally involve conversion of qualitative data into quantitative form, or vice versa (Tashakkori & Teddli 1998). While it is clear in principle that many of the approaches that involve 'quantitising' qualitative data lend themselves easily to subsequent analysis, few approaches that have dealt with qualitative synthesis have dealt directly or explicitly with how to incorporate quantitative evidence.

Should reviews start with a well-defined question and how many papers are required?

The issue of questions is an important one for syntheses. It will be clear that some of the methods described above will be more suited to some

questions than others: for example, questions concerning causality may be better suited to qualitative comparative analysis than questions concerned with the production of mid-range theory, which might be better suited to meta-ethnography. The issue of how questions should be identified and formulated is one on which there is much uncertainty. Estabrooks et al (1994) argue that review questions should be selected to focus on similar populations or themes. However, others (such as Glaser & Strauss 1967) point out that in primary qualitative research, definitions of the phenomenon emerge from the data. Whether one should start with an *a priori* definition of the phenomenon for purposes of a secondary synthesis is therefore an important question.

A related issue is how to limit the number of papers included in the review. One approach is to narrow the focus. An alternative strategy is offered by theoretical sampling, used in primary qualitative research with a view towards the evolving development of the concepts. Sampling continues until theoretical saturation is reached, where no new relevant data seem to emerge regarding a category, either to extend or contradict it (Strauss & Corbin 1990). It has been suggested that this approach would also be suitable for selecting papers for inclusion in reviews (Booth 2001, Paterson et al 1998a, Schreiber et al 1997). However, the application of this form of sampling has been rarely tested empirically, and some (Jensen & Allen 1996, Sherwood 1999) express anxiety that this may result in the omission of relevant data.

Appraising studies for inclusion

The CRD guidance emphasises the need for a structured approach to quality assessment for qualitative studies to be included in reviews, but also recognises the difficulties of achieving consensus on the criteria that might constitute quality standards. Some argue that weak papers should be excluded (Campbell et al 2003, Estabrooks et al 1994, Yin & Heald 1975). Others, however, propose that papers should not be excluded for reasons of quality (Jensen & Allen 1996, Sandelowski et al 1997), particularly where this might result in synthesisers discounting important studies for the sake of 'surface mistakes', which are distinguished from fatal mistakes that invalidate the findings (Sandelowski et al 1997). Published examples include reviews which have chosen not to appraise the papers (Garcia et al 2002) as well as those which have opted to appraise the papers using a formalised approach (Campbell et al 2003).

Conclusion

Methods for synthesis have been developing rapidly, informed by, amongst others, prominent nurse researchers. We have offered a review of a range of strategies for synthesising qualitative and quantitative forms of evidence. They vary in their ability to accommodate diverse forms of evidence. some have been developed within one paradigm for purposes of synthesising particular forms of data, and their suitability for other forms of data is potential rather than demonstrated. The likely appeal of the methods to researchers in different paradigms is variable. It will also be the case that the suitability and judgement of the strengths or weaknesses of any given approach will be very much context-specific, and dependent on the question being addressed. Registers of quantitative systematic reviews are available in the Cochrane Library and examples of qualitative and mixed methods reviews are available on the Cochrane Qualitative Research Methods Group, Joanna Briggs Institute and EPPI websites.

EXERCISE

Identify one published review that synthesises *qualitative* evidence only; one that synthesises *quantitative* evidence only; and one that synthesises *qualitative and quantitative* evidence.

1. Compare and contrast the scope, aims and research questions in each review.
2. Compare the search strategies, inclusion and exclusion criteria – what would you have done differently?
3. Identify whether studies have been quality appraised, and if not whether a justification was given.
4. Identify and critique the methods used for synthesising data.
5. Identify the strengths and limitations of each review – does the review provide new insights, new conceptual clarification or new theoretical developments?
6. Discuss the relevance and utility of each review design for your particular field of practice.

References

Abbott A 1990 Conceptions of time and events in social science methods: causal and narrative approaches. Historical Methods 23: 140–150

Barbour G 2004 Searching the Literature Guide. School of Health care Professions. University of Plymouth, Online. Available: http://www2.plymouth.ac.uk/millbrook/rsources/sealit/srchguid.htm#aim 31 Aug 2006

Barbour R 1998 Mixing methods: quality assurance or qualitative quagmire? Qualitative Health Research 8: 352–361

Booth A 2001 Cochrane or cock-eyed? How should we conduct systematic reviews of qualitative research? Paper presented at the Qualitative Evidence-based Practice Conference, Taking a Critical Stance. Coventry University, 14–16 May 2001. Online. Available: http://www.leeds.ac.uk/educol/documents/00001724.doc31 Aug 2006

Britten N, Campbell R, Pope C, et al 2002 Using meta-ethnography to synthesise qualitative research: a worked example. Journal of Health Services Research and Policy 7: 209–215

Bryman A 2001 Social Research Methods. Oxford University Press, Oxford

Campbell R, Pound P, Pope C, et al 2003 Evaluating meta-ethnography: a synthesis of qualitative research on lay experiences of diabetes and diabetes care. Social Science and Medicine 56: 671–684

Centre for Reviews and Dissemination 2001 Undertaking systematic reviews of research on effectiveness: CRD's guidance for those carrying out or commissioning reviews. CRD Report Number 4, 2nd edn. NHS CRD, York

Cress D, Snow D 2000 The outcomes of homeless mobilization: the influence of organization, disruption, political mediation, and framing. American Journal of Sociology 105: 1063–1104

Davies P, Boruch R 2001 The Campbell Collaboration. BMJ 323: 294–295

Dixon-Woods M, Fitzpatrick R 2001 Qualitative research in systematic reviews has established a place for itself. BMJ 323: 765–766

Dixon-Woods M, Shaw R L, Agarwal S 2004 The problem of quality in qualitative research. Quality and Safety in Healthcare 13: 223–225

Dixon-Woods M, Kirk D, Agarwal S, et al 2005 Vulnerable groups and access to health care: a critical interpretive review London: NHS SDO R&D Programme

Estabrooks C A, Field P A, Morse J M 1994 Aggregating qualitative findings: an approach to theory development. Qualitative Health Research 4: 503–511

Evans D, Fitzgerald M 2002 Reasons for physically restraining patients and residents: a systematic review and content analysis. International Journal of Nursing Studies 39: 735–743

Fairbank L, O'Meara S, Renfrew M J, et al 2000 A systematic review to evaluate the effectiveness of interventions to promote the initiation of breastfeeding. Health Technology Assessment 4: 1–171

Garcia J, Bricker L, Henderson J, et al 2002 Women's views of pregnancy ultrasound: a systematic review. Birth 29: 225–250

Glanville J 1999 Carrying out the literature search. In: Curran S, Williams C J (eds) Clinical Research in Psychiatry: A Practical Guide. Butterworth-Heinemann, Oxford, 57–58

Glaser B G, Strauss A L 1967 The Discovery of Grounded Theory: Strategies for Qualitative Research. Aldine de Gruyter, New York

Haggerty T R 1992 Unravelling patterns of multiple conjunctural causation in comparative research: Ragin's qualitative comparative method. Journal of Comparative Physical Education and Sport 14: 19–27

Henderson A 2005 The value of integrating interpretative research approaches in the exposition of healthcare context. Journal of Advanced Nursing 52: 554–560

Higgins J, Green S (eds) 2006 Cochrane Handbook for Systematic Reviews of Interventions 4.2.6. Cochrane Collaboration, Oxford

Jensen L A, Allen M N 1996 Meta-synthesis of qualitative findings. Qualitative Health Research 6: 553–560

Jensen J L, Rodgers R 2001 Cumulating the intellectual gold of case study research. Public Administration Review 61: 236–246

Kearney M 2001 Enduring love: a grounded formal theory of women's experience of domestic violence. Research in Nursing and Health 24: 270–282

Kelly M, Swann C, Killoran A, Naidoo B, Barnett-Paige E, Morgan A 2002 Methodological problems in constructing the evidence base in public health. Health Development Agency, London. Online. Available: http://www.hda-online.org.uk/evidence/meth_problems.html 14 Apr 2006

Larsson R 1993 Case survey methodology: quantitative analysis of patterns across case studies. Academy of Management Journal 36: 1515–1546

McNaughton D B 2000 A synthesis of qualitative home visiting research. Public Health Nursing 17: 405–414

Mays N, Roberts E, Popay J 2001 Synthesising research evidence. In: Fulop N, Allen P, Clarke A, Black N (eds) Studying the Organization and Delivery of Health Services. Routledge, London

Miles M B, Huberman M 1994 Qualitative Data Analysis: An Expanded Sourcebook. Sage, London

Morse J 2006 It is time to revise the Cochrane criteria. Qualitative Health Research 16: 315–317

Noblit G W, Hare R D 1988 Meta-ethnography: Synthesising Qualitative Studies. Sage, Newbury Park, CA

Oliver S, Harden A, Rees R, et al 2005 An emerging framework for including different types of evidence in systematic reviews for public policy. Evaluation 11: 428–446

Paterson B L, Thorne S E, Canam C, et al 1998a Meta-study of Qualitative Health Research. Sage, Thousand Oaks, CA

Paterson B L, Thorne S, Dewis M 1998b Adapting to and managing diabetes. Journal of Nursing Scholarship 30: 57–62

Pawson R 2002a Evidence-based policy: the promise of 'realist synthesis'. Evaluation; 8: 340–358

Pawson R 2002b Evidence and policy and naming and shaming. Policy Studies 23: 211–230

Pearson A, Wiechula R, Court A, et al 2005 The JBI model of evidence-based healthcare. Evidence in Healthcare Reports 3(8), Online. Available: www.joannabriggs.edu.au/pubs/systematic_reviews.php 31 Aug 2006

Popay J, Roberts H, Sowden A, et al 2006 Guidance on the conduct of narrative synthesis in systematic reviews. Report of the ESRC Methods Programme. Lancaster University, Lancaster. Online. Available: http://www.conted.ox.ac.uk/cpd/healthsciences/courses/short_courses/qsr/NSguidanceV1-JNoyes.pdf

Pound P, Britten N, Morgan M, et al 2005 Resisting medicines: a synthesis of qualitative studies of medicine taking. Social Sciences and Medicine 61: 133–155

Ragin C C 1987 The comparative method: moving beyond qualitative and quantitative strategies. University of California Press, Berkeley, CA

Ragin C C 2000 Fuzzy Set Social Science. University of Chicago Press, Chicago

Rees R, Harden A, Shepherd J, et al 2001 Young People and Physical Activity: A systematic Review of Research on Barriers and Facilitators. EPPI Centre, Social Sciences Research Unit, Institute of Education. University of London, London

Roberts K A, Dixon-Woods M, Fitzpatrick R, et al 2002 Factors affecting the uptake of childhood immunisation: a Bayesian synthesis of qualitative and quantitative evidence. Lancet 360: 1596–1599

Sandelowski M, Docherty S, Emden C 1997 Focus on qualitative methods. Qualitative meta-synthesis: issues and techniques. Research in Nursing and Health 20: 365–371

Schreiber R, Crooks D, Stern P N 1997 Qualitative meta-analysis. In: Morse J M (ed). Completing a Qualitative Project: Details and Dialogue. Sage, Thousand Oaks, CA

Schutz A 1962 Collected Papers, (vol 1. Martinus Nijhoff, The Hague

Sherwood G 1999 Meta-synthesis: Merging qualitative studies to develop nursing knowledge. International Journal for Human Caring 3: 37–42

Silverman D 2001 Interpreting Qualitative Data: Methods for Analysing Test, Talk and Interaction. Sage, London

Speller V, Learmonth A, Harrison D 1997 The search for evidence of effective health promotion. BMJ 315: 361–363

Strauss A L, Corbin J 1990 Basics of Qualitative Research. Sage, London

Strauss A, Corbin J 1998 Basics of Qualitative Research: Techniques and Procedures for Developing Grounded Theory, 2nd edn. Sage, Thousand Oaks, CA

Tashakkori A, Teddli, C 1998 Mixed Methodology: Combining Qualitative and Quantitative Approaches. Sage, Thousand Oaks, CA

Thorne S 1994 Secondary analysis: issues and implications. In: Morse J M (ed). Issues in Qualitative Research Methods. Sage, London

Walsh D, Downe S 2005 Meta-synthesis method for qualitative research: a literature review. Journal of Advanced Nursing 50: 204–211

Whittemore R, Knafl K 2005 The integrative review: updated methodology. Journal of Advanced Nursing 52: 546–553

Yin R K, Heald K A 1975 Using the case survey method to analyse policy studies. Administrative Science Quarterly 20: 371–381

Chapter 10

The Cochrane Database and Meta-analysis

Zena Moore and Seamus Cowman

Introduction

The cornerstone of evidence-based practice is the integration of high quality research evidence into clinical decision making. This evidence is used in combination with clinical judgement and experience to plan the most appropriate patient treatment (Sackett et al 1996). In striving to achieve evidence-based practice, the nurse is faced with an increasing dilemma. There is simply too much published literature and not enough time to appraise it all critically. There was a time when it was possible to read everything related to a particular speciality; however, currently over 6000 health-related articles are published each day (Levin 2001). The Cochrane Collaboration aims to be the medium through which this information is made accessible.

Background to the Cochrane Collaboration

A literature review forms the basis for further research through identification of the gaps in current knowledge (Burns & Grove 2001). On completion of a research project, each researcher's job is to identify the contribution of their research project to the body of knowledge (Burns & Grove 2001). The traditional literature review lacks a scientific approach to the selection and rejection of material for inclusion in the review (Egger et al 2003). The concern is that these reviews will be based on an inadequate or incomplete analysis of the evidence. For example, inclusion of only published material leads to bias in outcomes reporting as it is known that non-significant research findings take longer to appear in the literature (Misakian & Bero 1998). Non-significant research findings are just as important to be aware of as significant findings. Having only some of the information will result in bias in interpreting the strength, or direction, of the evidence base, leading to inappropriate clinical decisions.

Restriction of article inclusion to only those published in a particular language deliberately rejects important material. For example, in 36 meta-analyses published in leading English language general medical journals from 1991 to 1993, 26 had restricted their search to studies reported only in English (Grégoire et al 1995). These issues among others add bias to the review, reducing the confidence which can be placed in the results.

In essence, the problem lies in the fact that a different conclusion may be drawn if the whole body of knowledge was available. Rossouw et al (1990) noted, in their critique of a published review of cholesterol lowering after myocardial infarction, that inclusion bias led to a completely different meta-analysis than would have been achieved had other studies been included: although one study that met the inclusion criteria was available, it was excluded from the original review; along with 11 other studies where the reviewers had no clear rationale for their exclusion. The initial review found in favour of hormone treatment, whereas inclusion by Rossouw et al (1990) of the omitted studies, demonstrated the opposite.

A good example of the dilemma of trying to integrate a limited knowledge of evidence into clinical decision making was the use of anti-arrhythmic drugs postmyocardial infarction (Chalmers 2003). This treatment led to the deaths of thousands of people in the United States in the early 1980s. A previous systematic review of the treatment had sounded warning bells, but trials continued. Due to the lack of integration of the new trial evidence into the previous systematic review, the danger of these drugs went unrecognised. Thus, the

treatment continued to be used (Chalmers 2003). This lack of synthesis and dissemination of trial evidence was the inspiration for the development of the Cochrane Collaboration in 1993 (The Cochrane Collaboration 2005).

Cochrane realised that failure to use evidence appropriately from clinical trials was putting the lives of patients at risk, for example the use of steroids in women expected to deliver prematurely. The result of the meta-analysis of the available RCTs showed a reduction of the odds of death in the babies of these women by 30–50% (Antes & Oxman 2003). Before the publication of these findings, obstetricians were unaware of these outcomes; therefore, steroids were not widely used, resulting in unnecessary suffering and loss of life. The forest plot of this meta-analysis has become the logo for the Cochrane Collaboration (Antes & Oxman 2003).

Cochrane identified the requirement for high quality systematic reviews of literature and the importance of making such information readily available. For that reason, Cochrane began his mission for the development of a database of systematic reviews. The original systematic reviews focused on pregnancy and childbirth. Before his death in 1988, over 600 systematic reviews had been completed (Antes & Oxman 2003). Finally, in 1993 the Cochrane Collaboration was formally launched, bringing Cochrane's quest to fruition (The Cochrane Collaboration 2005).

What is the Cochrane Collaboration?

The Cochrane Collaboration is an international, not-for-profit organisation. It is established as a limited company and is registered as a charity in the UK. The collaboration is the largest organisation worldwide conducting systematic reviews (Bero & Rennie 1995). The aim is to provide individuals with up-to-date information regarding health care interventions. This is achieved through the production, dissemination and maintenance of systematic reviews, covering a wide variety of health care issues (The Cochrane Collaboration 2006). The work of the Cochrane Collaboration (2006) is based on 10 key principles (Box 10.1).

Box 10.1 – *The 10 key principles of the Cochrane Collaboration*

- Collaboration, by internally and externally fostering good communications, open decision-making and teamwork.
- Building on the enthusiasm of individuals, by involving and supporting people of different skills and background.
- Avoiding duplication, by good management and coordination to maximise economy of effort.
- Minimising bias, through a variety of approaches such as scientific rigour, ensuring broad participation and avoiding conflicts of interest.
- Keeping up to date, by a commitment to ensure that Cochrane Reviews are maintained through identification and incorporation of new evidence.
- Striving for relevance, by promoting the assessment of health care interventions using outcomes that matter to people making choices in health care.
- Promoting access, by wide dissemination of the outputs of the Collaboration, taking advantage of strategic alliances, and by promoting appropriate process, content and media to meet the needs of users worldwide.
- Ensuring quality, by being open and responsive to criticism, applying advances in methodology and developing systems for quality improvement.
- Continuity, by ensuring that responsibility for reviews, editorial processes and key functions is maintained and renewed.
- Enabling wide participation in the work of the Collaboration by reducing barriers to contributing and by encouraging diversity.

The Cochrane Collaboration Steering Group

The Cochrane Collaboration Steering Group (CCSG) is the governing body of the Cochrane Collaboration. The CCSG is divided into three subgroups and seven advisory groups (Hetherington 2005). The purpose of these groups is to ensure that the Cochrane Collaboration achieves its mission statement. For example, the handbook Advisory Group is responsible for the *Cochrane Handbook for Systematic Reviews of Interventions* and other handbooks, which are used as key sources of advice by reviewers in the preparing and maintenance of Cochrane reviews (Alderson et al 2004).

The format of the Cochrane Collaboration

The Cochrane collaboration is divided into a number of sections: Cochrane centres, review groups, methodology groups, fields, and a Cochrane Consumer Network (Alderson et al 2004). There are 12 Cochrane centres worldwide. The first Cochrane centre was established in Oxford, UK in 1993. Since then, centres have opened in South Africa, USA and many other countries, with the most recent being the Chinese Cochrane Centre which opened in 1999 (Alderson et al 2004).

The role and function of the Collaborative Review Groups

Currently there are 50 Collaborative Review Groups (CRGs) each focusing on a specific area of health care. The purpose of these groups is to produce and maintain systematic reviews (Alderson et al 2004). These systematic reviews are available from the Cochrane Library at http://www. thecochranelibrary.com.

One example of a CRG is the Cochrane Wounds Group, which has been in existence since 1995 (Cullum et al 2000). Their focus is on assessing the impact of interventions, including beds, dressings and bandages on both acute and chronic wounds including surgical and traumatic wounds, leg ulcers, pressure ulcers and diabetic foot ulcers. Evidence from randomised controlled trials using valid objective outcomes, such as healing rates or incidence of wounds, is the main source of data used in the development of the Wounds Group reviews (Cullum et al 2000).

Finding the evidence to appraise

A systematic review aims to summarise all the evidence available, published and unpublished, pertaining to a specific health care issue. Therefore, the reviewer needs to be able to access this evidence. The Cochrane Review Groups set out to make this goal possible. The Cochrane Collaboration has developed a search strategy for MEDLINE (Alderson et al 2004) and is working with the US National Library of Medicine to improve the identification of both old and new published trials through MEDLINE (Alderson et al 2004). The review groups can identify those journals that have been already or are currently being hand searched through a database maintained at the New England Cochrane Centre (Alderson et al 2004). The review groups also hand search journals and conference proceedings to identify further studies not available through the previous search strategies (Alderson et al 2004).

The Cochrane Methodology Groups

The expertise in conducting systematic reviews is growing and is supported by the work of the Methodology Groups which advise on different aspects of systematic reviews, for example, design, coding, analysis, dissemination or implementation. The purpose of the groups is to develop and improve the methodological quality of Cochrane reviews thereby ensuring that the reviews are conducted to the highest standards (Alderson et al 2004).

The Cochrane Fields

Fields differ from the review groups in that their focus is on aspects of heath care other than specific health care problems (Gotham 2005). For example, their interest is in the type of health care setting (e.g. primary or secondary) or the individuals involved (e.g. the very young or the very old). The purpose of the fields is not to conduct systematic reviews, rather it is to ensure that their specific area of interest is represented adequately in the work of the Cochrane Collaboration (Gotham 2005).

The Consumer Network

The Consumer Network was registered in 1995 (Jadad & Haynes 1998). The purpose of this network is to facilitate the dissemination of information from systematic reviews to patients, their carers and advocates. This purpose is achieved by sharing information and making the lay press aware of recent relevant additions to the Cochrane Collaboration review databases (Jadad & Haynes 1998).

Systematic reviews and nursing practice

The Cochrane Library has been traditionally linked to medicine due to its reliance on evidence from RCTs, the gold standard in research methodology. However, the practice of using high quality evidence as a basis for clinical decision making is also of fundamental importance in all aspects of nursing practice. More recently it has become clear that nurses have embraced the challenge of conducting systematic reviews evidenced by a search undertaken in the *Journal of Advanced Nursing*. The journal was searched for the years 1990–2006, using the term 'Systematic Review'. Systematic reviews began to appear in 1998 and since then the number included has increased steadily, indeed the search yielded 34 hits.

Further support for the role of the Cochrane database of systematic reviews (CDSR) as a source of evidence for nursing practice has been provided by Mistiaen and colleagues (2004). The authors conducted a search of the CDSR 2002 issue 3 and found 160 completed reviews.

Overall the authors found that 60% of the reviews were inconclusive (Mistiaen et al 2004). Either there was no evidence because no studies existed (8.1%), or there was insufficient evidence to support or refute the intervention (51.9%). Overall, the authors suggest that the outcomes of nursing interventions are well represented within the CDSR (Mistiaen et al 2004). Thus the CDSR is an important reference point for the development of clinical practice and research in the nursing arena.

What is meta-analysis?

Meta-analysis involves quantitatively combining the results from individual trials which have explored a similar research question (Naylor 1997). The origins of meta-analysis stem from the work of Pearson in 1902 (Naylor 1997). In an attempt to overcome the limitations of small sample sizes, Pearson developed a statistical method for combining the results of similar studies. The underlying premise is that the studies must be exploring a set of related research hypotheses. The purpose is to allow for greater accuracy in data analysis when using a group of studies rather than relying on the results of an individual study (Naylor 1997).

Undertaking a systematic review does not automatically imply that a meta-analysis will be conducted. Meta-analysis should only be carried out when it is appropriate, i.e. when the differences between studies have occurred by chance not due to factors such as study design or study quality (Greener & Grimshaw 1996). The rationale for this is that combining poor quality studies will still yield poor results even if the studies are similar (Deeks et al 2005).

Types of data

There are three types of data encountered in systematic reviews, dichotomous or binary data, continuous data and survival or time to event data (Deeks et al 2001). Dichotomous data are where there are two possible states, for example pressure ulcers healed versus pressure ulcers not healed. Continuous data are data arising through use of a scale, for example percentage reduction in wound size. Survival or time to event data are those where the outcome of interest is the time elapsing before an event is experienced; such data are commonly encountered during cancer studies (Deeks et al 2001).

How is meta-analysis conducted?

The process of conducting meta-analysis is undertaken in two steps.

Step one: calculate a summary statistic

Summary statistics are commonly reported for dichotomous data as the odds ratio or the risk ratio also called the relative risk and for continuous data as the weighted mean difference.

Odds and odds ratio. The odds are the probability of an event happening; for example pressure ulcer development, divided by the probability of the event not happening. The odds ratio is then calculated by dividing the odds of the event happening by the odds of the event not happening. An odds of greater than one suggests that the event is more likely to happen than not (Crichton 2001).

Relative risk. Relative risk is the rate of the event of interest; for example pressure ulcers healed in the experimental group divided by the rate of this event in the control group. It indicates the chances of pressure ulcer healing for people in the experimental treatment compared with the control group. As, by definition, the risk of an event occurring in the control group is 1 then the relative risk reduction associated with using the experimental treatment is $1 - RR$ (CLIB Training 2003).

Weighted mean difference. The mean difference, called the weighted mean difference, measures the absolute difference between the mean values in the experimental and control groups in a clinical trial. It estimates the amount by which the treatment changes the outcome on average and is used as a summary statistic in meta-analysis when all the studies are using the same scale. Interpretation of the result of this analysis is the same as for relative risk except the point of no effect is 0 rather than 1 (CLIB Training 2003).

Step two: calculate the overall treatment effect

The second step in the conduct of meta-analysis is to calculate the overall treatment effect of the studies included. This treatment effect is calculated as a weighted average of the summary statistics. However, before this is done it is of importance to establish the homogeneity of the studies. The purpose of this is to establish if there is a large variability in the studies, greater than one would expect to have occurred by chance alone (Deeks et al 2001). If heterogeneity is identified, the reviewer will need to decide whether or not the differences between the trials can be investigated or alternatively if it is better not to pool the results. Conducting a L'Abbe plot (Fig. 10.1) is a useful method of establishing homogeneity of results. By plotting the results of different studies against each other it is possible to assess the consistency of these results visually (Deeks & Altman 2001).

Lines are drawn for risk ratios (RR) and odds ratios (OR) of 0.2, 0.4, 0.6, 0.8, 1, 1.25, 1.67, 2.5, and 5 and for risk differences (RD) of -0.8 to $+0.8$ in steps of 0.2. The bold solid line marks the line of no treatment effect ($RR = 1, OR = 1, RD = 0$). The solid lines indicate treatment where the event rate is reduced (or the alternative outcome is increased). The dashed lines indicate interventions where the event rate is increased (or the alternative outcome is decreased).

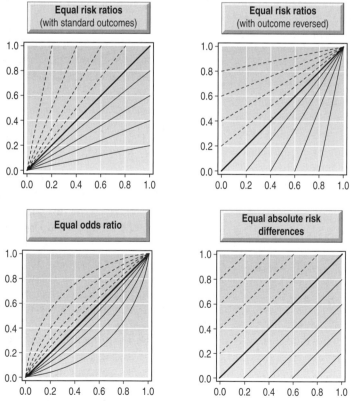

Figure 10.1 – *L'Abbe plots demonstrating constant odds ratios, risk differences and risk ratios for standard and reversed outcomes. (From Deeks & Altman 2001, with permission of the BMJ Publishing Group.)*

In each case, the further the lines are from the diagonal line of no effect, the stronger is the treatment effect.

Commonly the methods of meta-analysis for dichotomous outcomes are fixed effect methods and random effects method (Deeks et al 2001). For continuous data one fixed effect method and one random effects method are commonly used. Different weights are assigned to individual studies depending on the size and quality of the study. This means that all the data are not combined as if they arose from one large study; rather those studies with narrower confidence intervals are given greater weight (Deeks et al 2005).

Displaying the results of meta-analysis

The most common method used to display the results of individual studies and meta-analyses in a Cochrane review is a forest plot (Deeks et al 2005) in which each study is represented by a black square and a horizontal line. The size of the square is an indicator of the weight of the study and the horizontal line depicts the 95% confidence interval. The vertical line indicates the point of no effect, i.e. if the horizontal line touches, or passes through the vertical line, there is no statistically significant difference in outcome ($p > 0.05$) between the treatment and experimental group in the study (Deeks & Altman 2001).

Undertaking a systematic review

Using an example of a completed systematic review (Moore & Cowman 2005) the steps to undertaking a systematic review will be outlined.

Develop a review protocol

Initially a protocol for the review is developed and peer reviewed by the relevant Cochrane Review Group editors and other appropriate peer reviewers. Following the peer review, appropriate amendments are made to the protocol and it is then published in the Cochrane Library. The purpose of the protocol is to act as a map outlining the precise steps that will be taken during the completion of the full review. Development of a concise protocol is therefore invaluable as it makes the work of the review much clearer.

The review
Provide a background

The first step in undertaking the review is to provide a background and rationale for the requirement for a review of the chosen topic. Using the example of Moore and Cowman (2005) the authors argued that pressure ulcers are a significant health care problem and as such the wounds need to be managed effectively. Wound cleansing is necessary; however, there is confusion surrounding best practice, therefore a review of the evidence is required.

Outline the objective of the review

The exact objective of the study is outlined usually in the same format (the effect of X on Y). In this instance, Moore and Cowman (2005) wished to assess the effects of wound cleansing and techniques on the healing rates of pressure ulcers.

Outline the types of studies and interventions

The next part of the review is to outline the types of studies and interventions that will be considered for the review. In the main, randomised controlled trials (RCTs) are considered and controlled clinical trials are only considered in the absence of RCTs. Thus for the Moore and Cowman (2005) review the following were considered:

- RCTs comparing wound cleansing with no wound cleansing;
- RCTs comparing different wound cleansing solutions;
- RCTs comparing different wound cleansing techniques;
- no restrictions in terms of language or date of publication were applied.

Outline the type of participants

To appraise the relevancy of the review fully, it is important to make explicit the types of participants who will be included in the review. Moore and Cowman (2005) looked at studies involving people of any age, in any health care setting, with existing pressure ulcers (defined as a break in the continuity of the skin caused by pressure with or without shearing/friction forces).

Outline the type of outcome measures

Both the primary and secondary outcome measures are outlined to add clarity to the inclusion and exclusion of studies. In this instance Moore and Cowman (2005) identify the outcome measure as follows:

- Primary outcome measures – an objective measure of pressure ulcer healing such as:
  - time to complete healing
  - rate of change in pressure ulcer area or volume
  - proportion of pressure ulcers healed.
- Secondary outcome measures:
  - pain using a validated scale where reported
  - ease of use of the method of cleansing
  - secondary outcome measure would only be reported from studies which also reported the primary outcome measures.

Search strategy

The precise search strategy is identified including the search terms and the databases used. The detailed outline of the search undertaken by Moore and Cowman (2005) is available from http://www.thecochranelibrary.com.

Data extraction, validity assessment and synthesis

The next step is to conduct data extraction and to assess the methodological quality of each study. Following this, synthesis of the data is performed. In the initial search Moore and Cowman identified

111 potential studies; 33 letters were written to experts in pressure ulcer management to identify further potential studies; however, no further studies were found. Following review of the abstracts on the 111 articles, 12 were deemed possibly relevant. Finally having read all 12 papers, three papers were identified that met the inclusion criteria. Information pertaining to the reasons for exclusion of the nine papers is available from http://www.thecochranelibrary.com. Data were then extracted from these studies into pre-prepared data extraction tables. The two authors conducted the data extraction independently and any differences in opinion were resolved by discussion and reference to the Wounds Group editorial base. If data were missing from reports the trialists were contacted to obtain the missing information. Validity assessment of the papers was conducted using the framework suggested by Verhagen et al (1998) and Khan et al (2001).

Initially, a structured narrative summary of the studies was conducted. Data were then entered into the Cochrane RevMan 4.2 software and analysed with Cochrane MetaView. For dichotomous outcomes, relative risk (RR) plus 95% confidence intervals (CI) were calculated; for continuous outcomes weighted mean difference (WMD), plus 95% CI were calculated. Owing to the small number of diverse RCTs identified, meta-analysis was not conducted.

Results

The next step is to discuss the results of the analysis. Moore and Cowman (2005) discuss the results in terms of the initial interventions that they set out to explore, as follows:

- Comparison of cleansing versus no cleansing: No trials were identified for this comparison.
- Comparison of different cleansing solutions: Two trials were identified that compared different cleaning solutions (Bellingeri et al 2004, Griffiths et al 2001).
  - The first trial (Bellingeri et al 2004) compared saline spray with aloe vera, silver chloride and decyl glucoside against isotonic saline in

133 patients with pressure ulcers greater than grade 1 (NPUAP 1989). The primary outcome measure was the percentage reduction in pressure sore status. The mean percentage change from baseline to day 14 in the control group was −20.5 (SD 24.1, min −65.8, max 22.7), while the mean percentage change in the Vulnopur spray group was −27.8 (SD 31.3, min 69.8, max 123.5). The data from this study were skewed and the triallists used non-parametric tests that cannot be reproduced, because the raw data were not reported. As Rev-Man assumes a normal distribution, data were not entered into the 'Table of comparisons' section and the authors (Moore & Cowman 2005) have accepted the triallists' analysis, which found that there was a statistically significant improvement in healing in the intervention group (p value = 0.025).

– The second trial (Griffiths et al 2001) compared saline with tap water in 35 patients with 49 wounds – of which eight were pressure ulcers. The primary outcome measure was number of ulcers healed. Three wounds cleansed with tap water healed in the 6-week period, whereas none of the wounds cleansed with saline had healed at 6 weeks; the relative risk (RR) was 3.00 (95% confidence interval (CI) 0.21 to 41.89). The sample size was too small to draw any conclusions.

■ Comparison of different cleansing techniques: One trial was identified that compared different cleansing techniques (Burke et al 1998). Burke et al (1998) compared whirlpool versus no whirlpool in people with grade 3 or grade 4 pressure ulcers (no information about the pressure ulcer grading system was provided). Eighteen people with 42 ulcers were included in the study and were randomly allocated to the control group (non-whirlpool; $n = 18$ ulcers) or to the intervention group (whirlpool; $n = 24$ ulcers). The primary outcome measure was improvement in pressure ulcer condition. The wounds in the whirlpool group demonstrated improved healing

(number of wounds improved = 14) compared to the non-whirlpool group (number of wounds improved = 5). The authors conducted a t-test and found a statistically significant difference (p value = 0.0435). However, RevMan analysis identified no statistically significant findings; the RR was 2.10 (95% CI 0.93 to 4.76).

Review conclusion

The authors of systematic reviews finally draw conclusions from their analysis of the available data. Furthermore, where possible, they also outline the implications for practice and research arising from the review. Moore and Cowman (2005) conclude that overall there is no good trial evidence to support use of any particular wound cleansing solution or technique for pressure ulcers. Therefore, no firm recommendations for ways of cleansing pressure ulcers in clinical practice can be made. The authors also highlight that there is a need for further research in this area and any reports of such research findings should be made in accordance with the CONSORT guidelines (Moher et al 2001)

Conclusion

The requirement for the use of high quality evidence in nursing practice is now more important than ever. Traditional reviews lack a scientific basis and therefore have a tendency to lead to bias in outcome reporting. Clinicians need good quality information upon which to base clinical decisions, yet often lack the time and skills required to undertake detailed systematic reviews. The Cochrane Collaboration aims to bridge this gap and is now the world leader in the development, dissemination and maintenance of high quality systematic reviews. Indeed, the Cochrane Collaboration now includes more than 50 systematic review groups whose work spans over 4200 completed reviews. From a nursing perspective, the Cochrane Collaboration is a rich source of up-to-date information that can be used as a basis for clinical practice.

Acknowledgement

The section 'Undertaking a systematic review' in this chapter draws on material published in Moore and Cowman (2005), copyright Cochrane Library, reproduced with permission.

EXERCISE

- Log on to the Cochrane Collaboration and identify a Cochrane working group relevant to your own area of practice.
- Pick a review relevant to your area of practice and highlight within the review the steps taken in the production of the final work.
- Access a literature review relevant to your area of practice and highlight the components that differ from the systematic review you have read.
- Reflect on the relevance for your clinical practice, the recommendations made from the systematic review you have read.
- Discuss with your colleagues at work, the role and function of the Cochrane Collaboration.

References

Alderson P, Green S, Higgins J P T 2004 Cochrane Reviewers' Handbook 4.2.2. [updated March 2004]. In: The Cochrane Library, Issue 1. John Wiley, Chichester

Antes G, Oxman A D 2003 The Cochrane Collaboration in the 20th century. In: Egger M, Davey Smith G, Altman D G (eds) Systematic Reviews in Health Care – Meta-analysis in Context, 2nd edn BMJ Books, London, 447–458

Bellingeri R, Attolini C, Fioretti O, et al 2004 Evaluation of the efficacy of a preparation for the cleansing of cutaneous injuries. Minerva Medica 95: 1–9

Bero L, Rennie D 1995 The Cochrane Collaboration. Preparing, maintaining, and disseminating systematic reviews of the effects of health care. Journal of the American Medical Association 274: 1935–1938

Burke D T, Ho C H K, Saucier M, et al 1998 Effects of hydrotherapy on pressure ulcer healing. American Journal of Physical Medicine and Rehabilitation 77: 394–398

Burns N, Grove S K 2001 The Practice of Nursing Research, Conduct, Critique and Utilisation, 4th edn. Saunders, Philadelphia

Chalmers I 2003 Foreword. In: Egger M, Davey Smith G, Altman D G (eds) Systematic Reviews in Health Care – Meta-analysis in Context, 2nd edn. BMJ, London: iii–xviii

CLIB Training. 2003 CLIB Training Guide understanding the odds-ratio diagram in the CDSR. Online. Available: http://www.york.ac.uk/inst/crd/clibsec3.pdf2003;4 24 Jul 2005

Crichton N 2001 Information point: odds ratio. Journal of Clinical Nursing 10: 268–269

Cullum N, Bell-Syer S E M, Nelson E A 2000 About the Cochrane Collaboration (Cochrane Review Groups (CRGs)). Issue 1 Art. No: WOUNDS.

Deeks J J, Altman D G 2001 Effect measures for meta-analysis of trials with binary outcomes. In: Egger M, Davey Smith G, Altman D G (eds) Systematic Reviews in Health Care – Meta-analysis in Context, 2nd edn. BMJ, London: 313–335

Deeks J J, Altman D G, Bradburn M J 2001 Statistical methods for examining heterogeneity and combining results from several studies in meta-analysis. In: Egger M, Davey Smith G, Altman D G (eds) Systematic Reviews in Health Care – Meta-analysis in Context, 2nd edn. BMJ, London, 285–312

Deeks J J, Higgins J P T, Altman D G 2005 Analyzing and presenting results. In: Higgins J P T, Green S (eds) Cochrane Handbook for Systematic Reviews of Interventions 4.2.5 [updated May 2005]; Section 8. In: The Cochrane Library, Issue 3. John Wiley, Chichester

Egger M, Davey Smith G, O'Rourke K 2003 Rationale, potentials and promise of systematic reviews. In: Egger M, Davey Smith G, Altman D G (eds) Systematic Reviews in Health Care – Meta-analysis in Context, 2nd edn. BMJ, London: 3–19

Gotham T 2005 Cochrane Primary Health Care Field. About The Cochrane Collaboration (Fields). Issue 3, Art. No: CE000051

Greener J, Grimshaw J 1996 Using meta-analysis to summarise evidence within systematic reviews. Nurse Researcher 4: 27–38

Grégoire G, Derderian F, Le Lorier J 1995 Selecting the language of the publications included in a meta-analysis: is there a Tower of Babel bias? Journal of Clinical Epidemiology 48: 159–163

Griffiths R D, Fernandez R S, Ussia C A 2001 Is tap water a safe alternative to normal saline for wound irrigation in the community setting? Journal of Wound Care 10: 407–411

Hetherington J 2005 Cochrane Collaboration Steering Group. About The Cochrane Collaboration (The Cochrane Collaboration) Issue 4. Art. No.: COLLAB

Jadad A R, Haynes B 1998 The Cochrane Collaboration – advances and challenges in improving evidence-based decision making. Medical Decision Making 18: 2–9

Khan K S, ter Riet G, Popay J, et al 2001 Study quality assessment: undertaking systematic reviews of research of effectiveness. CRD's Guidance for those Carrying Out or Commissioning Reviews Report Number 4: 2–20

Levin A 2001 The Cochrane collaboration. Annals of Internal Medicine 136(4): 309–312

Misakian A L, Bero L A 1998 Publication bias and research on passive smoking: comparison of published and unpublished studies. Journal of the American Medical Association 280: 250–253

Mistiaen P, Poot E, Hickox S, et al 2004 The evidence for nursing interventions in the Cochrane database of systematic reviews. Nurse Researcher 12: 771–780

Moher D, Schulz K F, Altman D 2001 The CONSORT statement: revised recommendations for improving the quality of reports of parallel-group randomized trials. CONSORT group. Journal of the American Medical Association 285: 1987–1991

Moore Z E H, Cowman S 2005 Wound Cleansing for Pressure Ulcers. The Cochrane Database of Systematic Reviews. Issue 4, Art No.: CD004983.pub2. DOI: 10.1002/14651858. CD004983.pub2

Naylor D 1997 Meta-analysis and the meta-epidemiology of clinical research. BMJ 315: 617–619

Rossouw J E, Lewis B, Rifkind B M 1990 The value of lowering cholesterol after myocardial infarction. New England Journal of Medicine 323: 1112–1119

Sackett D, Rosenberg W, Gray M, et al 1996 Evidence based medicine: what it is and what it isn't. BMJ 312: 71–72

The Cochrane Collaboration. The Cochrane Manual Issue 1, 2006 [updated 16 November 2005]. Online. Available: http://www. cochrane.org/admin/manual.htm 23 Jan 2006

Verhagen A P, de Vet H C W, de Bie R A, et al 1998 The Delphi list: A criteria list for quality assessment of randomized clinical trials for conducting systematic reviews developed by Delphi consensus. Journal of Clinical Epidemiology 51: 1235–1241

Chapter 11

Evaluating the Literature

Geraldine McCarthy and Dawn O'Sullivan

Introduction

Evaluating the literature permits judgements to be made about the significance, merit and usefulness of a particular study (McCaughan 1999). Evaluation improves with practice and enhances comprehension and appreciation (Hek 1996). Critical evaluation entails objectively judging the strengths and weaknesses of research, systematically analysing each component in an unbiased and critical way thus reaching conclusions about the quality of the work.

The acknowledgement that nursing care should be evidence-based requires effective evaluation of the literature. With increasing numbers of nursing journals publishing research it becomes imperative for nurses to decide what they should read and what evidence to use in practice. Several questions should be considered before comprehensively reading a research publication and, once read, before deciding whether it is useful for purpose.

Getting started: is this paper worth reading?

With a vast amount of nursing literature available it is crucial to ascertain the appropriateness and quality of a research-based paper before engaging with it. Reviewing the title of the study is worthwhile as it usually reflects the content of the work. While it should not contain jargon, the title should stimulate the reader to continue reading. Some titles are misleading and it may not be worthwhile reading on. It is also worth checking the author's qualifications, as this should provide information on the experience of the researchers. Consideration of whether the study was published by a reputable journal is also advisable. The source of the article under review can provide valuable information on the quality of the study. Peer-reviewed journals, for example, acclaim a higher standard of publications than non-peer-reviewed journals as they are read by independent reviewers (Beeman 2002). However, if a study is published in a peer-reviewed journal this is not a non-disputable measure of its worth (Marshall 2005).

The abstract provides a concise summary of the study and careful evaluation is key to deciding its worth. Different journals request variations in the way abstracts are structured; however, the content is generally premised on similar requirements. The abstract should contain accurate, succinct information and must only include content which subsequently appears in the paper (Branson 2004). Appropriate evaluation of this can only occur once the paper is read. Reviewers should evaluate the provision of a concise summary of the aims, methods, subjects, main findings, conclusions and recommendations. It is necessary to evaluate whether the paper is an original piece of research or if it is simply reporting aspects of a study, which should be explicit having read the abstract (Hek 1996). Having accepted that the paper is worthwhile, it should be scanned in a structured way to answer specific questions regarding its quality (Makela & Witt 2005). If serious weaknesses or flaws are evident, it is advisable to abandon the paper.

It is necessary to examine, understand and evaluate each stage of the research independently. There are generic evaluation criteria that are applicable to both quantitative and qualitative research literature. However, the nature of the approaches means that specific criteria are also necessary. Generic evaluation criteria are presented in Table 11.1, and specific qualitative and quantitative criteria in Table 11.2.

Using generic evaluation criteria
Literature review

The literature review contains the researcher's appraisal of relevant literature associated with the research problem. It should include up-to-date references and provide a critical perspective of the existing literature. A combination of theoretical and research-based knowledge on the topic and sample population, where possible, should be presented. Biased opinions should not be evident and it is important that the researchers have provided evidence which supports as well as contradicts personal opinions (Marshall 2005). A good literature review draws from a wide range of sources, contains relevant information and provides a summary of current knowledge on the research topic (Carnwell & Daly 2001). It should begin broadly, narrow down to the specific problem and conclude with a clear justification for the research (Russell 2005). Secondary sources should only be used when absolutely necessary as the reader is subsequently analysing another's interpretation of the study. The review should highlight flaws in previous research methods that the current study will overcome (Summers 1991). The literature review, through identification of what is already known on a given topic, provides a rationale for the proposed study. The literature should not be presented as a descriptive narrative. Instead, conclusions should be drawn from individual research studies and analysed and compared to others. Research variables should be clearly defined to ensure consensus on what is actually being investigated. Overall the review should flow logically, include all major research previously conducted in the area and be consistently referenced. Word limitations in many journals mean that literature reviews are often very short, which can result in difficulties making balanced judgements about the review. Sometimes reviews are published separately and a quick look at the reference listing should confirm if this is the case.

Table 11.1   *Generic criteria for evaluating the literature*

Component	Key questions
Abstract	■ Does the abstract contain a brief description of aims, methods, data collection/analysis, sample, findings, conclusion? ■ Is a succinct, clear and comprehensive summary of the main text of the paper given? ■ Is the study original?
Literature review	■ Is the literature review critical, current, biased, relevant, structured? ■ Is the significance of the topic established? ■ Is there justification for the current study? ■ Are research variables/concepts clearly defined?
Aims/ objectives	■ Is the research question clear? ■ Are aims and objectives described? And are they capable of answering the research question?
Design	■ What is the research design and is it adequately explained? ■ Is the design appropriate and justified?
Sample	■ Is the sampling method explained including sample size and inclusion/exclusion criteria? ■ How were the subjects selected? ■ Are there sufficient descriptions of participants/respondents offered? ■ Will the sample allow limited or extensive generalisability? ■ Is there evidence of sampling bias?
Ethical approval	■ Was ethical approval obtained? ■ Were ethical principles upheld?
Data collection	■ What data were collected and by what methods? Were the methods described in sufficient detail? ■ Are the procedures used to collect data capable of providing the required information? ■ Was a pilot study conducted?
Data analysis	■ Is there a detailed description of the data analysis procedures? ■ Were data analysed in the most appropriate way?
Findings	■ Are the findings presented in a clear, concise and well-organised manner? ■ Are all relevant findings included? ■ What do the findings mean? ■ Do the findings answer the research questions? ■ How transferable are the findings?
Discussion	■ Are the results compared with previous findings? ■ Is there evidence of speculation? Or are the author's comments justified by the results? ■ Are major new findings clearly described and justified? ■ Are strengths and weaknesses of the study highlighted? ■ Are recommendations for future research provided? ■ Does the study enhance my knowledge of practice?

Table 11.2 – *Criteria for evaluating qualitative and quantitative research*

Qualitative criteria	Quantitative criteria
■ Is the design appropriate? Does it 'fit' the research question? ■ Have researchers documented their preconceptions? ■ Is the sample and setting described sufficiently? ■ Were sampling strategies suitable to identify participants and sources to inform research question? ■ Did researcher engage with participants and become familiar with study context? ■ Were multiple methods employed? ■ Was data collection capable of generating rich data? ■ To what extent did analysis inform subsequent data gathering? ■ Are the findings credible? ■ Was a member-check performed? ■ Were data analysed by more than one independent researcher? ■ Is a range of verbatim quotes provided? ■ Would interpretation of data be recognisable to those having experience in the situations described? ■ Has the research contributed to knowledge or theoretical advancement? ■ Can the findings be transferred to other patients or groups? ■ Were accurate records or an audit trail retained by the researchers?	■ Have the researchers used a theoretical or conceptual framework? If yes, is it adequately explained? ■ Are adequate descriptions of individuals provided? ■ Is there a control group? ■ Are instruments sufficiently described and is there a rationale for using each tool? ■ Are they reliable and valid? ■ Was the description of any interventions in sufficient detail to be repeatable? ■ Is data analysis described and appropriate? ■ Are statistical tests for analysing results stated and are they appropriate? ■ Are tables or graphs adequately labelled, explained and effective? ■ Are all respondents accounted for? ■ What claims are made for generalisability of findings? ■ Did the study give support for the theoretical framework (if one was used)?

Methodology

When evaluating the research methodology, ask the question 'could I replicate this study?' The provision of clear accounts on how the research was conducted is essential. In the methodology section there are a number of subsections, which mainly include the research design, sampling, data collection procedure, data analysis, results and ethical issues. A well-defined research problem is paramount to assessing whether the chosen design was able to address the problem appropriately (Rowan 1997). The aims, objectives, questions and hypotheses should be clearly stated and consistent with the research problem. Evaluation should be concerned with judging how capable the aims and objectives are of answering the research problem.

Research design/approach

The research design or approach should be explained sufficiently and include the identification of theoretical or conceptual frameworks used to underpin the study (Hek 1996). Evaluation of the design includes assessing the appropriateness of the approach to the research questions posed, the aims and objectives. For example, if the researcher is investigating 'lived experiences', then a phenomenological design is the most suitable; however, if exploring the relationship between variables, then a quantitative correlation design is appropriate (Polit & Beck 2004). In some instances a number of approaches may be suited to a particular study and evaluation should be concerned with how the researchers justify using the chosen design. The research design should be reflected in the research problem, sampling procedure and methods used in data collection and analysis (Benton & Cormack 1996).

Sampling

The sampling procedure should be described in detail, incorporating sample size and inclusion/exclusion criteria, as well as the rationale for the sampling procedure implemented. It is important to evaluate whether or not the sampling procedure was used appropriately by the researchers, i.e. was the sample type in keeping with the design. For example, in a quantitative experimental study, randomisation is the recommended sampling method (Burns & Grove 2001). Enough information should be provided to consider whether the sample selection method was valid. Questions surrounding the issue of sampling bias should also be raised. Sampling bias occurs when there is over- or under-representation of any characteristics of relevance to the research problem (Polit & Beck 2004). Consideration of whether the sample is large enough and representative of the population under investigation is important. While small samples may be appropriate in qualitative studies, a larger sample size is required for statistical analysis in quantitative research. Research reports should be specific about size and how researchers arrived at the number of subjects.

The sample should be sufficiently explicit to allow informed judgements about whether the findings can be generalised to others (McCaughan 1999).

Ethical approval

There are ethical issues in all research and it is necessary to evaluate whether appropriate ethical approval was obtained for the research. Normally, this is achieved after submission of a detailed proposal to a local ethics committee. Specific description of subject recruitment and retention should be provided. Subjects should be given adequate information, and be assured of their rights to confidentiality, anonymity and freedom to withdraw from the study at any time. It is also important to establish whether ethical principles such as informed consent were upheld throughout the research (Seals & Tanaka 2000) and whether data storage and disposal were addressed.

Data collection

Evaluating the methods used to collect data is important as any flaws in data collection may undermine findings. Procedures taken to collect data should be described in detail. How key concepts were defined is important. The relationship of this definition to method of data collection should be explicit. It is important to decide whether the way data were collected was appropriate to the specific data required. Irrespective of how data were collected, sample questions or interview topics should be provided so that the reader can make informed judgements concerning the relevance of the questions asked (Beeman 2002). Ascertaining whether a pilot study was conducted is a useful way of evaluating if potential problems with data collection methods were identified and altered (Polit & Beck 2004).

Data analysis and findings

The conclusions or results reached are largely dependent on the adequacy of data analysis. It is important to evaluate whether the researchers analysed the data in the most appropriate way (Seals & Tanaka 2000). Adequate descriptions of how data were analysed should be provided and in keeping with the research design. Owing to the different techniques quantitative and qualitative researchers use to analyse data, these issues will be dealt with separately below.

There should be no evidence of bias in the explanation of the results (Marshall 2005). All relevant findings should be presented in a suitable manner and their ability to answer the research questions carefully evaluated. Evaluate whether any vital information was missing or if the results represented the entire sample. Including details of response rates and incomplete data in results is important. Figures and tables should be well constructed and easily read. Once the findings are sufficiently evaluated, the implications of the findings should be considered. Interpreting the results into meaningful implications for practice is important. Although the discussion section usually deals with this, evaluating whether the findings are clinically significant is good practice as researchers may overestimate their relevance.

Discussion

In the discussion a summary of the study is presented and the authors present limitations and recommendations. The researcher should compare and interpret the findings in the context of the literature reviewed. It is necessary to consider whether the interpretation of the results follows the presentation of results. The possibility of inferring that results respond to the research problem is a pitfall and it is necessary to consider potential for speculation (Marshall 2005). The scope to which the findings can be generalised should be explored and evaluation of over- or under-generalisation is recommended (Burns & Grove 2001). Strengths and weaknesses of the study should be identified and recommendations on how to avoid future limitations provided (Hek 1996). New findings should be emphasised and recommendations for future research provided.

Conclusion

In this section, researchers draw conclusions from the main findings. The accuracy of the conclusions made is dependent on the quality of the research. Thorough evaluations of the conclusions are only possible once all other components have been analysed. Researchers should not speculate or overestimate the conclusions and should base them solely on the findings (Marshall 2005): how well the researchers justify the conclusions drawn is significant. Implications for further research, education or practice should be discussed.

Presentation and referencing

Presentation should be consistent and logical, with citations detailed properly in the text. Reports should be clearly written, well organised with a logical progression detailing each step of the research. Any sponsorship or support should be acknowledged and the author should write objectively. References should be current, extensive and focused.

Evaluating qualitative research

Cutcliffe and McKenna (1999) argue that there is no single accepted way of evaluating qualitative research. While there are overlaps in the evaluation of qualitative and quantitative research it is necessary to elucidate unique aspects of qualitative research evaluation. Qualitative researchers are concerned with gaining deep, meaningful, rich information from small groups that fulfil certain criteria (Ambert et al 1995). It is worth considering whether a qualitative design was appropriate or if a quantitative approach could have provided a more suitable exploration of the topic. Understanding what the researchers were striving to achieve is essential before meaningful evaluation can occur. If the aim of the research was interpretive, exploratory or premised on generating meaning or understanding, then qualitative methods are suitable (Greenhalgh & Taylor 1997). Additionally, qualitative research is recommended for the investigation of new topics, which have had little or no previous exploration.

Therefore, literature reviews in qualitative research can differ from those offered by researchers employing quantitative methods. New avenues of exploration will invariably have minimal literature associated with the topic so the review may not be extensive. However, some qualitative researchers do not engage extensively with the literature at the beginning as it may unduly influence the research question (Rowan 1997). It is important to establish whether the chosen design best suits the research problem. Ethnography, for example, is concerned with learning about individuals within their own culture whereas grounded theory seeks to understand various processes in social settings (Polit & Beck 2004).

A major challenge presented to reviewers of qualitative research is evaluating the truthfulness of the findings. In qualitative research validity is expressed in terms such as rigour, trustworthiness, credibility and believability (Russell & Gregory 2003).

The interpretive nature of qualitative research can threaten the credibility of findings and there is no way of totally eliminating bias in qualitative research (Greenhalgh & Taylor 1997). Nonetheless, this does not mean that qualitative research lacks rigour (Horsburgh 2003).

Qualitative researchers should document their preconceptions or biases before the study commences (Mays & Pope 2000). This ensures that the reviewer knows the researcher's views on the topic and observes for signs of influence on the study's outcomes. Although detailed descriptions of researchers' prejudices may not be permissible in journal articles, reviewers should evaluate whether or not some form of reference to them was made. Triangulation of methods is also regarded as a means of enhancing credibility and can include triangulation of data, methods, investigators or analysis (Byrne 2001). This process of using multiple methods 'enhances the completeness of data' (Brown & Lloyd 2001, p. 352).

The extent to which the data collection methods used have been described should be evaluated as the interpretation of findings is closely related (Greenhalgh & Taylor 1997). It is necessary to judge whether the methods used to collect data were capable of generating rich data. Qualitative researchers draw from a wide range of sources including individuals, documents, field notes and narrative stories (Ambert et al 1995). Prolonged engagement during interviews or observations is another way of promoting credibility as the researcher's understanding of the participant's world is enhanced (Cutcliffe & McKenna 1999). The setting, or the context in which the researchers engage with participants, is also an important aspect of data collection and evaluation should be concerned with the adequacy of the descriptions provided. Horsburgh (2003) stipulated that detailed accounts of the settings should be provided so that data can be contextualised and that researchers should highlight any factors, such as observations, which may affect the participant's actions.

It is difficult for novice researchers to understand fully the processes of data analysis in qualitative research. This difficulty is often compounded by the obscure language qualitative researchers use to articulate the process (Thorne 2000). How well the researcher explains the way data were analysed is significant. Different methods of analysis are more suitable to specific designs; for example, constant comparative analysis is more suited to grounded theory than ethnography. Irrespective of the methods of analysis employed it is vital to consider how well the analysis enabled the development of categories that articulated the participants' narrations or observations (Mays & Pope 2000). While statistical representations are not associated with qualitative data, it is not unusual for qualitative researchers to present frequencies and percentages in the findings (Parahoo 1997). If statistics are provided it is necessary to evaluate whether they were used to summarise certain data or if researchers relied inappropriately on their significance.

A member check, or returning to participants for verification of findings, is another strategy used to achieve credible findings (Cutcliffe & McKenna 2002). If findings were verified by a member check, researchers should divulge how the participants agreed and disagreed with the themes, categories or emerging theories (Cutcliffe & McKenna 1999). Therefore, it is important to evaluate whether opposing views were provided or cases that objected to the conclusions. Establishing whether more than one independent researcher, or peers not involved in the study but knowledgeable of the research design, were used to authenticate findings is also worthwhile. The more people that independently agree with the emerging findings, the more this enhances their believability and reduces the risk of researcher bias.

Another strategy often employed by qualitative researchers is the provision of verbatim quotes to substantiate interpretation derived from data. Findings from qualitative research should be presented in narrative form and data excerpts are usually offered (Fossey et al 2002). Evaluation involves assessing how clearly the data provided supported the main points. It is also necessary to observe whether theoretical assumptions were made without adequate supportive data or descriptions (Giacomini & Cook 2000a). The findings should substantiate an existing theory or generate new theory (Ambert et al 1995). Reviewers should question how well the findings were interpreted within the context of existing research. Furthermore, it should be evaluated whether researchers recommended questions or hypotheses to be tested by further research.

Qualitative researchers are not concerned with 'generalisation' of findings and evaluation is concerned with the extent to which the findings can be applied to other patients or groups, known as transferability. Evaluating the sampling method used can help the reviewer establish the scope for transferring findings. Sampling in qualitative research is usually purposive, which is recognised as a measure to improve transferability (Benton & Cormack 1996). Sampling is concerned with recruiting individuals who possess certain necessary traits for the research being conducted and should not be one of convenience (Brown & Lloyd 2001). When other methods of sampling are employed it is necessary to evaluate whether or not they were

justified and if participants were relevant to the research problem.

Confirmability of the research process is another aspect requiring evaluation. Qualitative researchers should retain a certain amount of information including data and analysis, which is referred to as an audit trail. Leaving a trail of data and analysis provides a way for other researchers to follow or audit the research (Giacomini & Cook 2000a). Evaluating how the findings enhance understanding of care, practice and relationships is also important (Giacomini & Cook 2000b).

Evaluating quantitative research

It is vital to have adequate comprehension of what quantitative researchers are trying to achieve before critical evaluation is possible. As well as research questions, quantitative researchers frequently present hypotheses for testing. Hypotheses are statements of the researcher's predictions on the relationships between variables (Russell 2005). While quantitative researcher's main intention is to measure, 'assessment', 'evaluation' and 'description' are often used as the former is not always possible (Parahoo 1997). Designs in quantitative research fall into one of two main categories, non-experimental and experimental. Non-experimental research includes descriptive and correlation designs, which are intended, simply, to describe or examine relationships. Experimental research is tightly controlled and should use random sampling, include a control group and an intervention (Parahoo 1997). If a study lacks one of these criteria, it is referred to as quasi-experimental. Designs in quantitative research can also be cross-sectional, longitudinal, retrospective or prospective. Evaluating the appropriateness of the design employed is crucial. For example, reviewers should question the use of a retrospective study when a prospective design could have been used. Retrospective studies are subject to recall bias whereas prospective designs collect data as they are produced, which are more reliable (Polit & Beck 2004).

It is necessary to establish whether a justified rationale for conducting the study was provided. Quantitative researchers use the existing literature to identify gaps and highlight the further research (Russell 2005). Theoretical or conceptual frameworks are often used in quantitative research. It is necessary to evaluate whether sufficient explanation of the concepts and their relationships within the framework have been provided. It is also important to establish whether the researchers have clearly defined the research variables and if they have identified them as independent or dependent.

To promote the genaralisability of statistical results quantitative researchers frequently use large random samples. Large numbers are required as they enhance the statistical power for data analysis (Marshall 2005, Seals & Tanaka 2000). Evaluation of the sampling process requires consideration of a number of factors. Sampling should be discussed in adequate detail. The researchers must clearly describe the sampling procedure, how respondents were identified, inclusion/exclusion criteria and sample size (Russell 2005). If a control group was used, assessing for the provision of adequate characteristics of both groups is necessary (Greenhalgh 1997a). Sufficient description should be provided to permit evaluation of the groups' level of comparability. For example, respondents in each group should have similar socio-demographic variables and disease or prognostic similarities. Significant variations in the characteristics of the groups can influence the results (Burns & Grove 2001).

In quantitative research data are generally collected in a structured objective way using questionnaires, instruments or bio-physiological measures (Russell 2005). It is important to evaluate how the researchers described the procedures followed. For example, reviewers need to understand how often respondents completed questionnaires, what happened between first and second measurements and what happened in treatment or control groups. Quantitative reviewers should evaluate whether the instruments used were sufficiently described and if their validity and reliability were established

(McCaughan 1999). It is necessary to assess whether the researchers clearly indicated which variables each instrument measured. Sufficient detail should be provided for each instrument, including what exactly was being measured, how the scores were calculated and previous use of the instruments discussed. Validity is the degree to which an instrument measures what it purports to measure (Polit & Beck 2004). Reliability is concerned with consistency and dependability. Reliability coefficients, such as Cronbach's alpha, should be provided as they offer objective estimates of the instrument's reliability (Polit & Beck 2004).

As with qualitative research, quantitative data analysis can seem daunting. However, there are certain ways of evaluating whether the methods used to analyse data were satisfactory. Firstly, verification that the results answered the research questions or problem is recommended (Beeman 2002). It is then worthwhile returning attention to the design. If a descriptive design was used then data analysis should yield descriptive results such as means and standard deviations, or medians and ranges. Alternatively, if the design used was correlational then the appropriateness of the use of inferential statistics such as Pearson's r or Spearman's rho should be evaluated (Russell 2005). If a control group was used it is important to establish whether data from both groups were analysed the same number of times (Greenhalgh 1997a). Evaluating whether the researchers justified the actual methods they used to analyse data is also important. There are different types of data in quantitative research; each data set is suited to specific analysis. For example, non-parametric tests are best suited to categorical data (nominal or ordinal) and parametric tests are more appropriate for interval or ratio data (Giuffre 1996).

Graphs and tables should be adequately explained and labelled, and discussed in the text (Branson 2004). Researchers usually present details of the sample group first. It is imperative to evaluate whether the researchers gave accurate details of response rates or incomplete data, which cannot be analysed. In addition it is necessary to note if any exceptional cases were removed from analysis, which may distort results. In effect, all respondents should be accounted for and any reasons for missing data should be highlighted (Makela & Witt 2005). In correlation research, it is crucial to consider whether the investigators have made assumptions about the causal relationships explored. For example, if it is established that two variables are closely related the direction of the relationship is not explicit and therefore cannot be assumed (Greenhalgh 1997b).

Evaluating the validity of the results is a crucial component of quantitative research. Both internal and external risks to the study's validity are possible. Internal threats to validity include analysing problems with the study design or its implementation (Russell 2005). Evaluating the risk of bias and how researchers minimise this risk is also recommended as sources of bias can falsify the interpretation of results. It is also possible that other variables, not identified by the researchers, could have influenced results. Reviewers should be observant for confounding variables (Marshall 2005). External threats to validity relate to the generalisability of results. The ability to generalise is closely related to the sample and settings used. Appropriate evaluation of the extent to which results could be applied to a different setting or population is therefore dependent on the adequacy of descriptions offered. A Hawthorne effect is another potential threat to the validity of quantitative research. The very fact that respondents know they are being studied may cause them to change behaviour to please, and reviewers should be alert for signs of this (Polit & Beck 2004).

The discussion section in quantitative research permits exploration of the results in the context of existing knowledge. If a theoretical framework was used, it is important to evaluate whether researchers discussed the findings in the context of the framework. If quantitative researchers make claims or offer interpretations of results it should be acknowledged as such (Branson 2004). Any limitations of the study must be emphasised and evaluated by reviewers. Evaluation of the researcher's appraisal of whether the study's aims and hypotheses were met is also warranted. Conclusions made should be consistent with the research question. Reviewers should evaluate whether questions for future research have been posed and if realistic implications for clinical practice have been offered.

Conclusion

Evaluating research is vital as nurses strive to provide evidence-based nursing care. It is also important as nursing develops as an academic discipline with increasing attention being paid to publications by nurses employed in academia. Nurses must decide what they should read, what evidence to use in practice and in the identification of research endeavours. This chapter proposes that several questions should be considered before comprehensively reading a research publication and once read, before deciding whether it is useful for purpose. A framework based on generic criteria for evaluation is firstly presented followed by two sections which focus specifically on evaluation strategies for both qualitative and quantitative research.

EXERCISES

1. Locate a research-based article on a topic of interest and evaluate the abstract using the criteria provided in this chapter. Having read and evaluated the abstract, decide whether or not you will read the full article. What are the factors which persuaded or dissuaded you from reading on?
2. Read a research-based article from a peer-reviewed journal and evaluate it using the evaluation criteria provided in the chapter. What are the merits and limitations of the study reviewed?

EXERCISES—Cont'd

3. Source two articles dealing with the same research problem – one using a qualitative design and one a quantitative design.

   - Evaluate each study independently, focusing specifically on the justification and appropriateness of the chosen design in each case.
   - Evaluate which approach was most appropriate to the research question posed or the problem under investigation.
   - Evaluate whether similar or opposing findings are emerging and the likely reasons for this.

References

Ambert A M, Adler P A, Adler P, et al 1995 Understanding and evaluating qualitative research. Journal of Marriage and the Family 57: 879–893

Beeman S K 2002 Evaluating violence against women research reports. National Electronic Network on Violence Against Women, Pennsylvania: 1–8

Benton D, Cormack D F 1996 Reviewing and evaluating the literature. In: Cormack D F (ed). The Research Process in Nursing, 3rd edn. Blackwell, Oxford

Branson R D 2004 Anatomy of a research paper. Respiratory Care 49: 1222–1228

Brown C, Lloyd K 2001 Qualitative methods in psychiatric research. Advances in Psychiatric Treatment 7: 350–356

Burns N, Grove S 2001 The Practice of Nursing Research Conduct, Critique and Utilisation, 4th edn. Saunders, London

Byrne M 2001 Evaluating the findings of qualitative research. AORN Journal 73: 703–706

Carnwell R, Daly W 2001 Strategies for the construction of a critical review of the literature. Nurse Education in Practice 1: 57–63

Cutcliffe J R, McKenna H P 1999 Establishing the credibility of qualitative research: the plot thickens. Journal of Advanced Nursing 30: 374–380

Cutcliffe J R, McKenna H P 2002 When do we know that we know? Considering the truth of research findings and the craft of qualitative research. International Journal of Nursing Studies 39: 611–618

Fossey E, Harvey C, McDermott F et al 2002 Understanding and evaluating qualitative research. Australian and New Zealand Journal of Psychiatry 36: 717–732

Giacomini M, Cook D J 2000a User's guide to the medical literature XXIII. Qualitative research in health care. A. Are the results of the study valid? Journal of the American Medical Association 284: 357–362

Giacomini M, Cook D J 2000b User's guide to the medical literature XXIII. Qualitative research in health care. B. What are the results and how do they help me care for my patients? Journal of the American Medical Association 284: 478–482

Giuffre M 1996 Reading research critically: Results-group data. Journal of Perianesthesia Nursing 11: 344–348

Greenhalgh T 1997a How to read a paper: Statistics for the non-statistician. 11: 'Significant' relations and their pitfalls. British Medical Journal 315: 422–425

Greenhalgh T 1997b How to read a paper: Statistics for the non-statistician. 1: different types of data needed for different tests. British Medical Journal 315: 364–366

Greenhalgh T, Taylor R 1997 How to read a paper: Papers that go beyond numbers (qualitative research). British Medical Journal 315: 740–743

Hek G 1996 Guidelines on conducting a critical research evaluation. Nursing Standard 11(6): 40–43

Horsburgh D 2003 Evaluation of qualitative research. Journal of Clinical Nursing 12: 307–312

McCaughan D 1999 Developing critical appraisal skills. Professional Nurse 14: 843–847

Makela M, Witt K 2005 How to read a paper: critical appraisal of studies for application in healthcare. Singapore Medical Journal 46: 108–115

Marshall G 2005 Critiquing a research article. Radiography 11: 55–59

Mays N, Pope C 2000 Qualitative research in health care: assessing quality in qualitative research. British Medical Journal 320: 50–52

Parahoo K 1997 Nursing Research: Principles, Processes and Issues. Macmillan, New York

Polit D, Beck C T 2004 Nursing Research: Principles and Methods, 7th edn. Lippincott, New York

Rowan M 1997 Qualitative research articles: information for authors and peer reviewers. Canadian Medical Association Journal 157: 1442–1446

Russell C 2005 Evaluating quantitative research reports. Nephrology Nursing Journal 32: 1–5

Russell C, Gregory D 2003 Evaluation of qualitative research studies. Evidence Based Nursing 6: 36–40

Seals D, Tanaka H 2000 Manuscript peer review: A helpful checklist for students and novice referees. Advances in Physiology Education 23: 52–58

Summers S 1991 Steps in reviewing literature. Journal of Post Anaesthesia Nursing 6: 188–192

Thorne S 2000 Data analysis in qualitative research. Evidence-Based Nursing 3: 68–70

Chapter 12

Research Governance and Research Ethics

Carol Haigh

Introduction

The aim of this chapter is to examine the dual concepts of research governance and research ethics. The first part of this chapter will be concerned with the international development of research governance frameworks, followed by an exploration of the fundamental elements that go to make up the concept of governance. The subsequent section of the chapter will explore the essential concepts inherent in an ethical approach to research and how these translate into the ethical issues that researchers must consider if they are to achieve a successful ethical review prior to commencing their study. The evolving nature of both research ethics and research governance is highlighted in the concluding part of the chapter. For the purposes of this chapter the term research participants is widened to include both the individuals who form the study sample and the research teams themselves.

Why have governance guidelines developed?

The earlier development of research governance guidelines was driven by specific failures in research supervision systems which resulted in public scandals. In the USA a review of the systems available for protecting the public participants of research trials was initiated by the (unrelated) deaths of Jesse Gelsinger in 1999 and Ellen Roche in 2002. In the UK the Alder Hey organ retention scandal which was beginning to unfold in 1999 likewise prompted a review of the systems that were in place to ensure the safety of research volunteers. The results, from both sides of the Atlantic, highlighted serious and widespread deficiencies (Steinbrook 2002). This led the US and UK governments to examine the research culture more closely and to develop frameworks and guidelines that addressed more issues than the traditional ethical review. Other countries were quick to see the implications of such an approach and began to consider the concept of research governance with the same degree of urgency they had once applied to the concepts of ethical inquiry. The approach to research governance is slightly different across the world, with some countries such as Australia (NHMRC 2004) and the OECD countries (2003) taking an integrated approach to ethics and research governance while others, notably the UK (2005), prefer to set out researcher obligations to governance in a separate document designed to complement existing ethics guidance. Nevertheless, the fundamental principles are the same. Since the UK has articulated these governance principles most clearly, it is appropriate to consider the elements of good research governance within the UK definitions and framework.

Fundamentals of research governance

Research governance is a framework through which institutions are accountable for the ethical quality, scientific acceptability and management of participant safety in the research that they sponsor or permit. Although there is a variety of approaches to the application of good governance strategies, fundamental elements can be expressed as falling within one of five domains (Fig. 12.1). These are:

- ethics;
- science;
- information;
- health and safety and employment;
- financial and intellectual property (Department of Health 2001).

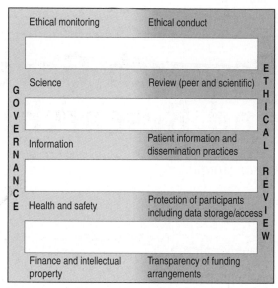

Figure 12.1 – *How research governance and ethical review link together.*

Ethics

In the UK, ethics and governance are closely intertwined. Historically, once ethical approval had been obtained from the appropriate committee there was no monitoring of the subsequent research study, which rendered the system open to abuse. Governance processes are designed to promote monitoring of all aspects of research studies, in particular methods of obtaining consent, data protection and data storage. In the UK, governance departments must review 10% of all studies they approve each year.

Science

This governance domain is concerned with ensuring that the research that is carried out in the health and social care arena is scientifically robust, subject to expert review in its early stages and based as far as is practicable upon existing sources of information. This ensures that research is seen as a linear process with new work building upon that which has gone before. It requires potential researchers to show a thorough examination of the literature when submitting proposals for both ethical review and governance approval.

Information

Research that is not disseminated in the public domain is 'dead' research. Nonetheless a significant amount of research projects are completed without the results being made available to the interested parties. This is a particular concern with post-graduate research (Teacher Training Agency 1998). Even more projects are lodged in the public domain but are only accessible to a highly specialised or technical audience. Many grant-making bodies are now insisting that researchers should provide information for both the professional and the lay readership (Joseph Rowntree Foundation 2005). The governance province of 'information' helps to address the issue of research which is wasted through failure to disseminate, which in turn leads to failure to implement research findings. In an effort to ensure that research findings are implemented in health care practice, all proposed research projects must have considered how the anticipated findings will be disseminated across all interested parties. In the UK, the National Research Register records all NHS Trust research activities. This provides the public with information about ongoing and completed research projects.

Health and safety

This area of governance can be seen to address two significant areas. Firstly, it is connected to protection of participant well-being. Informed by the EU Clinical Trials Directive (2001/20/EU), published in May 2001, governance became part of UK legislation in 2003, and was fully implemented by 2004; the health and safety domain of governance frameworks requires that researchers have the protection and safety of participants in mind at all times. Prior to the development of governance frameworks and, for European countries, the drafting of the EU clinical trials directive (European Commission 2001), researchers were not obliged to report or disclose the health and safety issues inherent in their research. Additionally, in the UK, researchers who are not NHS employees, but who are carrying out research on NHS user/employee populations are required to obtain an honorary contract from the participating trust prior to commencing data collection. Concerns have been mooted that this often protracted process has the overall effect of, at best, slowing down research and, at worst, acting as a disincentive to health service research (Howarth & Kneafsey 2004). However, it does act as an additional protection for participants since it allows NHS establishments to satisfy themselves about the credibility and ability of the researcher who wishes to undertake research within their organisation.

The second area of health and safety concern addressed by this aspect of governance is focused upon the safety of the researchers themselves. This may mean assessing whether the researcher is likely to be exposed to ionising radiation or noxious substances during the course of the research study (not usually an issue for the majority of health and social care research studies for which nurses are likely to be responsible) or, more importantly, may concentrate upon issues such as visiting research participants in their own homes, or late night working. For the first time, researchers are encouraged to think about their personal safety.

Finance

Organisations involved in research activity must be able to demonstrate that research funds can be managed appropriately in line with any financial legislation. This includes compliance with audit requirements and the ability to compensate research participants in the event of negligent harm. In the UK, there is no strategy for the provision of compensation in the event of non-negligent harm. However, if the researcher is employed by an organisation which does provide indemnity against non-negligent harm, the organisation must also be able to demonstrate that they can offer that compensation.

Other considerations within the 'finance' governance domain overlap with the domain of intellectual property (see below) in that arrangements must be in place to protect and exploit any commercial benefit that may accrue from research studies.

Intellectual property

The UK, and the NHS in particular, has a poor record in terms of the exploitation of potential commercial benefits and opportunities that can be developed from research carried out within health care settings compared with other countries and organisations. The research governance framework is designed to ensure that the NHS benefits from new technologies and patentable materials that are generated by research within its environs by setting up monitoring processes and strategies for the protection of intellectual property rights.

Quality research culture

The creation of a quality research culture can be seen to have direct links to the research 'incidents' that drove the development of governance procedures. The UK government describe such a research culture as having the following characteristics:

- respect for participants' dignity, rights, safety and well-being;
- valuing the diversity within society;
- personal and scientific integrity;
- leadership;
- honesty;
- accountability;
- openness;
- clear and supportive management (Department of Health 2001).

This aspect of research governance focuses upon clear identification of responsibility amongst the research team. The UK model proposes that strong research leadership should be allied to the promotion and support of research studies that reflect the national research agenda and the local priorities of the trust. Research governance frameworks set out definitions of the various roles within the research process such as:

- *Principal investigator:* the person responsible for the day-to-day management of the study who,

by definition, has the skills and expertise to plan, direct and report the project.
- *Sponsor:* usually a representative of either the trust or the researcher's employing organisation. Their role is to guarantee the quality of the research environment and the competence of the research team.

Responsibility for the safe, robust conduct of the research lies with the principal investigator; however, the investigator's employing institution is also responsible for ensuring that the appropriate quality monitoring mechanisms are in place. Thus, the intention of research governance strategies is to improve research quality and safeguard the public by giving due consideration to all aspects of research project management via these five domains. Inherent to this intention are a number of prerequisites which are key conditions if the twin goals of improvement and protection are to be achieved. These are outlined in Table 12.1.

These prerequisites form the basis of most of the approaches that have been taken to the management of research governance. For example, the European Forum for Good Clinical Practice overtly incorporated them into its recommendations and

Table 12.1 – *Prerequisite conditions mapped against the five governance domains*

Prerequisite	Governance domain
Enhancement of ethical and scientific quality	▪ Ethics ▪ Science ▪ Financial and intellectual property
Reduction of adverse incidents and ensuring lessons are learned	▪ Health, safety and employment ▪ Information
Prevention of poor performance and misconduct	▪ Health, safety and employment

guidelines for European ethics committees (EFGCP 1997) whilst the OECD (2003) have taken a broader approach, using these concepts less explicitly as a framework for recommendations. The National Health and Medical Research Council of Australia (NHMRC 2004) have, in a draft document, produced governance guidelines that closely mirror those of the UK but which are far more directive.

The scope of research governance is comprehensive; as can be seen from Table 12.2, research

Table 12.2 – *Scope of research governance*

Governance applies to...	This includes...
All who participate in research	■ Patients/service users ■ Patients' relatives ■ Carers ■ Carer/patient organisations ■ The general public ■ Charities ■ Health and social care professionals
Organisations that host research	■ Hospitals ■ Community health centres ■ Local authorities
Organisations that fund research	■ Research Councils ■ Charities ■ Government departments ■ Professional organisations
Organisations or individuals that manage research All who undertake research	■ Universities ■ Academics ■ Student supervisors ■ Researchers ■ Universities ■ Commercial organisations and industry ■ Students (and their supervisors)

governance guidelines apply to managers and staff, in all professional groups, no matter how senior or junior and in all aspects of health and social care, primary, secondary and tertiary care.

Fundamentals of research ethics

The majority of research projects in the health and social care domain require both research governance approval and satisfactory ethical review before they can begin. Novice researchers and, occasionally some experienced researchers, often find ethical and moral reasoning the most challenging part of their research project (Haigh & Jones 2005). Beauchamp and Childress (2001) suggest a hierarchy of moral reasoning which can be helpful in that instance. At level 1 of the hierarchy, morally based judgements and actions are justified by the rules which form the hierarchical level and also define which actions are acceptable. For example, the decision to be open and honest with a patient (level 1) is supported by the ethical rule 'it is wrong to lie' (level 2). Ethical principles, the third level of the hierarchy, are seen as more general and often serve as a form of justification for the application of the rules in specific situations. Thus the 'wrong to lie' rule is supported by the moral principle of autonomy. Finally, these bodies of rules and principles are organised into ethical theories such as utilitarianism, which evaluates the worth of actions (or research projects) by their ends or consequences, and deontology, which argues that acts (or, again, research projects) are right or wrong independent of their consequences.

Different countries tend to adopt different theoretical stances when considering the ethical elements of a research proposal. For instance, European ethical review is underpinned by a strong deontological stance so, for example, a study that used placebos would have to be strongly and robustly justified since the implied deception of participants inherent in placebo administration is not acceptable from a deontological viewpoint. Conversely the USA is known to view research ethics from a more consequentialist (utilitarian) viewpoint which would

Table 12.3 – *Hierarchy of moral and ethical reasoning (Beauchamp & Childress 2001)*

Hierarchical levels	Examples
4. Theories	■ Utilitarian ■ Deontological
3. Principles	■ Autonomy ■ Justice ■ Beneficence ■ Non-maleficence (not causing harm)
2. Rules	■ Wrong to kill ■ Truth telling
1. Judgements and actions	■ Respect for life ■ Being honest

balance such deception against the outcome of increased good for the majority.

Ethical review of research projects is generally based upon the four key principles of 'practical ethics' as outlined in Table 12.3. Although it must be acknowledged that other ethical approaches exist, practical, principle-focused ethics as described by Beauchamp and Childress (2001) are seen as particularly useful to health and social care researchers since they attempt to apply general norms and ethical principles to specific research problems or contexts. In Europe, this principalist approach is widespread, with ethical review focusing upon key specific issues that are grounded in these main principles (Fig. 12.2).

To contextualise the ethical requirements of a successful research project with this principalist approach it is appropriate to examine each of the four main ethical principles in detail to assess what impact they have upon the elements of the research process that require ethical review.

Autonomy

Beauchamp and Childress (2001) note that numerous and diverse philosophers have argued that

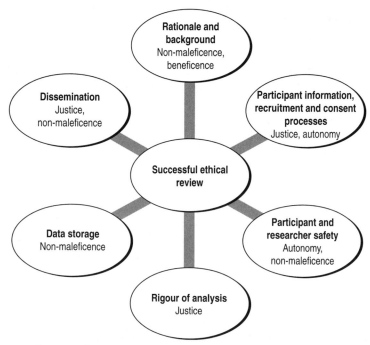

Figure 12.2 – *Elements of successful ethical review.*

morality and ethical reasoning requires that individuals are autonomous. Autonomy implies that an individual chooses their own course of action, usually in accordance with a plan that they have decided for themselves. It is very easy for a novice researcher inadvertently to undermine the autonomy of their potential study participants, usually from the best of intentions. It is crucial that the recruitment process is as open to as many volunteers as is practicable. For example, often significant sections of society are excluded from research studies for no good reason. The groups may include, so-called, vulnerable groups such as individuals with learning disabilities or mental health problems or members of ethnic groups who are not fluent in the language of the researcher's home country (Involve 2004). Whilst there may be a tension between wishing to avoid marginalising certain sections of society and subjecting the same sections to significant over-researching (as is often the case with palliative care patients, for example), the final decision to participate or not in any research project lies with the individual. Johnson (2003) has suggested that the research community has replaced an indisputable obligation to protect from genuine harm with a need to protect everybody at all costs and that this is a redundant attitude when dealing with individuals who can say 'no thank you' for themselves. It must also be emphasised that being a member of a vulnerable group does not necessarily mean that saying 'no thank you' is impossible – vulnerable people may not be vulnerable is every aspect of their lives and to assume that they are is a significant erosion of their autonomy.

The responsibility of the researcher is to ensure that recruitment, information and consent procedures are such that participation in their proposed study is equally available to all members of their identified population. This may mean reviewing consent forms and information literature to ensure that it is understandable and accessible to everyone. As a guide, the researcher is advised to find out what the average reading age is in their country (for example, in the UK the average reading age is

that of an educated 9-year-old) and write all such literature to that level.

Non-maleficence

The ethical principle of non-maleficence is concerned with the concept that one should not inflict evil or harm (Beauchamp & Childress 2001). For the researcher this principle is first addressed at the start of their project when setting out the background and justification for their approach. If it has been shown that previous, similar studies have been seen to cause discomfort or distress to participants there is a moral imperative upon the researcher to minimise that harm. A successful ethics application would acknowledge this difficulty and ensure that ways of managing potential harm are identified. Pragmatically, this may mean minimising invasive procedures or ensuring that support mechanisms are in place for participants who become distressed during or after data collection.

The ethical principle of non-maleficence also applies to data that have been collected. Most ethical guidelines and review panels insist that researchers are required to make explicit how data will be stored and who will have access to it. In this instance, data may be anything from biological materials to interview transcripts. It is essential that the data are stored in such a manner that no harm could accrue to the individual from whom that data originated. This is particularly important when the data concern sensitive activities. The practical issues that researchers need to consider are anonymity, confidentiality, country-specific data protection guidelines and any national legislation that affects biological material, especially that which would allow genetic identification of an individual.

The final stage of any good research project is that of dissemination. At this point the principle of non-maleficence is also key. The need to protect participants from harm has already been emphasised but, in some cases, that responsibility also extends to participating institutions. The researcher's obligation to ensure that institutions are not harmed sites itself in two key areas. First, protecting the confidentiality or anonymity of participants is futile if they can easily be identified from the institutional or group data which are presented. Secondly, if the reputation of a specific body or institution would be harmed from being disclosed, the researcher would not be acting in an ethically acceptable manner if their dissemination strategies make such identification possible.

Beneficence

If the principle of non-maleficence places an obligation upon the research to do no harm, beneficence requires the promotion of good. Although the distinction between these two concepts may seem obscure, they are extremely different since one is passive (non-maleficence) and one is active (beneficence) in nature. The earliest stages of the research process allow researchers to evaluate their overall aim to decide whether one of the aims of the study is to be the prevention of harm or the active promotion of good. Of course, this is never as clear as this rather simplistic view may imply. For example, testing a new drug via a randomised controlled trial may subject the intervention group to highly unpleasant or debilitating side effects. If this is going to be the case, the researcher should ensure that they have provided a robust and detailed rationale and justification for their proposed approach which allows for the potential harm that participants may experience to be contextualised into the overall good that may accrue from the study. Likewise using children in research, childhood diseases, and childhood development and drug reactions can only be studied in children. The children who participate may accrue no benefit but the wider understanding is that such studies translate into an overall 'good' for the wider population.

Justice

Generally, in the health care environment, the principle of justice is concerned with access to and allocation of resources. However, Beauchamp and Childress (2001) also note that the ethical principle of justice incorporates the concept of 'fair opportunity', which does have an impact upon the ethical construction of a research project. The importance of including all eligible individuals regardless of gender, language, age etc. has already been discussed as an element of autonomy. However, providing the opportunity for participation to all groups can been seen as an example of the ethical principle of justice.

Furthermore, the principle of justice can also be applied to the analysis of data. It is ethically inappropriate to 'cherry pick' elements of data for either analysis or dissemination. Whilst it is accepted, particularly when writing for publication, that a researcher may have to select certain elements of their work to be presented, all data should be represented in any final reports.

Ethical evolution

Although each of these ethical principles has been considered separately, in the real world of research they do overlap and have a synergistic impact upon each other. It must also be acknowledged that ethical concepts are dynamic and evolve and develop in conjunction with the changes in the boundaries and norms of society itself. To illustrate the impact changes in societal knowledge and mores have on ethical thinking, consider the following examples which discuss, first, changes to attitudes towards recognising the vulnerable research participants and second, the development of the internet as a research tool.

Example 1 – vulnerable groups

It has already been emphasised that ethical review committees exist for the protection of the public and that this obligation is taken extremely seriously. Occasionally, inadvertently, this can develop into a paternalistic attitude. This occurs when beneficence is elevated to such a level that, not only is the proposed project jeopardised by excess protective restrictions, the autonomy of participants is also compromised in that they are prevented from exercising their own judgement with regard to the level of potential risk they are willing to accept. This is often the case if the proposed research requires the participation of, so-called, vulnerable groups, such as children or people with learning disabilities. However, in Western societies, particularly over the past two decades, it has been increasingly acknowledged via challenges to existing laws, changes in legislation and changes in both health care and social opinion that such groups, in certain situations, can and do act autonomously. This is not to say that these groups are not deserving of extra consideration in many circumstances, However, both children and people with learning disabilities can make informed decisions and give consent to their participation in some research projects. This consent should be subject to the provision that the information offered to potential participants is done so in an age/cognitive appropriate manner and this should be the key responsibility of the researcher. However, it can be argued that the definition of which sections of society are viewed as vulnerable has changed to give more control and inclusion to groups who, in the past, were 'protected' from research participation.

On the other hand, as one vulnerable group obtains greater autonomy in the research arena, another section of society finds that its vulnerability has increased. The rapid expansion of knowledge that is attendant upon the sequencing of the human genome means that vast amounts of information on the molecular pathogenesis of diseases has become available, as has the amount of individual information that can be gained from simple biological research materials such as blood or tissue samples. This has had an impact upon the ethics of biomedical research to varying extents across the planet, from the creation of protective legislation (Council of the European Union 2004, Australian Government 2002, US Food and Drug Administration 2005) to an urgent review of the number and nature of ethics committees (Shirai 2003). This means that nurses who are involved in obtaining biological samples from research volunteers must be aware that such participants

are in potentially vulnerable situations and should be fully informed of the fate of any biological materials they offer.

Example 2 – internet research

Generally, health care has been slower than other disciplines to exploit the World Wide Web as a research tool. It is further conceded that many of the concerns that exercise cyber-ethicists are those of real world research (Jankowski & van Selm 2001). Nonetheless, as international or even global collaborative research is facilitated by use of the World Wide Web, certain issues require greater ethical consideration in cyberspace than is generally expected from real world human subject research (Association of Internet Researchers (AoIR) 2002). For example, the AoIR maintain that there are greater ethical challenges surrounding privacy and confidentiality and informed consent.

In contrast to the USA, European citizens enjoy stringent levels of personal data security thanks to the European Union Data Protection Directive (1995). This means that participants should be protected from having their data transferred to countries with less rigorous level of protection of privacy (AoIR 2002). This includes non-identifiable data that may be electronically transferred to another country for the purpose of data analysis. For the online researcher there is an augmented obligation to consider, in some detail, how the data are to be acquired and with whom the data will be shared.

As with the real world, so with cyberspace – consent is not optional. It may be obtained electronically if the respondent is over 18 but this is only appropriate if the risk to participants is low and if the online consent form takes potential participants through the documentation a step at a time. Additionally, the consent process must not be perceived as disruptive to discourse in the virtual world that the techno-researcher inhabits (Haigh & Jones 2005). If consent is being sought from minors, parental consent must be obtained in paper format (via surface mail or fax) or verbally if the research is low risk. If the online researcher wishes to interview minors online then parental consent must be obtained in a face-to-face interview (Bruckman 2002).

Conclusion

The main focus of this chapter has been upon the protective role that both governance and ethical review procedures play in the planning and management of all research projects. The principalist approach to ethical thinking as outlined by Beauchamp and Childress (2001) has been suggested as a framework for evaluating the ethical components of any proposed research project. It must be emphasised that ethical considerations (and, by association, governance processes) are reflective of societal norms and mores and are dynamic and changing to reflect the demands of progress of the global community.

EXERCISES

1. Seek out examples of 'Lone Worker Policies' on the internet. Identify examples of good practice.
2. Compare two research papers. Evaluate the strength of the ethical considerations within the paper. Attempt to categorise the theoretical ethical approach that the researcher used.
3. Review the challenges and changes in health care related legislation over the past decade. How will these changes have an impact upon the ethical planning and management of research projects?

References

Association of Internet Researchers 2002 Ethical Decision Making and Internet Research. Recommendations from the AoIR ethics working committee. Online. Available: www.aoir.org/report/ethics/pdf 6 Aug 2003

Australian Government 2002 Regulatory framework for human tissues and biological therapies. Online. Available: http://www.tga.gov.au/docs/html/humantiss.htm 12 Dec 2005

Beauchamp T L, Childress J F 2001 Principles of Biomedical Ethics, 5th edn. Oxford University Press, Oxford

Bruckman A 2002 Ethical guidelines for research online. Online. Available: http://www-static.cc.gatech.edu/~asb/ethics/ 7 May 2007

Council of the European Union 2004 Directive 2004/23/EC Setting standards of quality and safety for the donation, procurement, testing, processing, preservation, storage and distribution of human tissues and cells. Online. Available: http://europa.eu.int/eur-lex/pri/en/oj/dat/2004/l_102/l_10220040407en00480058.pdf 7 May 2007

Department of Health 2001 Research Governance Framework for Health and Social Care. Department of Health, London

European Commission. 2001 Directive 2001/20/EU. Good clinical practice on the conduct of clinical trials. Online. Available: http://www.corec.org.uk 20 June 2005

EFGCP 1997 Guidelines and recommendations for European Ethics committees. Online. Available: http://www.nus.edu.sg/irb/Articles/EFGCP-Guidelines%20and%20Recommendations%201997.pdf 7 May 2007

Haigh C, Jones N 2005 An overview of the ethics of cyber-space research and the implication for nurse educators. Nurse Education Today 25: 3–8

Howarth M L, Kneasfey R 2004 The impact of research governance in healthcare and higher education organisations. Journal of Advanced Nursing 49: 675–683

Involve 2004 Involving marginalised and vulnerable people in research. Online. Available: http://www.invo.org.uk/pdfs/Involving%20Marginalised%20and%20VullGroups%20in%20Researchver2.pdf 31 Sept 2005

Jankowski N, van Selm M 2001 Research ethics in a virtual world: some guidelines and illustrations. Online. Available: http://oase.uci.kun.nl/~jankow/Jankowski/publications/Research%20Ethics%20in%20a%20Virtual%20World.pdf 7 May 2007

Johnson M 2003 Research ethics and education: a consequentialist view. Nurse Education Today 23: 165–167

Joseph Rowntree Foundation 2005 Publication and Dissemination. A guide for JRF reports. Online. Available: http://www.jrf.org.uk/funding/research/projectholders/default.asp 26 Aug 2005

NHMRC 2004 Consultation Draft #1. The Australian code for conducting research. Online. Available: http://www.nhmrc.gov.au/publications 31 Aug 2005

OECD 2003 Governance of Public Research. Towards Better Practices. OECD Publishing, Paris

Shirai Y 2003 The status of ethics committees in Japan. Eubios Journal of Asian and International Bioethics 13: 130–134

Steinbrook R 2002 Protecting research subjects – the crisis at Johns Hopkins. New England Journal of Medicine 346: 716–720

Teacher Training Agency 1998 MA and PhD Dissemination. Off the Shelf Consultation Report. Online. Available: www.tta.gov.uk/php 26 Aug 2005

US Food and Drug Administration 2005 Questions and Answers Human Cells, Tissues, and Cellular and Tissue-Based Products; Donor Screening and Testing, and Related Labelling; Interim Final Rule. Online. Available: http://www.fda.gov/cber/rules/hctdnrq&a. htm 12 Dec 2005

Chapter 13

The Research Proposal

Renzo Zanotti and Seamus Cowman

Introduction

A research proposal is the means by which research panels and commissioners assess whether the writer knows how to plan a piece of research and whether the study will lead to important new knowledge (Reif-Lehrer 2005). Proposals for historical or philosophical study must reflect aspects unique to those areas of inquiry, and plans for ethnographic research will begin with assumptions that are consistent with the qualitative paradigm. Whether qualitative or quantitative, ethnographic or experimental, a research study must begin with questions, identify data sources, and present plans for analysis.

Functions of the proposal

A proposal has at least three main functions:

1. Communication – the proposal serves to communicate the investigator's research plans to those who provide consultation, give consent, or approval for funding agencies.
2. Plan – the proposal serves as a plan for action. Empirical research consists of systematic, rigorously pre-planned observations of some restricted set of phenomena. An adequate proposal outlines the research plan in systematic detail. The hallmark of a good proposal is a level of thoroughness and detail sufficient to permit another investigator to replicate the study.
3. Contract – an approved grant proposal is a contract between the investigator and the funding source. Once a contract has been made, all but minor changes should be supported by

arguments for absolute necessity or compelling desirability.

The common difficulties in proposal preparation arise from the most basic elements of the research process: What is the proper question to ask? How to underline the unique contribution of the study? How best to describe the data analysis? Determining the best answers to these questions constitutes a common difficulty through the endeavour of having a good proposal ready to submit (Gitlin & Lyons 2004).

The problem in writing a proposal is essentially the same as in writing the final report. Preliminary discussion with colleagues and faculty members may lead to a series of drafts that evolve toward a final document presented to a funding source (Locke et al 2000).

Elements of the proposal
The title

A title should describe accurately the main variables of the phenomena investigated, free of jargon and unnecessary technical terms. In other words, a title should send a clear message to the reader about the research focus. Therefore, the elements best considered for inclusion in the title are the dependent and independent variables, performance component by criterion task, the experimental treatment, the model underlying the study or the purpose of the study.

Any aspect of the study that is unique, particularly unusual, or representing a unique contribution to the literature may also be considered for inclusion in the title (Reif-Lehrer 2005).

Research design and instrumentation are not appropriate for inclusion in the title unless they represent an unusual approach to measurement or analysis (New & Quick 2003).

Summary or abstract

An abstract includes a brief summary of a much larger document. All indexed journals in electronic databases (MEDLINE, CINAHL) have to provide an abstract of the published articles; that abstract will be retrieved by the search engine and outlined with titles and authors. Those abstracts are written in simple past tense since they describe a study already accomplished; an abstract for a grant proposal is written in the future tense and summarises work that will be done.

An abstract may serve several purposes: (a) to focus the thinking by establishing an explicit goal to which all investigators involved subscribe; (b) to develop a concise prospectus for internal purposes to negotiate administrative approval and needed resources; (c) serve as a summary in order to obtain preliminary consensus by potential recruiters. Finally, funding agencies usually require a 'Letter of Intent', the content of which may be mostly derived from the abstract. An abstract prepared prior to the development of the full proposal must be frequently revised. That will be necessary to maintain the perfect consistency between abstract and the other sections of the proposal. The abstract is what is often read first and, frequently, the reading of those few paragraphs provides the reviewers with a clear image of the objectives, method and justification.

The anticipated results and conclusions can also be included to underline their importance for the granting agency, the institution and the discipline.

Starting from the abstract, the proposal must communicate the impression that the study contains something of special interest and fully deserves to be considered. Thus, a well-written abstract must convey a concise but clear picture of the study while also highlighting its unique characteristics. Language should be as plain as possible, avoiding constructs that require definition, keeping to a minimum the use of adjectives, and the use of slogans. Overall, economy and clarity are the essential features of a good abstract (Gitlin & Lyons 2004).

Investigators and collaborators

Concise information is required about the principal investigator, co-investigators, research assistants, research coordinator, administrative personnel and scientific consultants. Usually, a CV in the form of a biographical sketch of each investigator must be included. The reviewers will look for key information about researchers' credentials and specific experience as well as the number of grants obtained for conducting research in the field. Reviewers want to assess the capability of the investigators to conduct the proposed study, not only in a scientific manner, but also within the dedicated resources and administrative support.

Introduction

Proposals, like any other form of communication, are better introduced by a short, clear statement that declares the subject matter of the research, arouses interest and communicates information essential to the reader and provides a general outline of what is to follow.

The most effective way to introduce the study is to identify and define the abstract concept (or construct) that symbolises the central phenomenon of interest. It is appropriate to make the first sentence more general than the question, just to introduce the idea.

The fundamental question is 'What is this study about?' and the best approach, without too much detailed discussion, is to present the key concept and explain how it will be represented in the investigation. Some indications of the importance of the study to increase or validate the available theory or to improve the quality of practice may be used to underline the benefit of the study. Unnecessary technical language should be avoided since it requires more ability and focused attention to grasp the main idea (Gitlin & Lyons 2004). Similarly, an unnecessary use of quotations and extensive references are often perceived as intrusions into what should be a clean and simple preliminary outline.

Rationale and research question

The specific phenomenon of interest or the related question should be explicitly stated early in the proposal. The importance of the question lies in the fact that it sets the direction of the investigation (Henson 2004). Therefore, the statement should not include subtopics nor should it be confused with a formal research question. Instead, the opening question addresses the primary target and should ensure an easy understanding of the subsequent exposition and topic development. It should be noted that funding agencies assess to determine if the topic is germane to the mission of the agency.

The significance of stating the specific question is to indicate why the study deserves to be done and what benefit derives, for the development of the scientific knowledge and the quality of practice, from the study's results (New & Quick 2003). The form of the question should be stated after accurate reflection. In fact, the structure of the research question will help in understanding why those relationships and variables have been identified for the study.

Research questions should be simple, direct and should invite an answer. The specificity of the question should provide an indication of the depth of the analysis contained in the study.

Background to the problem

A research problem has to be well supported by a comprehensive critical review of the existing knowledge. The review is the backbone of all the conceptual and methodological decisions that have to be taken in the research process. A good review should address the following three questions:

1. What is already available in the scientific literature?
2. What is already known that leads to the study's question or hypothesis?
3. Is the selected research method appropriate to the investigation?

In discussing the background to the study, the investigator's task is to provide a comprehensive overview, reviewing the main theoretical and methodological issues that have arisen.

An applicant must be able to insert the proposed study into a line of inquiry and a developing body of knowledge. Therefore, the study's framework must be devised from the structure of the existing knowledge and the research questions and hypothesis where appropriate should emerge from the matrix of answered and unanswered questions; the choice of contingent method should arise from previous results (Kenner & Walden 2001). Discussing a volume of interesting but irrelevant information acquired in the process of a literature search should be avoided. Limiting the discussion to what is essential to the main topic has to be adopted throughout the proposal. When possible, the quoted studies should be grouped for analyses according to their framework, specific methodological features, or their results.

It is useful to create a schema that helps to grasp the meaning in similarities and dissimilarities in the past work of others in relation to the present proposal (Ogden & Goldberg 2002). An approach of conceptual ordering often leads to an assumption about causal relationships and thus can serve as a precursor of the explanatory theory to be tested with an experimental design. In fact, a well-written research proposal may be perceived as an elegant bridge between existing knowledge, a proposed theory, and the theory-based hypotheses to be empirically tested.

The conclusion of the critical review should be kept short and concise since it serves as an introduction to the other stages of the proposal (Ogden & Goldberg 2002). The conclusion always draws together the various elements and it should end with the research question, written either in the form of a question or as a statement. The conclusion may rephrase the introduction, expanding and explaining, and thus underlining the same statement with authority. A systematic and well-focused critical review demonstrates the investigator's mastery of the current knowledge in a field.

Purpose and hypothesis

In this section, the 'aim and key objectives of the research' may be delineated simply and clearly. Specific and achievable objectives provide the reader with clear criteria against which the proposed research method can be assessed. In quantitative studies a hypothesis (often referred to as an educated guess) is adopted when the interest is about predicting a relationship between variables and there is theory available for making predictions. Furthermore, other elements of a good proposal will help the reader to understand the connections between variables and how scientific theory underpins the study's testable hypotheses. Generally, in qualitative studies, the investigator does not directly state a hypothesis most often because little is known about the topic to justify it. In developing an hypothesis there are a number of essential features to be considered. Specificity is the key to making a research question or hypothesis clear (Locke et al 2000). The best way to introduce the hypotheses is simply to say: 'The purpose of this study is to test the following hypotheses...' Questions and hypotheses in quantitative studies should meet three criteria: clarity, brevity and inclusiveness; they are exemplified as follows:

1. Is the question free of ambiguity?
2. Is the relationship among variables expressed?
3. Does the question/hypotheses lead to the selection of an empirical test?

Applying these three criteria to the question 'Is a person's way of coping with cancer a modulator of chemotherapy effectiveness?', the relationship between the variable 'Way of coping' and 'Effectiveness of chemotherapy' in a person with cancer is reasonably clear, as is the target population (people with cancer undergoing chemotherapy).

A relationship is focused and a correlation test between ways of coping and level of effectiveness of chemotherapy is implied as the appropriate statistics. However, the potential ambiguity in the concept of 'modulator' should be addressed, identifying what aspects of the variable 'Ways of coping' should be observed so that its relationships with level of 'effectiveness' can be measured. If more clarity is required, then the question should be more specific without endangering the simplicity of the question itself.

Research hypotheses predict the answer to the questions, in testable form. A clear question is easily transformed into an hypothesis in the form of an affirmative statement that can be tested for being true or false. An hypothesis exerts a direct influence on each step of the research process, until the final report. The hypothesis states a relationship between variables bridging from the leading theory to the statistical tests and answers to the question (Miller & Salkind 2002).

A good hypothesis, as well as predicting a relationship, should also indicate the specific direction of the hypothesis (Coping Way X increases Effectiveness; Coping Way Y decreases Effectiveness).

A directional hypothesis has the added advantage of ensuring an investigation of the specific effect of the relationship not just the existence of a relationship. A good principle is to employ directional hypotheses when pilot data or previous studies are available clearly indicating a direction, or when the theory from which the hypotheses were drawn is sufficiently robust to include evidence of directionality.

Terms and definitions

The variables to be observed in the investigation should be operationally defined. The definitions should follow the elements of the proposal where the purpose of the study is discussed, so the reader follows the logical links with the key terms in the purpose statement. It has to be very clear, in the definitions, what is going to be observed and, therefore, measured. It is crucial to maintain high consistency between concepts, definitions, and derived empirical variables from the operational process.

Thus, a clear description requires that all necessary operational definitions about concepts to be measured are described in order to achieve maximum clarity (Miller & Salkind 2002).

Research design and sampling

It is often helpful to introduce the design with a general statement about what it will encompass. Frequently, the introduction states the direction

the research will take: exploratory, descriptive or experimental. Consequently, the chosen design of the study will be reflected in the amount of detail that has to be considered in the research proposal. Compared with an exploratory study, an experimental design requires a highly detailed proposal since the literature review should be exhaustive and even a small detail must be carefully planned in advance.

Following the introductory statement on the research design, the sampling should be described. When describing the sample, the starting point is to describe the population in as much detail as possible considering who and where they are, and when they can be accessed. A reader has to be clear about what is known about the target population and, therefore, how representative the sample may be.

The level of generalisability of the study depends on the quality and size of the sample and the power of the adopted statistical tests. The larger the sample, the more representative of the population the findings are likely to be. Power analysis is a means of establishing how large the sample should be for an adequate test of the research hypothesis.

In qualitative research the aim is to discover meaning and unfold realities and generalisation is normally not a guiding criterion. Therefore, there are no solid criteria for sample size in qualitative research and the starting point in sampling is often the selection of the setting where informants can be contacted.

The term 'delimiting' refers to defining the limits within which the results may be applied maintaining their validity; thus, the scientific power of the study itself. Limitations, in the context of a research proposal, address the main weaknesses. Causes of limitations may be restrictions in design, control on confounding variables, or constraints in measuring. The investigator should approach this part carefully and make it clear that limitations have been carefully considered and weighted but, nevertheless, making it clear that the study will provide valid and useful information.

Procedures and instruments

A research proposal is in itself a rational and a fully described plan for careful and systematic observation of events in order to test hypotheses or answer questions. Procedures to be used to collect data must be described in detail as well as the instruments adopted for data collection (Coley & Scheinberg 2000).

Therefore, a detailed description should include sources of data, data collection methods and instruments as well as statistical procedures for data analysis. Furthermore, how subjects' rights will be protected must be outlined in great detail. Overall, the specific techniques must maintain consistency with the chosen framework, nature of variables and empirical indicators, and finally with the sample.

Usually, the procedures section of the proposal provides specific explication of the following aspects:

- target population and sampling methods;
- instruments and measurements techniques;
- design for the data collection;
- procedures for data recording and collection;
- tests and procedures for data analysis;
- plans for counteracting contingencies such as lower recruitment or high mortality.

It is important to provide a rationale for the choice of methods of investigation when the method is introduced as part of the investigation plan. Figures and diagrams with few sentences of accompanying text will help to increase clarity and attractiveness and avoid pages of boring detailed descriptions, often confusing the reader. Particularly when data are to be collected from many subgroups, pages of explanatory text about how the variables are going to be related may be confusing. An explanatory graph with a brief introduction will clarify the relationships with no need of further explanations.

The methods section should present the order and timing for the tasks. It might make sense to provide a Gantt chart so that readers can map out the sequencing on their own.

On the basis of the methods selected, a discussion of the chosen instruments should follow, describing strengths and weaknesses. An outline of the tests done for instruments' reliability and validity, referring to the specific population, should be provided.

In the case of an instrument developed by the investigator, the same type of rationale must be discussed, making absolutely clear on the basis of literature review that a self-made instrument is the best available choice, followed by a description of how it is going to be tested for reliability and validity and a discussion of any shortcomings and limitations (Burr 2004). Using existing instruments is desirable, whenever possible, because their psychometric qualities will already have been established.

Data analysis

The data analysis follows directly from sample selection and data collection techniques. Therefore, it should be clear which statistical tests need to be used for which set of variables in relation to the measurement scales adopted. One should be careful not to include an unrelated test or to include statistical techniques only because they look sophisticated.

In qualitative research, a data analysis proposal should identify the strategy and a rationale for the particular approach taken.

Ethics and human rights

It is essential to describe in full detail how the rights of persons included or excluded from the sample are going to be protected since ethical approval of the study is required by funding agencies and publication journals.

Some statements must be included on how understandable information will be provided to eligible subjects, informed consent obtained, and how anonymity will be protected for subjects and their records (Coley & Scheinberg 2000). When informed consent is going to be used, a copy of the consent form should be included in an appendix to the proposal. In that form it has to be clearly described, in lay language, the goal of the study, risks and benefits, alternative to participation, confidentiality, rights of the subjects and name of the reference person to be contacted for queries or dropout.

Institutions such as universities and hospitals have an Institutional Review Board (IRB), or Research Ethics Committee, for the protection of human rights to which the proposal has to be submitted. If ethics approval has not been obtained in advance of submitting a proposal, it is considered acceptable to indicate that ethics approval is pending and send a copy of the approval letter when available.

Budget and resources

The budget may be discussed in subsections related to activities and products specified for each year of the study plan. A proposed study may last several years. Therefore, it is possible that funding agencies will ask for a detailed budget for the first year, a budget for the remaining period, and the budget justification. The researchers should provide a detailed breakdown of their budget, especially for making valid estimations of the total cost and maintaining control of the flow of daily expenditure during the course of the study.

Typical items included in the budget are personnel, consultants, technical equipment and supplies. Personnel expenses include the costs for all the people who will work on the project. They may be employees of the organisation or independent contractors. If they are employees, the portion of time to be dedicated to the project has to be calculated.

Direct project expenses are non-personnel expenses that arise due to the project. They can be almost anything: travel costs, printing, space or equipment rental, supplies, insurance, or meeting expenses such as food. Travel expenses for meetings, data collection, and related conference participation are included, plus indirect administrative costs.

Administrative or overhead expenses are non-personnel expenses that will also be incurred. For example, the use of part of an office by the research assistant. A quote for use of facilities, utilities and administrative costs, such as phone, copying, postage and office supplies, may be considered in the research budget.

Not all funding agencies allow unrestricted type of expenditures; some do not support indirect costs or the purchase of generic equipment such as computers or software. To avoid errors and technical hitches, it is important to read the rules and regulations of the selected funding agency carefully.

It is becoming common practice for funding agencies to ask for letters of support from key stakeholders declaring their commitment to participate and eventually to cover part of the cost. Supporting letters can be announced in this section and included in appendices to the proposal. If costs are straightforward and the numbers are congruent and clear, any further explanation is redundant. However, if a budget narrative is needed, it can be structured as 'Notes to the Budget', with footnote-style numbers on the line items in the budget keyed to numbered explanations. If an extensive or more general explanation is required, then the structure of the budget narrative should be straight text.

Conclusions

Every proposal should have a concluding paragraph or two. This is a good place to call attention to the future, after the grant is completed. If appropriate, it should outline some of the follow-up activities that might be undertaken. This section is also the place to make a final appeal for the project. The important strengths and uniqueness of the study can be reiterated and can be presented in a final appeal for financial support for the project.

References and appendices

The final reference list should contain only literature cited, not all the literature used; that is a quite different notion. In general, it is better to avoid using too many quotations and to limit the citations (Locke et al 2000). Reviewers deem the use of unrelated references as an indicator of poor scholarship and an inappropriate way to increase the weight of the proposal.

The same is valid for lengthy quotations: It may be suggested that, if the substance of a quotation can be conveyed by a careful paraphrase, followed by the appropriate credit of a citation with all the clarity and persuasive impact of the original, then a quote should be avoided (Kenner & Walden 2001).

Many items are attached in appendices in order to maintain clarity and avoid distraction throughout the presentation. The following items are generally placed as appendices:

- equipment specifics;
- instructions to subjects;
- letters of support and other relevant documents;
- consent form to be signed by subjects;
- tabulated data from pilot study;
- forms, questionnaires for data collection;
- grid or questions for in-depth interviews;
- credentials of personnel to be employed in the study;
- diagrams of statistical analysis;
- schematics for equipment;
- supplementary bibliographies.

Writing style

The writing style of the research proposal is one of the most important factors in conveying the ideas to funding agencies. The researcher must ensure clarity and coherence in presentation. The following are some useful suggestions which may alleviate the necessity to rewrite numerous drafts of the proposal.

Some inexperienced researchers use exhortative language to underline the importance of the study for the development of professional practice. Generally, it is much better to maintain the focus on the topic and to avoid the temptation to manipulate the reviewer using supposed 'positive' aspects, not essential or not related to the investigation. If asking the question 'Is this point making things

clearer?' provides the answer 'No', then that point should be deleted (Burke 2002).

When the proposal is sent to a funding agency it has to be in the specifically defined format with no opportunity to re-edit or make last-minute corrections. Every sentence must be previously examined for its clarity, grammar and relationship with the previous and following sentences. If a statement must be read twice to understand the content, then it should be rephrased. The use of a spellchecker and the help of a few colleagues external to the study will greatly increase the likelihood of a clean, proofread final draft.

Proposal review and funding agencies

A proposal should not be submitted to more then one agency. Nevertheless, some funding agencies allow a double application (to two different agencies) when duly informed about the possible split or sharing of the cost between the two.

The proposal writer must have a good understanding of the review process, though each funding agency has its own review process, usually updated or slightly modified each year. It is important to find and select the appropriate agency for funding. Always verify the procedure described in its grant application, and make sure that it is the most recent version.

These guidelines must be followed meticulously (Henson 2005). In a typical university, an application has to pass several formal approvals, committee and signatures, depending on the level of financial commitment. That takes a considerable amount of time. The personnel in the institution's Grants and Contracts (or Research) office usually have experience with funding agencies and they can be a valuable resource in order to identify the agency that, for characteristics and mission, provides the best chances of being accepted for a grant. Via the internet it is easy to find sources of information about funding agencies; fishing with the keyword 'grant' or 'research grant' will catch almost a hundred web pages and reference addresses.

Finally, the procedure for proposal evaluation is based on (a) assessment of the scientific merit, and (b) overall ranking for funding. From the step (a) the proposal may receive an 'Approval' with a score number that defines also its priority, (b) the proposal will then be assessed for relevance in comparison with all the other proposals and the resources available. If rejected, a summary will be provided with the main critical aspects identified by reviewers of the grant application. The priority scores of all proposals are rank ordered to form a single list of approved applications. In particular cases, reviewers will recommend that particular proposals be given special consideration for funding or recommend a reassignment of an application (Barber 2002).

At the final step, when ranking for funding has been done, the grants are approved in that order as far as funds permit. If the proposal is approved and funded, notification is sent to the investigator and the sponsoring institution. In the case of the European Commission for Research, the grant usually covers 40% or 60% of the total cost in the budget. For that reason, in the application it is truly important to provide evidence of an institution supporting the investigator, committed and willing to support the project in the strongest possible way.

EXERCISES

It is of foremost importance to practise in order to develop skills in proposal writing, therefore:

1. Select research articles reporting that they have been supported with a grant.
2. Compare those articles with a comparable selection of articles (by topic, study design, and type of journals) that have not been supported: identify if differences exist in methods, style, and level of detail provided.
3. Search the web for European and American guidelines about submitting a research proposal: identify agencies, rules, and procedures.
4. Classify agencies and procedures of interest to a novice nurse researcher.
5. Develop an initial sketch of a nursing research proposal meeting the guidelines of the selected agency.

References

Barber D M 2002 Finding Funding: The Comprehensive Guide to Grant Writing, 2nd edn. Bond Street Publishers, Long Beach

Burke M A 2002 Simplified Grantwriting. Corwin Press, Thousand Oaks, CA

Burr P L 2004 Internationalizing Your Campus: Fifteen Steps and Fifty Federal Grants to Success. Information Age Publishing, Greenwich, CT

Coley S M, Scheinberg C A 2000 Proposal Writing, 2nd edn. Sage, Thousand Oaks, CA

Gitlin L N, Lyons K J 2004 Successful Grant Writing: Strategies for Health and Human Service Professionals, 2nd edn. Springer, New York

Henson K T 2004 Grant Writing in Higher Education : a Step-by-Step Guide. Allyn and Bacon, Boston

Henson K T 2005 Writing for Publication: Road to Academic Advancement. Allyn and Bacon, Boston

Kenner C, Walden M 2001 Grant writing tips for nurses and other health professionals American Nurses Association, Washington, DC

Locke L F, Spirduso W W, Silverman S J 2000 Proposals That Work: A Guide for Planning Dissertations and Grant Proposals, 4th edn. Sage, Newbury Park, CA

Miller D C, Salkind N J 2002 Handbook of Research Design and Social Measurement, 6th edn. Sage, Thousand Oaks, CA

New C C, Quick J A 2003 How to Write a Grant Proposal. John Wiley, Hoboken, NJ

Ogden T E, Goldberg I A 2002 Research Proposals: A Guide to Success, 3rd edn. Academic Press, San Diego, CA

Reif-Lehrer L 2005 Grant Application Writer's Handbook. Jones and Bartlett, Sudbury, MA

Chapter 14

Managing a Research Project

Richard Whittington

Introduction

Managing a research project successfully from start to finish involves many skills including, for instance, combining an ability to keep a close eye on detail with the capacity, at times, for highly creative and lateral thinking. It involves looking forward to anticipate the unknown and looking back to summarise the essential achievements of the project at the end. It can combine periods of isolation and working alone with episodes of meeting and coordinating large or small groups of people committed in some way to the delivery of the project. The depth to which these various skills are required depends entirely on the scope of the project being managed. Every project is unique and involves new challenges which can only be partially anticipated. The diversity of demands faced by those planning and managing a research project makes the task challenging and potentially difficult but, with sufficient foresight, ingenuity and luck, it will also be enjoyable and rewarding.

Research projects differ in terms of their complexity and, more importantly, in terms of the level of support available from others. Researchers also differ in terms of experience. They can include the undergraduate student doing research for the first time for a dissertation with the close support of a supervisor, the postgraduate student who has completed such a dissertation but now has to take the lead in the conduct of a larger, more innovative project over several years, and the experienced researcher who will have learned from these previous experiences but who has a particular set of additional demands to consider when managing funded research. In addition, research projects should be unique in their focus in that they are attempting to produce new knowledge. Whatever the level, no two research projects are the same and it is not possible to reduce research project management to a simple routine (Meredith & Mantel 2000). A 'cookbook' with effective research project management menus cannot be offered and the creative satisfaction of the activity itself would be lost if this approach were adopted. Despite all these differences, there are certain core research project management skills and these will be considered below. Other skills such as budget management are specific to the more advanced types of study and these will be considered afterwards.

Project management for beginners

A research project is like any other sort of discrete, time-limited project and the principles of good project management can be used to steer towards the delivery of a successful outcome (Lock 2003, Meredith & Mantel 2000). Most projects have clear, specified outcomes which may be educational (e.g. learning outcomes) or scientific. These objectives may be fixed by outside parties, such as external funders or those setting the learning outcomes for a dissertation module, and thus they may be non-negotiable. Alternatively, the researcher may have a free hand to set the objectives, as is often the case with postgraduate research. Whichever situation applies, the first, and most important, requirement for researchers is to make absolutely sure that they know what the objectives of the project are and that these objectives are clearly defined and understood by all the relevant stakeholders. With no idea of the endpoint, navigation through the project will quickly become impossible.

All projects have a life cycle and activity over that life cycle is inevitably variable, with periods of low activity punctuated by times of high demand and effort. This means that the successful researcher must have a clear sense of the deadline

for completion of the objectives and what is needed along the way to get to that point. Every project is composed of sub-tasks (sometimes known as work packages) and these can be further broken down into more specific activities (sometimes known as work units). Each of these activities can be given a deadline for completion and thus the researcher can start to see when the periods of high demand are likely to occur and to plan accordingly. Box 14.1 lists some of the sub-tasks which might need to be considered in working towards an overall project objective.

Lock (2003) identifies four types of project which need to be managed in some way. Of these four types (industrial, manufacturing, management and

Box 14.1 – *Some typical research project management tasks*

1. Draw up deadlines for work packages and sub-tasks
2. Establish responsibility for each sub-task
3. Write and submit REC application
4. Attend REC meeting and make necessary revisions
5. Submit update reports to REC
6. Write and submit application for access to health care organisation
7. Liaise with individual health care staff with access to potential participants
8. Obtain copies of questionnaires and other instruments
9. Obtain necessary equipment, e.g. tape recorders
10. Draw up and arrange testing of new instruments
11. Operationalise recruitment procedures
12. Administer data collection instruments
13. Check data quality as collected and make preliminary interpretations
14. Transcribe textual data
15. Load data into analysis software
16. Check quality of loaded data (data cleaning)
17. Conduct data analysis
18. Prepare and circulate draft final report

research) the research project is viewed as the type carrying the highest risk of failure. The best way of dealing with this risk is always planning ahead, constantly anticipating likely problems and mapping out some potential solutions to the potential problems if and when they occur. Having identified what needs to be done by when, it is a good idea to have Plan B ready in case Plan A fails, as it often does! It is always best to operate with the expectation that the worst case scenarios will actually happen and, thus, be ready to deal with them. This imagining and working through takes considerable mental effort and creativity but it is the best way of avoiding the sense of panic which inevitably descends when the worst happens and the project is facing failure.

Health or nursing research projects have quite specific aspects which make them different from projects generally (e.g. construction) and even from other types of research project. Most projects in this area are concerned with investigating people and many are concerned with people who are ill or vulnerable in some way. Some projects, like those testing a new nursing intervention, involve doing things to people which may cause pain, distress or carry some other sort of risk. Therefore, health research projects always carry an extra level of ethical and political demand which is absent in other disciplines where, for instance, research takes place exclusively in laboratories or libraries. This is particularly a challenge for new researchers in health who, as a result, have to start off at the deep end having to navigate ethical and organisational contexts before the data can be collected. Some of the necessary tasks to be considered prior to data-collection are listed in Box 14.1.

Stakeholders, roles and responsibilities

Any project will have a number of people involved who contribute to its successful completion. There will be a researcher and one or more study participants but very few projects involve only these, and health research projects always involve a wider array of stakeholders. One approach (Department

Box 14.2 – *Potential stakeholders in a research project (Department of Health 2005)*

- Participants (and potential participants)
- Researchers
- Investigators
- Chief investigators
- Research funders
- Sponsors
- Universities and others employing researchers
- Organisations providing health care
- Health care professionals
- Research Ethics Committees

of Health 2005) identifies ten different types of stakeholder who may need to be consulted or need to give permission for a study to take place (Box 14.2). Some of these are 'core' stakeholders in that almost all projects will involve them, i.e. participants and researchers. More advanced projects will involve many stakeholders who must be engaged in the project in some way including investigators, funders, sponsors, researchers' employers, care providers and care professionals.

With regard to participants, clearly any study involving collecting data from human participants generates the need to make moral and ethical decisions which may be highly complex. Any approved project will be governed by strict ethical principles established by the local Research Ethics Committee (REC) or equivalent. The researcher (or their supervisor) will have steered the proposal through the relevant REC prior to starting and must ensure that the delivery of the project fits within the specification approved by the REC. The REC will expect regular updates on progress and any variations to the protocol which become necessary after the study has started will need to be approved. The researcher, as defined by the Department of Health (2005), is the person with day-to-day responsibility for conducting the research by, for instance, conducting interviews or distributing questionnaires, and part of their role is to adhere to the protocol, report adverse events and keep the data confidential, safe and secure.

It is worth distinguishing studies in which project managers are the 'hands-on' researcher (as defined above) from those in which they have a more supervisory role for students or research assistants. These more senior researchers are designated as investigators if they are responsible for the research activity at one particular site or as chief investigators if they coordinate across several sites (Department of Health 2005). Of course, the two roles can be combined in one person and, at different times and during different components, an investigator may take the 'hands-on' role themselves. There is a push in some countries to tighten up these role definitions to clarify who is responsible for what and thus who is accountable if things go wrong. This 'managerialism', it is argued, improves the overall standards of research and the experience of participants. Certainly, the person designated as the chief investigator in some research governance systems has the primary responsibility for the effective delivery of the project and the longest job description with over twenty specific responsibilities for which he or she is accountable (Department of Health 2005).

At the heart of the chief investigator's role is the management of the student or junior researchers within the team. If this relationship does not work properly the project is likely to be seriously jeopardised. The skills of effective person management and the principles governing recruitment of appropriate staff are beyond the scope of this chapter but they include regular face-to-face meetings, clear specification of sub-tasks, joint inspection of collected data and encouragement to report problems. If the relationship is between a research student and supervisor, the same principles apply but the emphasis is much more on the student taking the initiative in identifying problems, although the supervisor remains responsible if identified problems are not dealt with appropriately.

Beyond the research team, most health researchers will need to negotiate with a care provider such as a hospital or community service to gain access to participants and then will need to talk to individual care staff within that organisation who may be acting as gatekeepers or facilitators of direct access. In some countries, formal application to the service provider's research governance committee is required alongside the REC application and the service provider must weigh up the potential benefits of the research to their specific population against the potential costs such as staff time (e.g. to escort patients) and other resources (e.g. paperwork). These costs must be estimated by the researcher as part of the application and, whilst the direct cost of the project to a funding organisation may have already been calculated as part of a bid, it may be a surprising challenge to specify, for instance, how long ward nurses will have to take out of their clinical time to accompany patients to a research interview and how much each trip will cost. The project manager needs to be aware of any requirements regarding honorary contracts for those who are doing the research in the host organisation. Such contracts may need to be established and, since this can only be done after the researcher has been appointed to a funded project, the extra time to achieve this requirement needs to be factored into the project plan. Health care organisations are inherently complex entities who view research at best as a secondary priority and at worst as a distraction. With such complexity it is a good idea, if operating from outside the organisation, to have one or two key contacts on the inside who are enthusiastic and supportive and can keep things moving in the right direction. It is important to be aware of the likely impact of the project on the resources of the organisation and to be sensitive to how this might be viewed. As the project progresses it is important to stay in touch with the research and development (R&D) department of the host organisation. Regular reports on progress will be requested by the R&D team including information on recruitment against the targets set out in the proposal and notification of any adverse events related to the conduct of the project. The latter should be reported as they occur anyway, rather than waiting for a formal report request. More complex studies may involve collecting data from two or more different care providers and, until a coordinated system of approval is established, this will probably involve liaising with R&D teams in several organisations simultaneously. This can add significantly to the time lag in getting the project up and running and should be thought about at the planning stage.

The same principles of awareness and sensitivity apply when establishing relationships as a researcher with the individual staff who are either caring for the potential participants or are going to be asked to be participants themselves. The research project is not going to be a priority for them and may, indeed, be experienced as a significant burden in a busy working life. Some projects have incentives such as prizes, raffle tickets and free beverages built into their budget and, whilst there are ethical issues to be examined around such inducements, they undoubtedly help in creating a sense of being appreciated. Even if incentives are not used, it is vital to advertise the project as widely and energetically as possible through any available media such as newsletters and notice boards and to include the details of a person who can be contacted to talk about the project further. It is also important to stress the anticipated benefits of the project for the participants and/or the staff caring for them. The concrete and direct nature of these benefits should be stressed rather than referring to idealistic 'cloud nine' benefits with little practical relevance to the bedside.

All these stakeholders relate to the successful delivery of a particular project but it is important to remember that the effective research project manager, whilst responsible for their individual project, often operates within their own larger organisation and should have certain expectations of what that organisation can provide for them 'in-house'. This is particularly true when the employing organisation is a university. These expectations will vary according to their own management responsibilities on the project (i.e. if they are a student or researcher) but, ideally, some key entitlements can be specified. The organisation should be promoting a healthy research culture in which the project can be located and to which the project contributes. This culture should be supportive whilst also being clear about accountability through the development of codes of practice (Department of Health 2005). The culture of a research organisation should have certain values embedded in it including intellectual freedom, enthusiasm for new and 'off-the-wall' ideas and encouragement of interaction between researchers from different disciplines. Access to an institutional seminar programme is fundamental to the development of such cultures. The project manager needs somebody to turn to for advice and supervision whatever level they occupy in the organisation and their current project should fit, where possible, within an overall career plan. In addition, peer-support groups can be established to enable sharing of problems and potential solutions. Ideally, for career researchers, the projects allocated to or bid for by a particular person should follow a consistent theme so that skills and knowledge in a specialist area can be built up. This is not to say that a 'top-down' managerial approach should be adopted, though, as such an approach will stifle creative thinking and sap the culture of the organisation. Researchers should have training opportunities communicated to them regularly so they can upgrade and fine-tune their research skills.

Scheduling

All successful projects are based at least partly on effective planning so that each component of the overall study is completed at around the right time. If the project is based on a proposal there will have been some requirement to plan how long it will take to achieve the overall objectives and each step along the way. Once the project is up and running, this plan needs to be thought about in some detail and operationalised. Each work package should be split into the necessary sub-tasks and an indication made of when these sub-tasks should be completed. It is best not to make these estimates over-optimistic.

Various rules of thumb can be used to guide this process. For a quantitative study, the time available can be split into thirds: one third for preparation, one third for data collection and one third for data analysis and report writing. In qualitative studies, more time is usually needed to deal with the complexities of data analysis and up to half of the available time should be allocated for this and the subsequent tasks. It is very easy to make the mistake of devoting too much time to data collection and not enough time for other tasks. Preparation time is particularly important as it can involve REC and health authority applications followed by several meetings with relevant staff. Setting up such meetings with busy health care staff can be very time-consuming and a planned start date can be delayed significantly if this has not been considered. It is important to bear in mind the issues around recruitment of participants (Usherwood 1996), especially if a large number are required for a quantitative study and if the topic is sensitive or embarrassing. Estimates of refusal rates should be built in to the planning process as early as possible to ensure that sufficient people are approached early enough to meet the targets for the study. Alternatively, there can be unforeseen problems with loading and cleaning data before

the analysis can begin. These difficulties become magnified when a project involves coordinated input from several sites.

Software packages are available to aid scheduling. At a more basic level techniques for visualising the project plan are available, with the most common being the Gantt chart (Fig. 14.1). This chart lists all the work packages and sub-tasks on the left side and the months or weeks available across the top. The time to be devoted to each activity is represented by lines clearly indicating when the activity starts and finishes. Activities may overlap and the overall chart gives a good sense of the demands associated with each stage of the project life-cycle.

Project management when externally funded

Research projects can be divided into those where external funds are provided to carry out the project (e.g. government, industry, charity) and 'unfunded' projects where the people doing the project (i.e. researcher, supervisor, investigator) do it as part of their normal job and/or an educational qualification.

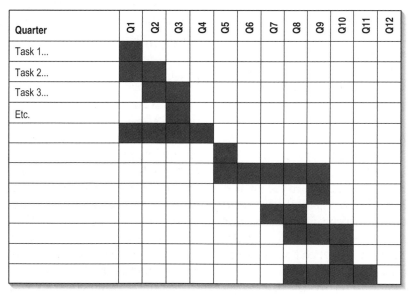

Figure 14.1 – *Example of a Gantt chart.*

Planning and conducting a funded research project adds another layer of complexity to the core skills of project management discussed so far. Now the standard research proposal sent to the REC and local health care provider for approval must be supplemented with a detailed projection of the financial costs likely to be incurred in running the project to a successful conclusion. There is little room for error here as the project must not cost more than the funding potentially available from the funder and, once agreed, no more funding will be made available if things go wrong and the estimate proves to be too low. Therefore extreme care needs to be taken in drawing up a budget and advice should be sought from as many people as possible before submitting the application. Most universities require funding applications to be approved by them before submission and this approval will include detailed scrutiny of the anticipated salary costs. A typical project budget will cover salary costs (including 'on-costs', such as national insurance) of one or more people to be employed to work directly on the project for its duration; consumables such as the cost of photocopying or purchasing questionnaires; travel costs if this is necessary for the project, including accommodation and daily subsistence allowances; and special items such as consultancy fees. Any application passing through a UK university for approval will be subjected to a new system of Full Economic Costing (FEC) in which the 'true' cost of the project (defined as the cost when invisible staffing elements such as accommodation and time have been added in) is calculated and specified in the application. Funders vary with regard to what they will consider as legitimate costs but most funders will view the headings above as legitimate as long as they are justified in relation to the scope of the project. Other costs which might be considered by some funders would include equipment, specialist software, payments or other rewards to participants, conference fees, conference travel and accommodation, student bursaries and student fees.

Usually the salary cost is by far the largest component of a budget unless, as in basic medical sciences, large items of equipment need to be bought to run the project but this is not common in health or nursing research. Much thought must be given to the salary point at which the staff will be appointed dependent on how much money is available and what the responsibilities of the person will be. Researchers employed by a university and seeking or working on externally funded projects can expect institutional assistance from a dedicated research support office (Hogan & Clark 1996). This office should proactively disseminate funding opportunities around the organisation, and work with researchers in developing applications. It should then be involved in negotiating the contract with the funder including clarification of copyright and intellectual property issues. This contract is usually between the institution, rather than the individual researcher, and the funder to maximise insurance and other benefits.

If funding is obtained, the golden rule is to keep a very close eye on the expenditure of the project as it goes along to ensure that no overspend occurs. This will require regular statements from the finance office to be inspected and sometimes adjustments to the projected costs as the completion date for the project approaches. Usherwood (1996) discusses various techniques for monitoring expenditure on a budget and staying within the limits imposed.

Case study

Cathy Smith is a mental health nurse consultant working on an acute admission unit who has become interested in the management of self-harming behaviour. Based on an application prepared with the help of her MSc project supervisor, her employer has awarded her funding for a one-year full-time secondment plus additional costs to interview service users who self-harm and the staff who care for them using a structured interview schedule. She breaks the 12-month period into quarters and establishes what needs to be achieved at the end of each quarter. She defines herself as responsible for achievement of each of these objectives as nobody else is involved in running the project but she does arrange fortnightly meetings with her supervisor. She has reviewed the literature and started the REC application before the funding was released so is able to submit the application early on in the project. After she has attended the relevant meeting and explained various aspects of the study, it is approved, and the hospital approves the study as well before the end of the first quarter. The second quarter is taken up with bedding in the project on the participating wards, piloting the interview and starting formal data collection. Some time is spent explaining the project generally to ward managers and staff, especially with regard to how service users and staff become eligible for the study so that she can be notified when this happens. She aimed to have 50 participants recruited by the end of the second quarter but for unknown reasons only 30 participants have taken part at this point. She obtains agreement to expand the number of wards participating to enable capture of more incidents. At this point also she needs to submit a progress report to the hospital which includes discussion of this issue. Data loading for statistical analysis starts as soon as the early interviews are completed and continues in parallel to avoid a backlog developing. Responses to open questions need to be content analysed before they can be entered into the software, which was unanticipated but unavoidable as they relate to key variables in the study. Data

loading is completed by the end of the third quarter but then the statistician with whom she had arranged to work to carry out the more complex parts of the analysis goes off sick. A preliminary report involving basic analysis is completed by the end of the 12 months to meet the project requirements. The report is used as the basis for service improvements to self-harming users. A fuller report is completed at 18 months and is published three years after the start of the project.

Conclusion

People often think of research as a very abstract and rarefied activity divorced from the realities and practicalities of clinical work. It is true that much of the thinking and talking by researchers is concerned with these theoretical concerns and that these must of course be got right from the start. However, it must never be forgotten that health research is also an intensely practical and concrete activity that takes place in the real world of health care with real people experiencing real problems and it only works properly as an activity when the practical challenges discussed above are anticipated and successfully overcome. Whilst it may or may not be true that there is nothing as practical as a good theory, it is certainly true that no theory can be tested successfully without considering the practical problems that might be encountered.

EXERCISES

1. Draw up a Gantt chart for the activities set out in the case study using the information provided and the task list set out in Box 14.2. Are there any additional tasks that need to be added to the list? When is the time of highest activity?

2. Calculate the cost of this hypothetical study based on the assumptions below (Fig. 14.3).

   Assumptions:
   Pay employer pension contributions @ 13%
   Pay employer National Insurance contributions @ 7%
   Cost photocopying @ 5p per sheet
   Cost the laptop computer @ £600

EXERCISES—Cont'd

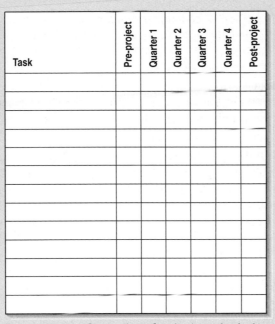

Task	Pre-project	Quarter 1	Quarter 2	Quarter 3	Quarter 4	Post-project

Figure 14.2 – *Gantt chart for the hypothetical case study.*

		Sub-total
Basic salary per annum	22 111	
Employer pension contributions		
Employer National Insurance contributions		
TOTAL SALARY		
10 page self-designed interview schedule to be completed by 100 participants		
TOTAL CONSUMABLES		
Laptop computer		
TOTAL EQUIPMENT		
1 visit per month for 12 months to a hospital 10 miles away		
1 visit per month for 12 months to a hospital 300 miles away		
TOTAL TRAVEL		
TOTAL ACCOMMODATION		
TOTAL SUBSISTENCE		
2 consultants for 18 1-hour meetings		
TOTAL COST		

Figure 14.3 – *Assumed costs of the hypothetical study.*

Continued

EXERCISES—Cont'd

The nearby hospital can be visited in a day's round trip but the distant hospital requires train travel, an overnight stay and subsistence

Pay car travel @ 30p per mile

Pay £150 return for train travel

Pay £100 per night for a hotel

Pay £20 per day for subsistence

Pay consultants £75 each per hour (including travel).

3. Choose a recently published nursing research study in one of the leading journals such as the *Journal of Advanced Nursing* or *Journal of Psychiatric and Mental Health Nursing*. Take the list of stakeholders in Box 14.2 and try to identify who the stakeholders were in your selected study. Who were the participants? What were the criteria for inclusion in the study? Are they explicitly stated? Were any eligible participants excluded? Who was the hands-on data collector? Were they also the study investigator? Was data collected from multiple sites? Not all of the stakeholders will be obvious from the way the study is written up but some of them should be. The funder may be mentioned in an acknowledgement at the start or end of the paper.

References

Department of Health. 2005 Research Governance Framework for Health and Social Care, 2nd edn. Department of Health, London

Hogan J, Clark M 1996 Postgraduate and research organization and management. In: Warner D, Palfreyman D (eds) Higher Education Management. The Key Elements. Open University Press, Buckingham

Lock D 2003 Project Management, 8th edn. Gower, Aldershot

Meredith J, Mantel S 2000 Project Management. A Managerial Approach, 4th edn. Wiley, New York

Usherwood T 1996 Introduction to Project Management in Health Research. A Guide for New Researchers. Open University Press, Buckingham

Chapter 15

Supervising Research Students

David Thompson

Introduction

Supervising research is an important but often under-valued activity. It has traditionally been a bit of a 'hit-or-miss' affair, depending to a large extent on the calibre of the student, who has to have a great deal of enthusiasm and commitment to drive the project and overcome the whims of the supervisor and the vagaries of funding. With limited availability of expertise and resources, considerable variation in institutional practices and little empirical evidence from which to draw guidance, there is a pressing need for some guiding principles for research supervision. This chapter draws heavily upon a recent position paper (Thompson et al 2005) referring to a consultation document, *Improving standards in postgraduate research degree programmes* (Higher Education Funding Council for England 2003), incorporated in the Quality Assurance Agency for Higher Education (2004) *Code of Practice* which proposed a framework of minimum threshold standards and good practice guidelines for postgraduate research degree programmes in the UK.

Supervising research

Many nurses undertaking research do so as part of a higher degree programme. Success or failure to a large extent depends on the quality and experience of supervision that research students receive. Neophyte researchers can learn a great deal from an experienced research supervisor, especially in relation to designing and conducting a project. Indeed, trying to ensure that research students complete their programme of study and improving the quality of their experience of the research process often hinges on the supervisor, who has a responsibility for providing guidance to the student and fostering an environment in which research is seen as a creative and exciting activity. However, although supervising research can be a rewarding experience which improves with experience, it can also be laborious or stressful; therefore, it is important for both the student and supervisor to develop an informed and shared understanding of the supervision process. This is particularly pressing with increased competition for research awards, an emphasis on completion times and submission rates, and limited availability of resources and expertise in supervision.

A code of good practice for research supervision is available in many universities, the main purpose being to set down the broad expectations the institution has of those involved with research training and its perceptions of the specific roles and responsibilities of various parties, including the student and the supervisor, in ensuring that the research experience is as valuable as possible.

Selecting the student

Selecting the right student is essential to the success of the research and the student–supervisor relationship. Many aspiring candidates, who have an excellent idea, are naïve or ignorant about the demands the proposed research can place upon them, particularly regarding their family and social life. Without dampening enthusiasm and commitment, the student needs to be fully apprised of what is expected, especially the time involved, and account needs to be taken of the degree of enterprise, initiative and intellectual autonomy that the student displays. The student should be able to reflect critically and take a creative approach to issues in and beyond their field of expertise and be expected to have a positive attitude to the acquisition and advancement of knowledge. In essence, the student should be imbued with a commitment to scholarly values.

In the UK, the Higher Education Funding Council (HEFCE) minimum threshold standard for selection, admission, enrolment and induction of students specifies a normal entry requirement to be either an upper second class degree in a relevant subject, a Masters degree or institutionally defined equivalent accreditation of prior learning (APL) or experiential learning (APEL) equivalent. In addition, it recommends that the selection process and admission decisions involve at least two research active academics trained in selection and admission procedures. To obviate the problem of students registering and subsequently discontinuing, some UK universities require at least a year of preparation prior to registration during which a sound research proposal can be drawn up and scrutinised. At this pre-proposal stage a small committee (three to five people) may be required to decide whether or not the student's proposal is feasible. Clearly, this adds to the length of time the student spends on the study with no commitment, initially, from the university (Thompson et al 2005).

Selecting the supervisor

Selecting the right supervisor is also important. Many students are allocated a supervisor who is ill-equipped to perform the function of supervision. The supervisor should be familiar not only with the subject area and/or appropriate methodology but also with policy issues such as research degree regulations, admission process, intellectual property, ethics and occupational health and safety guidelines, induction and orientation programmes, and submission and examination processes. Institutional guidelines often refer to the minimum expectations and describe them only in broad terms, but a good and successful supervisor will be able to bring much more to the supervisory relationship and practice.

The HEFCE standard for supervision states that all new supervisors should undertake mandatory institutionally specified training. There should be a team of at least two active researchers with relevant knowledge and skills, of whom one should be designated as the main supervisor with overall responsibility for the student. The main supervisor should have had experience of at least one successful supervision of a student through to a research degree award. The main supervisor should normally take responsibility for a maximum of six students. The team should meet regularly with the student to report, discuss and agree academic and personal progress, with outcomes of all such interactions being recorded (Thompson et al 2005).

Having two supervisors has benefits for all parties: the student to see different perspectives and the supervisor, particularly the novice, learning 'on the job' from the experienced one. Also, each supervisor might bring a different, but complementary, specialist perspective, such as clinical or research method expertise. The supervisors should possess not only recognised subject expertise, but also the skills and experience necessary to monitor, support and direct the student's work (Thompson et al 2005).

The student–supervisor relationship

The relationship that develops between the student and supervisor, which is in essence one that combines formal instruction and interpersonal support, is lengthy and demanding intellectually, and potentially emotionally, of both parties. The expectations, roles and responsibilities of both should be clarified early in the partnership, which should operate in an atmosphere of respect, commitment, collegiality and maturity (Thompson et al 2005).

The early stage of supervision is vital to establishing mutual understanding and rapport, factors that contribute to the quality of the relationship and to the likelihood of successful completion. The research student and supervisor should negotiate and agree what is expected from each. This will require clarification of the student's interests and may include refining the research topic, taking into account feasibility in terms of resources and facilities. It will also require drawing up draft time frames, diagnosing the student's knowledge and identifying training needs.

In establishing a rapport, several issues should be considered. For example, are there relevant personal circumstances that might make the supervision or completion of the research thesis difficult? What is the time frame for the study and writing up? With joint supervision, what will be the roles and responsibilities of each supervisor? What access does the student have to facilities and resources?

The student should expect to be provided with at least a desk, a computer and access to a library and appropriate databases. A programme of research training that includes the use of information technology, project management, literature searching, database management, statistical and qualitative data analysis, personal effectiveness, communication skills (written, oral, listening), networking and team-working, and career development should be available. This should be determined by a training needs analysis and reviewed to ensure that it is meeting the needs of the student. The student should be encouraged to attend seminars, conferences and discussion forums and participate in presentations, teaching and demonstrations, maintaining a portfolio of these activities.

Regular face-to-face meetings between the student and supervisor should be arranged and each meeting carefully planned and structured to make efficient and effective use of time so that both parties benefit. Each meeting should review plans and progress, making notes to check perceptions of decisions made, recall previous discussions, inquire into progress towards goals and exchange pertinent information. The content of meetings should include an exchange of written lists of queries or areas to be discussed prior to the scheduled time as well as a discussion and submission of regular progress reports. The student and supervisor may wish to keep a diary or record notes about each supervision session, such as on the topics covered, problems that may have arisen, decisions made and time estimates discussed. Feedback is important and involves summarising, evaluating, advising, motivating and facilitating understanding, and can be given in formal or informal meetings. Telephone, fax or email communication can be a particularly important mode of interaction, especially with part-time students, but these should not be regarded as a complete substitute for face-to-face meetings.

Either the student or supervisor should be responsible for keeping a record of the meetings and what was agreed, such as plans, timescales and deadlines, and this should be filed and easily accessible to all relevant and interested parties such as postgraduate admission tutors. Such documents are invaluable for the process of monitoring progress and this is increasingly expected of universities. It is important that mapping of the task ahead occurs. This involves setting out what a research degree is and what is expected in terms of originality (Phillips & Pugh 2000) and contribution to knowledge and scholarship. These meetings provide important opportunities for exploring ideas, thinking the project through, agreeing the prerequisites the student should bring and preparing the research.

The frequency of meetings should be mutually agreed and will depend on the stage of the student's research and the needs of the student. It is important, at each meeting, to make firm arrangements for the next. Although the amount of contact between the student and supervisors can vary, it is largely via this route that the student is given guidance, especially on thesis content, organisation and timescale. The student and supervisors should agree sensible and realistic periods for the supervisors to read and comment on work, otherwise tensions will inevitably occur. Meeting too frequently will not allow time for progress and can be dispiriting for the student (and supervisor); meeting too infrequently usually leads to difficulties.

The need to foster independence and instil confidence is a key step in the maturation of the research student. However, the student should be assured of support and help with any difficulties that may arise. During this period the degree of responsibility and control should shift gradually from the supervisor to the student, who should be prepared for the long duration and the demanding and sustained effort a research degree entails,

and to expect periods of comparative inactivity such as waiting for research data to be returned and obtaining ethical permission. The student and supervisor should evaluate progress against the research plan, discuss an annual progress report and negotiate any follow-up action.

The student and supervisor should be provided with clear criteria to guide the process. The HEFCE standard for initial review and subsequent progress includes a formal annual review by a panel, including at least one person independent of the supervisory team (Thompson et al 2005).

Role and responsibility of the student

The student must have a capacity for taking the initiative and an ability to accept and discharge responsibilities, to work autonomously and to take responsibility in complex and unpredictable situations. It is the student's responsibility to establish, in consultation with the supervisor, a plan for the conduct of the research and to monitor and review his or her progress against that plan. The student should also submit work to an agreed timetable and maintain an agreed schedule of meetings with the supervisor and a jointly agreed record of personal progress. Importantly, the student has a responsibility to commit to complete the research and submit the thesis in good time.

The student should discuss with the supervisor the type of guidance required, agree a schedule of meetings and take the initiative in arranging further meetings if necessary, and maintain progress as required and agreed, including, in particular, the presentation of written material in sufficient time to allow for comments and discussion. The student should expect the supervisor to read and comment on work in a timely fashion, giving good reasons for any delay.

A learning plan may be prepared by the student, in consultation with the supervisor, for each year and be formally reviewed annually. Developing a personal learning plan provides a structured process to help the student think about key areas essential to the success of the research and identifies the student's desired learning outcomes, the learning opportunities the student will seek in order to achieve them and a timeline for this.

Role and responsibility of the supervisor

The supervisor is responsible for the overall academic direction of the student's research project and for the conduct of the student and must be available for advice, assistance and direction and should have sufficient expertise and experience. The supervisor should provide intellectual expertise, bolster the student's confidence and morale, and act as a guide, intellectual critic and general counsellor (Hockey 1994). This includes guidance about the nature of the research and the standard expected, the formulation of the research question, the planning of the research project and the searching of the literature. Thus, the supervisor will assist the student to identify specific research-related hypotheses or questions, methodologies, resources and facilities leading to the development of a detailed research plan, and will advise on structure, style and thesis format.

The supervisor should ensure that the student is aware of the standards expected and identify with the student training needs such as the particular research skills that will need to be acquired and what are the most appropriate data gathering and analysing techniques to be used.

The supervisor and student should monitor progress made within the context of the overall research plan. The supervisor is also responsible for advising the student of applicable guidelines for the conduct of research, including those covering ethical and intellectual property requirements.

The supervisor should be accessible to the student at appropriate times when the student may need advice on academic (and personal) problems and should give detailed advice (verbal and written) on the necessary completion dates of successive stages of the work, and expected targets and timetables so that the work may be submitted within the normative time schedule. This necessitates providing the student with timely, critical and constructive comment on the content and drafts, returning work within a reasonable length of time, and advising on matters relating to the presentation of work for publication, including the avoidance of plagiarism and the process of due acknowledgement (Thompson et al 2005).

The supervisor should identify skills required for successful completion of the research project and recommend remedial action as appropriate. This may include arranging for the student to present and discuss their work in graduate seminars, conferences and in other forums to expose it to peer review and encourage and assist them to develop or improve their skills.

The supervisor should take the major responsibility for the supervisory process and, though all supervisors should be bound by duty, obligation and commitment, the degree to which this is enacted should be carefully balanced. There is a real danger of spoon-feeding and over-commitment on behalf of the supervisor, who can sometimes become too emotional, intimate and subjective. Reassurance, encouragement and enthusiasm are necessary to maintain the student over such a prolonged period of arduous study, for example helping the student overcome a research barrier such as 'writer's block' or rekindling enthusiasm when a severe disengagement or loss of motivation has occurred. Thus, problem-solving is an important area of the supervision process and the supervisor often has to be prepared to deal with unexpected and difficult scenarios, including handling difficulties in the student's conduct. The supervisor is not expected to be a parental substitute but should be concerned with the general welfare of the student.

Although research supervision is an important academic function it is often accorded too little value, preparation or recognition. For example, it should be formally recognised in workloads as student contact time using an appropriate formula. Increasingly, it is recognised that training and staff development should be offered. Sharing experiences with other supervisors from different disciplines may also be valuable. This is now becoming mandatory for universities in the UK before certain bodies will fund research students.

Ethics, authorship and intellectual property

Important issues in research supervision include ethics, authorship and intellectual property. These are often vague areas that can, if not anticipated and informed, give rise to serious problems for all concerned. The whole process of research supervision should be operated within an ethical framework. Honesty, integrity, consent, confidentiality, data protection, intellectual property and copyright are all issues that should be addressed. At the outset it should be acknowledged that intellectual ownership be invested in the research student.

Authorship and acknowledgement guidelines are important and agreement should be reached between the student and the supervisor concerning authorship of publications and acknowledgements of contributions during the research study. Ethically and legally, all who have made a substantial contribution to the production of work should be acknowledged. It is suggested that the question of acknowledgement, including the likelihood of co-authorship, be discussed at the beginning of a project with all who are likely to participate. Agreement should be reached then, but decisions may need to be reviewed as the project proceeds. As a guiding principle, a co-author would have an excellent mastery of the subject. Academic rank should neither preclude nor necessitate co-authorship. Guidelines are provided by many journals and authorship credit should be based only on substantial contribution to: conception and design, or analysis and interpretation of data; drafting the article or revising it critically for important intellectual content; final approval of the version to be published.

It is often university policy that students own any intellectual property that they create pursuant to their studies, although their opportunities to exploit their intellectual property commercially may be limited. Important issues for intellectual property arise in the consideration of copyright, inventions and involvement with confidential research projects (Thompson et al 2005).

Examination process

The student and supervisor will need to determine when enough work has been completed to meet the thesis requirements. In preparation for the examination, there should be transparency and accountability in relation to how examiners (internal and external) are selected, with the choice and role being determined by academic credentials, experience and independence (Tinkler & Jackson 2000). The supervisor will need to identify and propose potential examiners taking account of their perspectives and expectations. To avoid compromising the examination and to enable it to be conducted in a fair manner, both the student and supervisor should refrain from communicating with the external examiner during the examination process.

Agreeing and nominating appropriate examiners in plenty of time is essential. This allows the student to become familiar with the work of the examiner. Examinations will be determined to a large extent by university regulations but should comprise the student, supervisor (as observer only) and the internal and external examiners.

It is increasingly difficult to persuade academics to be examiners in view of the amount of time and effort this function entails and the modest financial recognition for their knowledge and expertise. The HEFCE standard for selection of examiners is that there should be an independent panel of at least two examiners who are research-active in relevant fields, at least one of whom is an external examiner (both in the case of staff candidates). Each examiner should provide an independent report on the thesis before any viva, but it may be unreasonable to expect this more than a few days in advance.

A vital aspect of research supervision is the examination process, both at the transfer stage and as a final evaluation of the student's training and completed thesis. Although there is considerable diversity in policy regulating all aspects of the examination process (Tinkler & Jackson 2000), maintenance of and commitment to high academic standards and integrity should be paramount, and the examiners should be the final judges of quality as well as ensuring fairness and transparency. Examiners should normally be supervisors in their own right. They should be sufficiently aware of the intellectual frontiers in their subject that they can judge whether the thesis makes an original contribution to the advancement of knowledge or scholarship sufficient to justify the award. The hallmark of a PhD, for instance, is originality and the student and thesis need to convince the examiners that this criterion is met. It is usually stated that a PhD thesis should make a substantial and original contribution to knowledge. Examiners will have certain criteria they use and levels of student performance they expect. For example, they are likely to be influenced by previously published work in the area, the views of the other examiners, and their knowledge of the student's supervisor and/or department and the level of perceived responsibility between the student and supervisor (Mullins & Kiley 2002). A key message is that first impressions count and influence an examiner's frame of mind for the rest of the thesis. Experienced examiners make judgements about the quality of the thesis after reading the first few chapters. Positive indicators include: sparkle, elan, cohesiveness, clarity, style and sophistication; negative ones include: poor referencing, typographical errors, carelessness and lack of attention to detail. The final, substantive judgement is determined by: the student's confidence and independence, creativity, structure of argument, coherence of theoretical and methodological perspectives, and critical self-assessment (Mullins & Kiley 2002).

Characteristics of a poor thesis include: lack of coherence, lack of or confused understanding of the theory and/or methodology, lack of confidence and lack of originality. In contrast, those of an outstanding thesis include: elegance of design, synthesis and execution, coherence and creativity (Mullins & Kiley 2002). To achieve this, supervisors should be willing to read and comment on draft chapters and to read the whole work over prior to submission. (Examiners sometimes find it hard to believe that supervisors have done this!) The student should be encouraged to employ the services of an independent proofreader and to make use of electronic referencing systems.

Although the viva voce is a standard feature of the doctoral examination in the UK, guidelines outlining practice suggest that its significance in the overall assessment varies among institutions (Morley et al 2002, Tinkler & Jackson 2000). The viva voce is probably the most stressful component of the PhD and there is wide variation in how far students are prepared for it, how long it will last and what form it will take.

The student and supervisors should be encouraged to participate in practice viva voce examinations (Tinkler & Jackson 2004). This provides opportunities and experiences to demystify the viva examination and to identify and plug any gaps in knowledge. It also helps to focus the student in terms of gauging the audience and analysing the purpose and target the communication (Murray 2002). For the newer supervisor, it provides an opportunity for training and development. It may be helpful if examiners' reports were made available to potential examiners and if inexperienced examiners sought advice from more experienced colleagues.

The presence of supervisors, the balance between the thesis and the viva voce, the purpose, length and impact of the viva voce and the mode and timing of the release of the decision are all issues that vary between institutions. However, the examination process should be a worthwhile and developmental experience for the candidate, irrespective of the outcome. The candidate should be recognised as the expert in their work, treated accordingly and expected to behave accordingly.

Conclusion

The recent threshold standards proposed by HEFCE are intended to represent an essential minimum for the provision of high quality research degree programmes. They are likely to improve significantly the performance of research supervision in nursing, where the situation is in need of development. Systematic and transparent supervisory arrangements are needed. In nursing, too often, students who have completed a research degree feel, or are led to believe, that they are fully fledged researchers. Undertaking research training is akin to an apprenticeship. It should be seen as the beginning of a research career, not the end. It is important that the experience has been positive and that the student has a strong commitment, enthusiasm and intention to continue to undertake research. Finally, the student should ideally have a career aspiration in relation to research (Thompson et al 2005).

EXERCISES

- Identify a supervision training programme in your institution.
- Review best practice in research supervision in your institution.
- Ask your research student to consider developing a personal learning plan.
- Discuss with at least one experienced supervisor how to provide feedback and constructive criticism.
- Participate in a meeting between a student and a supervisor as an observer.

References

Higher Education Funding Council for England 2003 Improving standards in postgraduate research degree programmes. Formal consultation, London Department for Employment and Learning, Northern Ireland, Higher Education Funding Council for England, Higher Education Funding Council for Wales, Scottish Higher Education Funding Council, London

Hockey J 1994 Establishing boundaries: Problems and solutions in managing the PhD supervisor's role. Cambridge Journal of Education 24: 293–305

Morley L, Leonard D, David M 2002 Variations in vivas: Quality and equality in British PhD assessments. Studies in Higher Education 27: 263–273

Mullins G, Kiley M 2002 It's a PhD, not a Nobel Prize: How experienced examiners assess research theses. Studies in Higher Education 27: 369–386

Murray R 2002 How to Write a Thesis. Open University Press, Buckingham

Phillips E M, Pugh D S 2000 How to Get a PhD: a Handbook for Students and Their Supervisors. Open University Press, Buckingham

Quality Assurance Agency for Higher Education 2004 Code of Practice for assurance of academic quality and standards in higher education. Section 1. Postgraduate research programmes QAA, Gloucester

Thompson D R, Kirkman S, Watson R, et al 2005 Improving research supervision in nursing. Nurse Education Today 25: 283–290

Tinkler P, Jackson C 2000 Examining the doctorate: Institutional policy and the PhD examination process in the UK. Studies in Higher Education 25: 167–180

Chapter 16

Publishing and Dissemination of Research

Mi Ja Kim and Heeseung Choi

Introduction

This chapter describes the components, process, strategies, and ethical guidelines to facilitate the publishing and disseminating (P&D) of nursing knowledge.

Components of a nursing research paper

Academic papers generally include four sections: Introduction, Methods, Results findings, and Discussion/Conclusions.

Introduction

The primary purpose of the introduction is to draw the attention of readers and inform them what to expect in the paper. The significance, uniqueness, and timeliness of the topic under study should be presented at the beginning of the introduction to invite readers' attention. It usually includes a statement of the problem or research question, the purpose of the study, significance of the study, conceptual or theoretical framework that guided the study and hypotheses (if applicable). A brief review of relevant literature along with identification of the gap in the current knowledge that the present study intends to fill are also included. It is important to include a concluding paragraph that summarises the introduction section and addresses how the new knowledge acquired in the study will contribute to nursing (Table 16.1).

Table 16.1 – *Sample paragraphs for the introduction section*

	Quantitative	Qualitative
Research questions	The research questions were as follows: (1) What are the demographics, health characteristics, and family histories of women with and without breast cancer who are scheduled to be seen for genetic cancer risk assessment (GCRA)? ... (5) Are there differences between the unaffected and affected groups regarding these questions? (MacDonald et al 2005, p. 373; Lipincott Williams & Wilkins ©)	Specific aims of the study were to seek answers to the following questions. 1. How do these elderly people define their health? Do they define health in ways other than by reference to illness and disease, disability and dysfunction? ... 3. What behavior and/or activities do these elderly respondents describe as contributing to their health? (van Maanen 2006, p. 55; Blackwell Publishing)
Purposes	Specifically, we intended to: ■ determine whether RNs were aware of their need for information and the importance of using evidence (including research) in practice ... ■ define, from the RN's point of view, the individual and institutional barriers to using research and other evidence in practice that are present in the clinical environment (Pravikoff et al 2005, p. 43; Lipincott Williams & Wilkins ©)	The purpose of the present study was to determine the most frequently perceived benefits of and barriers to medication and dietary compliance among two samples of patients with heart failure (Heilemann et al 2005, p. 953)
Significance of the study	Presently, there is paucity of empirical data on Nigerian nurses' overall knowledge of and attitude towards AIDS. This study is part of a larger study on the knowledge about AIDS among Nigerian nurses, their attitudes and level of comfort (LOC) in providing services to surviving patients with AIDS (Oyeyemi et al 2006, p. 197; Blackwell Publishing)	The concept of patient advocacy has in recent times become enshrined in nursing practice. The International Council of Nurses calls on nurses and nursing organizations to promote advocacy as 'a key nursing role' ... Despite this adoption of the role of nurses as advocates, difficulties arise when precise definitions of the concept are sought, which, in turn, make it difficult to enact in practice ... This study is aimed to investigate general nurses' perceptions of the role in Ireland, where notably there are no published articles to date, and compare these with the existing literature on the subject (O'Connor & Kelly 2005, p. 454; © 2005 Edward Arnold (Publishers) Ltd. (www.hodderarnoldjournals.com))
Conceptual framework	Roy's Adaptation Model (1984) was chosen as the conceptual framework for this exploratory study... Roy's theoretical model is particularly well suited to this study as	Explanatory models are beliefs and knowledge that individuals use in response to a specific experience of illness ... Kleinman's (1980) explanatory models of

Table 16.1 – *Sample paragraphs for the introduction section Cont'd*

Quantitative	Qualitative
verbal abuse in this case is an external, focal stimulus to which the pediatric nurse is exposed. The environment is the unit in which the pediatric nurse has to work, and the pediatric nurse represents the adaptive system that responds to this external stimulus . . . (Pejic 2005, p. 272; reprinted with permission of the publisher, Janetti Publications, Inc., East Holly Avenue, Box 56, Pitman, NJ08071–0056; (856)256–2300; Fax (856)589–7463; Website: www.pediatricnursing.net; For a sample copy of the journal, please contact the publisher)	illness guided this study; Kleinman's model captures both individuals' and cultural groups' understandings of disease and illness and identifies five themes common across explanatory models: (a) etiology, (b). . . Understanding the explanatory model shared by a group can be used to develop culturally sensitive diabetes prevention programs targeted to the needs of the community (Skelly et al 2006, pp. 10–11)

Sample extracts reproduced with permission of the publishers.

Methods

Information provided in this section should be detailed enough for readers to picture each step of the study process and to replicate or critique the study. Included in this section are research design, sample, setting, measurement, data collection procedure and data analysis. The following subsections are likely to be presented in a section on methods.

Research design

In this subsection, authors concisely address what type of study design was selected for the study and justify the reasons for the design. Authors may provide more detailed information, such as for how long and how often the subjects were examined (longitudinal study), how the subjects were assigned to groups (experimental study) and in what context the study was conducted (qualitative study).

Sample and setting

This subsection includes demographic characteristics of the target population, selection criteria for the sample and sample size, the method used to determine this and the setting/context. Power analysis is often used in quantitative studies to estimate the size of the sample needed to obtain a significant result. Special recruitment strategies used to increase the response rates along with the actual response rates are discussed in this section.

Instrument, measures and data collection procedure

Detailed information about the psychometric properties of the instruments and a rationale for their choice are required. A description of how study variables were defined, measured and scored by using the instruments is necessary. Conceptual and/or operational definitions of study variables are included as appropriate. When authors used instruments that required translation, they need to specify how they ensured the equivalency of the translated instrument. If equipment was used to measure physiological variables, authors should describe data collection procedures including the accuracy of the measures using the equipment.

Data collection procedures include the consent process; steps taken to collect data; amount of time, effort and risk involved; description of any incentives; and time frame for the data collection. Written informed consent is secured before collecting any data and it involves explanation of the purpose and the procedure of the study and question/answer period.

For qualitative studies using interview methods, it is necessary to present an interview guide, a training protocol for interviewers and the context in which the interviews were conducted. For focus groups, it is important to address the characteristics of group members, the nature and sequence of questions and the main role of a moderator (Morgan 1993). Also, authors need to elucidate how confidentiality was assured in the group and how the group dynamics and ground rules were managed. When any equipment (e.g. audiotape) was used to collect data for qualitative studies, the use of the equipment needs to be clearly stated in the consent form as well as in the methods section. Authors need to describe how the audiotapes were transcribed and how data were analysed. Helping readers to understand the detailed study process as well as the sociocultural and historical context of a study is essential in a qualitative study. Sample paragraphs for a methods section are outlined in Table 16.2.

Ethical considerations

Authors need to state that the study received the approval of the institutional review board (IRB) or institutional ethics committee (IEC). Some journals require evidence of IRB approval prior to publication, and retrospective approval by the IRB is neither allowed nor accepted (Cleary & Horsfall 2002).

Data analysis

This section should describe how data were analysed along with the names of statistical tests used for each research question. For a qualitative study, one describes how the quality check was performed; how the coding scheme was developed; how data were sorted, summarised, coded, and organised; and how themes were identified and synthesised. Any software program used to manage data should be specified.

Results/findings

The main goal of the results/findings section is to display what the study found. Research findings are presented in reference to the research questions or hypotheses proposed in the introduction. When presenting the findings, specific statistical tests

Table 16.2 – *Sample paragraphs for the methods section*

	Quantitative	Qualitative
Research design	This study represents baseline assessments of homeless participants engaged in a randomized clinical trial of an intervention designed to assess completion of TB chemoprophylaxis among homeless adults. Participants were randomized into a nurse case-managed program versus a standard program (Nyamathi et al 2005, p. 899)	This study used ground theory method. 'Ground theory is an approach to qualitative research informed by symbolic interactionism... An assumption of grounded theory is that individuals and groups share social circumstances, generating common meaning and understanding' (Lutz 2005, p. 804)
Sample/ Setting	Strata in the quota sampling were ethnicity (Hispanic or non-Hispanic), and previous expression of Advance Directives (ADs) (either stated or not expressed prior to enrollment). Equal numbers of Hispanics and non-Hispanics ($n = 60$ each) were targeted for enrollment. Within each group, equal numbers of adults with and without expressed ADs at the point of enrollment were sought. Finally, subjects within the four	In each of 2 years, 12 women were to be recruited. In the three-stage sampling strategy, convenience sampling was used first; volunteers were sought within a 50-mile radius of the university. Social service agencies distributed 300 brochures (with attached postcards that volunteers could return) to women who might qualify or know of someone who might qualify. The second sampling stage was purposive.

Table 16.2 – *Sample paragraphs for the methods section—Cont'd*

	Quantitative	Qualitative
	groups were divided randomly to receive either the increased AD information condition (the LSPQ), or the attention control condition (an irrelevant survey). Thus, the research design created eight comparison groups. A power analysis, assuming a medium effect size, power of 0.80, and an alpha of 0.05, indicated a required sample size of $n = 120$. A total of 123 patients were initially enrolled; 106 were successfully retained with complete, usable data sets (Froman & Owen 2005, pp. 401–402; © 2005, reprinted with permission of John Wiley & Sons, Inc)	During a telephone call, volunteers were screened for 'predefined traits' that were typical of older women or linked to home-care use: (a) being age 80 or older; (b) ... Finally, quota sampling was done to bolster representativeness (Porter 2005, p. 297; Lipincott Williams & Wilkins ©)
Instrument or measures	The Brazelton Neonatal Behavioral Assessment Scale is a means of scoring interactive behavior for both full-term and stable preterm infants. The scale consists of 27 behavioral items, each scored on a 9-point scale, and 20 elicited responses, each scored on a 3-point scale. In most cases, the infant's score is based on the best performance, not an average performance. Areas of assessment include infant state, orientation... and smiling. A mean test–retest stability of all items was 0.592, with a range of 0.293 to 0.967. Reliabilities for independent tests range from 0.85 to 1.00. Testers can be trained at a 0.90 level of reliability, with this level remaining for long periods of time (Medoff-Cooper & Ratcliffe 2005, p. 358; Lipincott Williams & Wilkins ©)	Group sessions were audiotape-recorded. Tabletop microphones were placed to ensure that all comments were recorded clearly and accurately. Tapes were immediately labeled and stored for subsequent verbatim transcription. The group discussions were focused on the following topics: ... Demographic data were collected. ... All participants were asked about age, gender... and annual income. Questions initially were broad and open-ended. A flip chart was used at times in the session to make lists of responses and to validate for participants that their opinions mattered (Rose et al 2004, p. 41; Blackwell Publishing)
Data collection process	Blood pressure (BP) was measured with a Colin tonometric monitor, which noninvasively records BP with each heartbeat. Data collection occurred in a quiet room adjacent to a clinic setting, which was convenient for both inpatients and outpatients. Participants sat quietly and rested for 5 minutes before beginning the protocol. After the rest period, the protocol included four 4-minute segments (baseline; quiet #1; talking; quiet-time #2). During the quiet tasks neither the researcher nor the	We initiated the focus group discussions with an introductory message, thanking participants for volunteering and recounting the aims, purpose, and issues of confidentiality and anonymity. We informed participants of the scope of the discussion by introducing the topics under consideration. Ground rules were stated... Subsequent procedure depended on the dynamics and progression of each particular discussion, requiring the moderator to be responsive to the changing

Continued

Table 16.2 – *Sample paragraphs for the methods section—Cont'd*

	Quantitative	Qualitative
	participant talked. During the 4 minutes of talking, participants were asked to describe what health means to them. Specific prompts included 'How do you know you are healthy?' ... The entire protocol required a minimum of 21 minutes including the 5-minute rest period before beginning (Liehr et al 2002, p. 29; Blackwell Publishing)	demands of the group... Following the discussion, a debriefing session took place. Participants were thanked for their contribution and informed of the subsequent stages of analysis (Adams et al 2005, p. 1298; Blackwell Publishing)
Data analysis	Path analysis was conducted in order to determine the goodness of fit of the model. Criterion for examining the goodness of fit included a chi-square probability greater than or equal to .05 with a Comparative Fit Index (CFI) of at least .90. Based on this criterion, the model provided an exceptional description of the relationships between the study variables in the dataset ($\chi^2 = 26.2$, $p > .10$, CFI $= .968$). Regression analysis was used to compute the path coefficients (Steele & Porche 2005, p. 335; Lipincott Williams & Williams ©)	The approach for data analysis was adapted from the steps described by Collaizzi. Initially, all transcripts were read to develop an overall understanding of the experience. Then, significant statements were identified, coded, and grouped into broad topical areas... A number of measures that address issues of trustworthiness of qualitative data, as described by Lincoln and Guba and applied to phenomenological research, were performed. First, peer debriefing, which is interaction of the investigator with other professionals, was used... Second, thick descriptive data were collected, which is the process of providing a detailed description of the participants to allow for transferability of findings. Third, the investigators established an audit trail, which is a mechanism of maintaining extensive notes that reflect the investigators' analytical thought process during the course of the study ... (Kavanaugh & Hershberger 2005, p. 598; Blackwell Publishing)

Sample extracts reproduced with permission of the publishers.

used for each of the findings should be stated, including the level of significance (usually $p \leq 0.05$ is used).

Compared with a quantitative study, qualitative reports often have lengthy results/findings sections (e.g. narratives) because the findings and interpretation are discussed together. Charts, diagrams and graphs can be used in a qualitative study to communicate complicated concepts and arguments effectively (Meadows 2004). Statistical analysis should be avoided in a qualitative study because 'participants of the qualitative study have not been selected to be statistically representative of the population being studied, but to provide variations in the nature of their views and experiences' (Meadows 2004, p. 39).

Table 16.3 – *Sample paragraphs for the results section*

	Quantitative	Qualitative
Results/ Findings	To answer the first research question, the dataset at time 1 was submitted to cluster analysis, and a three-cluster solution was obtained … To determine how the clusters differed in the specific problem behaviours, research question number three, the group means for the three clusters at Times 1 and 2 were graphically represented. These can be found in Figures 1 and 2 (Bartlett et al 2005, p. 233; © 2005, reprinted with permission of John Wiley & Sons, Inc)	A number of themes emerged. In response to the questions and the ensuing discussion, young women spoke about the connotations of smoking, smoking initiation, …, and experiences of quitting. Smoking was seen as meeting a number of needs, which varied according to the age groups of the women. Young women referred to the role of smoking in helping adolescents (themselves or peers) to fit in at the crucial time of starting high school (Lennon et al 2005, p. 1350; © 2005, reprinted with permission of John Wiley & Sons, Inc)

Summarising findings in tables or figures in a quantitative study is a useful strategy for presenting ideas clearly and concisely. However, tables and figures should be simple, understandable by themselves and the content in the tables should not be repeated in the text. See sample paragraphs for a results section in Table 16.3

Discussion/Conclusions

The discussion section is one of the most challenging sections to write because it requires a significant amount of synthesis of the findings and good writing skills. Authors present interpretation of the main findings, make inferences, deliberate what they have learned from the study and suggest implications for clinical practice and/or future research. In addition, authors need to discuss whether or not the findings from the study are consistent with previous studies. If the findings are not consistent, possible explanations for the differences should be presented. The discussion section also provides an opportunity to evaluate the study as a whole and to explore the possible directions for future work. See sample paragraphs for a discussion section in Table 16.4.

Authors should address the possible limitations of the study. It is also important to emphasise the significance and the strengths of the study and to offer suggestions on how to overcome the limitations in the future. In a conclusion section, authors highlight major findings and reinforce the message that they intended to deliver based on the findings of the study. Particularly for a qualitative study, authors should resist the temptation to end the paper with an inspiring, powerful, but irrelevant message that was neither based on the findings of the study nor discussed in the previous sections (Wolcott 2001).

Steps in writing for publication
Planning phase

This chapter focuses on writing research journal articles primarily for the academic and scientific community. Authors need to select the journal that is most appropriate for the study including the fit of the research project to the type of journal. Factors to consider are: a refereed journal; the portion devoted to research articles; acceptance rate; review time; level of citation in the Social Citation Index or Supplemental Social Citation Index; frequency of publication; and circulation number.

Once the journal is selected, it is advisable to send a query letter to the editor of the journal

Table 16.4 – *Sample paragraphs for the discussion*

	Quantitative	Qualitative
Discussion	Memory, learning, and sleep were impaired in this group of older Off-Pump Coronary Artery Bypass (OPCAB) patients. This is the first study (of which the author is aware) to evaluate both sleep and the cognitive function of memory and verbal learning in OPCAB patients... The findings of this study demonstrated that many older OPCAB patients exhibit difficulties in memory and learning in the early postoperative period. The hypothesis that sleep is related to memory and learning was not supported. This may have several explanations (Hedges 2005, pp. 469–470; © 2005, reprinted with permission of John Wiley & Sons, Inc)	The findings of the focus groups confirmed that nurses face both personal and professional issues related to smoking cessation... Thus, in addition to the previously identified need to increase tobacco-related content in the curricula of nursing schools, it is important for nursing schools to provide support for students who want to quit... Despite the limitations of a small sample size and the nature of focus group methodology, the findings from the study provide insights and information about the attitudes of nurses who are either smokers or former smokers... This information was used to develop the Tobacco Free Nurses Initiatives, the first ever national program to support nurses' smoking cessation efforts (Bialous et al 2004, pp. 393–394; Lipincott Williams & Wilkins ©)

Sample extracts reproduced with permission of the publishers.

asking about the appropriateness of your manuscript. You can send query letters to multiple journals, but you can submit a manuscript to only one journal at a time. If the response to your query letters is encouraging, you may want to select the journal using the criteria mentioned above.

Writing phase

Beginning the writing can sometimes be the hardest part. Many experience 'writer's block' when they force themselves into a writing style with which they are not comfortable. If you prefer a highly ordered approach to writing, writing an abstract of the study would be the first thing to do (Happell 2005). If you prefer to write now and organise later, pouring all your thoughts out, without concerns about the format of the manuscript is the thing to do. Putting your ideas and main points on the paper is the essence of the first draft. Write

clearly using simple terms. Research articles are not used to show 'an aura of intellectual prowess and erudition' (Fairbairn & Carson 2002, p. 10). Communicating contents of the studies clearly with readers is as important as conducting clinically relevant research studies (Forman 2005, Hegyvary 2005). Whenever possible, use an active tense instead of a passive one (Meadows 2004).

Revise the first and later drafts, focusing on the content for logical flow. Then revise for grammar, spelling, punctuation and writing style. Revise the manuscript deliberately and slowly. Revising up to 10 drafts for a manuscript is not unusual. Number the pages. Use the primary source for references; quote other people's work only if unusual circumstances dictate. It is advisable to synthesise what another author has written, rather than secondary quoting. If this is unavoidable, cite the quoted work with quotation marks followed by a statement, 'cited in [use the reference that you are using]'. When citing information from websites, include the web address with the date of your retrieval (American Psychological Association (APA) 2001). Follow the Instructions to Authors specified in the journal regarding the font size, line spacing, page margins, word limits, the reference format and length, and number of copies to be submitted.

Before submission, ask experienced researchers to critique your manuscript for scientific merit and your clinical peers to critique it for clarity of presentation and the impact it may have on the nursing discipline, including clinical practice and/ or theory development. Verify the accuracy of the text and the references. Citations must be complete, accurate and current (Valente 2005).

Write a title page for the manuscript including the title of your paper with the list of authors, their affiliations, corresponding author and any acknowledgements. The corresponding author is responsible for follow-up correspondence, including response to the queries and galley or page proofs. The senior author (usually the first author) normally assumes this role. Acknowledgement usually includes the funding source, if applicable, and other notable services such as consultation and editorial assistance.

Submit a cover letter with the manuscript to a journal. The cover letter should be addressed to the editor of the journal, and should include the title of the paper and a request for review for consideration of publication in the journal. Submission may be done electronically, as an increasing number of journals request submission online. You should receive a notice that your article is under review. Follow up with an inquiry letter if you have not heard from the journal for more than four months.

You will receive one of the following responses from the editor:

(a) Accepted for publication with no changes required.
(b) Accepted for publication subject to minor or major revisions.
(c) Not acceptable for publication.

If you received a letter in the 'a' category, congratulations! If your paper is accepted with revisions ('b' category), follow the reviewers' comments and questions carefully, completely and faithfully. It is important not to take their constructive criticism personally. Do not be defensive, but address each point with factual information. If you disagree with their points, you may do so respectfully, again with factual information and/or theoretical rationale.

You need to respond to each question or comment by each reviewer so that the reviewers understand how you responded to each of the concerns. You may respond by using the MS Word 'track changes' tool and submit both with and without tracked changes to facilitate their understanding.

Once your revision is accepted, you will receive a query letter that asks for more clear and complete information before the galley or page proof stage. Reviewing the proofs is the final stage of publication, and changes are allowed only if absolutely necessary. Your final joy is to see it in the journal. Celebrate!

If your paper is rejected do not give up. Give yourself some time to regroup yourself and co-authors (if any) and reformat it to meet the requirements of another journal. You may need to update the literature before the second submission. It is well worth remembering that there is no one who has not had a rejection letter. Persistence is very important, as publishing is a long process.

Ethical practice of publication and dissemination

Publication of research must observe the guidelines for publication such as those of the Committee on Publication Ethics (COPE) in the United Kingdom (http://www.publicationethics.org.uk/guidelines). Authors must avoid plagiarism and this could be prevented by using the website turnitin.com (http://www.turnitin.com).

Authors should seek permission from the copyright owner(s) if more than 500 words of the original journal text were quoted (APA 2001), but it may vary between publishers. Publication of fraudulent research is not acceptable, nor is redundant publication. Authorship should be granted when authors make a substantial contribution to all of the following areas: conception and design of the research study, analysis and interpretation of the research findings, writing and revising significant contents of the manuscript and approval of the final version of the manuscript (American Medical Association 2006). All listed authors are expected to share 'public responsibility' and assure the scientific integrity of the work (Anderson et al 2005, para 4).

Conclusion

Publication of nursing research is the responsibility of every researcher, to disseminate new knowledge to nurses, other health professionals and consumers. For publication of a research article, authors need to pay attention to the process of publication and dissemination, selection of journal and the components of a research article. Following the guidelines of the journal to which they submit is imperative for authors, as is following the ethical guidelines for publication. Steps for writing an article for publication using ethical guidelines mentioned in this chapter may facilitate the publication efforts of nurse researchers. Last but not least, researchers should be mindful of the end result of the publication. That is, the new knowledge should benefit patients and the health of people whom the nursing profession serves.

Acknowledgement

The authors wish to acknowledge editorial assistance given by Kevin Grandfield.

EXERCISES

1. Choose a clinical problem of interest to you, perform a literature review, and develop an introduction section.
2. According to the guidelines presented in this chapter, write strengths and weaknesses of the methods section of a qualitative study of your choice.
3. Do the same as Exercise 2 on a quantitative study.

References

American Medical Association 2006 JAMA authorship responsibility, financial disclosure, copyright transfer, and acknowledgement. Journal of the American Medical Association. 295: 111

American Psychological Association 2001 Publication Manual of the American Psychological Association, 5th edn. American Psychological Association, Washington DC

Anderson E, Ayachi S, Boisaubin E V, et al Suggested authorship guidelines. Online. Available: http://research.utmb.edu/starline/integrity/guidelines.htm 13 Dec 2005

Adams J, Rodham K, Gavin J 2005 Investigating the 'Self' in deliberate self-harm. Qualitative Health Research. 15: 1293–1309

Bartlett R, Holditch-Davis D, Belyea M 2005 Clusters of problem behaviors in adolescents. Research in Nursing and Health. 28: 230–239

Bialous S A, Sarna L, Wewers M E, et al 2004 Nurses' perspectives of smoking initiation, addiction, and cessation. Nursing Research 53: 387–395

Cleary M, Horsfall J 2002 Quality improvement projects: finding a pathway through policies. International Journal of Mental Health Nursing 11: 121–127

Fairbairn G J, Carson A M 2002 Writing about nursing research: a storytelling approach. Nursing Research 10: 7–14

Forman H 2005 A plea for relevance in scholarly writing. Journal of Nursing Scholarship 37: 195

Froman R D, Owen S V 2005 Randomized study of stability and change in patients' advance directives. Research in Nursing and Health 28: 398–407

Happell B 2005 Disseminating nursing knowledge – a guide to writing for publication. International Journal of Psychiatric Nursing Research 10: 1147–1155

Hedges C 2005 Sleep, memory, and learning in off-pump coronary artery bypass patients. Research in Nursing and Health 28: 462–473

Hegyvary S T 2005 Writing that matters. Journal of Nursing Scholarship 37: 193–194

Hellemann M V, Lee K A, Kury F S 2005 Strength factors among women of Mexican descent. Western Journal of Nursing Research 27: 949–965

Kavanaugh K, Hershberger P 2005 Perinatal loss in low-income African American parents. Journal of Obstetric, Gynecologic, and Neonatal Nursing 34: 595–605

Kleinman A 1980 Patients and healers in the context of culture. University of California, Berkeley

Lennon A, Galloia C, Owen N, et al 2005 Young women as smokers and nonsmokers: a qualitative social identity approach. Qualitative Health Research 15: 1345–1359

Liehr P, Takahashi R, Nishimura C, et al 2002 Expressing health experience through embodied language. Journal of Nursing Scholarship 34: 27–32

Lutz K F 2005 Abuse experiences, perceptions, and associated decisions during the childbearing cycle. Western Journal of Nursing Research 27: 802–824

MacDonald D J, Sarna L, Uman G C, et al 2005 Health beliefs of women with and without breast cancer seeking genetic cancer risk assessment. Cancer Nursing 28: 372–379

Meadows K A 2004 So you want to do research? 6: reporting research. British Journal of Community Nursing 9: 37–41

Medoff-Cooper B, Ratcliffe S J 2005 Development of preterm infants: feeding behaviors and Brazelton Neonatal Behavioral Assessment Scale at 40 and 44 weeks' postconceptional age. Advances in Nursing Science 28: 356–363

Morgan D L 1993 Successful Focus Groups: Advancing the State of the Art. Sage, Newbury Park

Nyamathi A, Berg J, Jones T 2005 Predictors of perceived health status of tuberculosis-infected homeless. Western Journal of Nursing Research 27: 896–910

O'Connor T, Kelly B 2005 Bridging the gap: A study of general nurses' perceptions of patient advocacy in Ireland. Nursing Ethics 12: 453–456

Oyeyemi A, Oyeyemi B, Bello I 2006 Caring for patients living with AIDS: knowledge, attitude and global level of comfort. Journal of Advanced Nursing 53: 196–204

Pejic A R 2005 Verbal abuse. A problem for pediatric nurses. Pediatric Nursing 31: 271–279

Porter E J 2005 Older widows' experience of home care. Nursing Research 54: 296–303

Pravikoff D S, Tanner A B, Pierce S T 2005 Readiness of US nurses for evidence-based practice. American Journal of Nursing 105(9): 40–51

Rose L E, Mallinson R K, Walton-Moss B 2004 Barrier to family care in psychiatric settings. Journal of Nursing Scholarship 36: 39–47

Skelly A H, Dougherty M, Gesler W M et al 2006 African American beliefs about diabetes. Western Journal of Nursing Research 28: 9–29

Steele S K, Porche D J 2005 Testing the theory of planned behaviors to predict mammography intention. Nursing Research 54: 332–338

Valente S M 2005 Tips for success: matching journals and topics. Nurse Author and Editor 15(2): 3–4, 7

van Maanen H M 2006 Being old does not always mean being sick: perspectives on conditions of health as perceived by British and American elderly. Journal of Advanced Nursing 53: 54–61

Wolcott H F 2001 Writing up Qualitative Research, 2nd edn. Sage, Thousand Oaks, CA

Section 3

Research Designs

Chapter 17

Surveys

Ingalill Rahm Hallberg

Introduction

A survey involves gaining an overview of a specific phenomenon or situation directly from those concerned (Polit & Hungler 1999). Thus it allows one to obtain a description of the phenomenon or situation under study. Correlations can be established as well as relationships of various kinds, although no interpretations of causal relationships can be established. Surveys can be used in cross-sectional or in longitudinal research (see Chapter 25), including the same people several times and over time to study how their views change (studying trends). They can also be repeated over time with different people, but the same population (trend study). Also, various types of data can be collected at different points in time but from the same people (panel study).

The other meaning often connected with the term survey is self-report, which refers to a way of collecting data rather than a design. Self-reports can be obtained in other designs also. Self-reports refer to information given to the researchers directly by the people belonging to the target sample. This can be done through personal interviews or in response to questionnaires distributed in various ways.

In this chapter, survey as a design for research will be addressed, as will the data collection method self-reports. It seems worthwhile to keep these two senses of the term survey separate, i.e. when it is used in the sense of research design or when it refers to the data collection method (see also Chapters 25 and 29).

Areas or phenomena suitable for a survey design

Research questions suitable for a survey design are those where the researcher wants a broad overview of a certain phenomenon or a certain situation. This design can also be used as a platform for further in-depth studies of a certain aspect. Before going into depth in a study of fatigue, for instance, in patients with Parkinson's disease, you may want to know how prevalent the problem is in such a sample compared with people of the same age who are healthy. You may also want to know more about the circumstances in which it is more or less prevalent, age-related, gender-related or related to the severity of the disease. The survey design may be useful in giving this broad overview of the problem and the conditions under which it may vary. This can, for instance, be an overview of a certain opinion as, for instance, that of patient satisfaction, or a certain attitude, for instance how to prioritise in the public health care system (Werntoft et al 2006), or a certain behaviour, for instance how people act in an emergency situation. Other areas that can be addressed by surveys include people's knowledge in a certain situation, for example patients with diabetes and their knowledge of lifestyle factors contributing to control over the HbA1c level.

As for behaviour, the survey design may be useful to investigate practice in nursing care. An example of this may be the sedation of patients cared for using a ventilator and the techniques used to establish the depth to which the patient is sedated. Also, people's living conditions can be investigated in this type of design. Thus, what is common to the questions used in a survey is that people's views, experiences, attitudes, knowledge or the like (Polit & Hungler 1999) are elicited in a systematic and standardised manner so that the response from respondent A addresses the same issue as the response from respondent B. The internal validity (Kazdin 1998) depends, among other things, on the

questions being phrased in a manner that prevents ambiguity, and it must be possible to understand the questions, free from arbitrary interpretations.

It is of utmost importance for the response rate that people included in a survey study view the issue as being important to them. People's motivation to participate in surveys of various types has decreased over the years (Herzog & Kulka 1989). This calls for care when choosing this research design and the sample to be studied.

Methods for carrying out a survey study

Various techniques can be used for data collection in survey studies. In general there are two different ways: personal interviews or some kind of self-administered questionnaire (Baker 1994). Personal interviews can be conducted in a face-to-face situation or as telephone interviews. The self-administered questionnaire can be sent by post or by handing over the questionnaire, for instance in a waiting room, on admission or when leaving hospital. The questionnaire can also be distributed at, for instance, a class meeting, or a meeting of an interest organisation such as a pensioners' or asthma patients' association or a group of people discussing, for example, living with heart disease. Also, it is becoming more common to use the internet for distributing questionnaires, either by attaching them to an electronic mail or by giving the respondents an internet address and a login code to respond to the questions directly on the web.

Survey techniques: advantages and disadvantages

Surveys serve many purposes and have their pros and cons. Among the strengths is the fact that a large group of respondents can be reached relatively easily. If sampling is carefully planned and performed, sufficiently strong conclusions can be drawn. Among the disadvantages is especially that only superficial knowledge of a certain aspect or phenomenon can be obtained. Thus no in-depth understanding can be obtained. Other drawbacks of this design depend on the method of data collection; for instance, if it is done through personal interviews or through postal questionnaires. In both cases the dropout can be substantial. Conducting personal interviews is costly and may suffer from interviewer effects (see Chapter 27) stemming either from avoiding a specific subject in a face-to-face interview or from the fact that different interviewers phrase or rephrase the questions in different ways. Personal interviews may contribute to more reliable responses but they are very costly in terms of man-power and travelling. If several interviewers are involved they may approach the questions in differ-ent ways, thus biasing the results. There may also be a problem with some questions that may be more sensitive to respond to face-to-face.

The advantages of the personal interview is that, by establishing contact and working through an interview schedule with fixed response alternatives, the interviewer can make sure that there will be no internal dropout. The interviewer can also clarify questions that the respondent may have difficulties with. The interviewer can facilitate the respon-dents' interest in the study by explaining its purpose and how it can be used.

Alternatively, telephone interviews may be less expensive but not as personal. They may work very well if personal contact has been established before the interview, for instance in discharge planning, or if the clinic is known to the person.

Self-administered questionnaires may be less expensive but there is a risk of a low response rate and steps need to be taken to prevent dropout. This can be done in various ways, one of which is to call the respondents and inform them about the study, asking for consent and explaining what is expected of them and how data will be treated. Sending reminders after a few weeks is another way of encouraging people to respond, as well as providing some token of gratitude, for instance a gift voucher. The benefits of a self-administered questionnaire are that it is less costly, and it allows for the inclusion of a sample large enough to respond to the research questions with satisfactory power (Kazdin 1998). It also allows for the inclusion of a larger geographic area. The respondents can reflect on the questions and take the time needed to respond in a satisfactory manner. Interviewer effect is eliminated but there is no one to correct misunderstanding of a question or response format.

Another shortcoming of using self-administered questionnaires is that it is hard to know whether the respondent has responded independently, received help from family members or if a different person has responded. Another limitation when a self-administered questionnaire is used is that people who have difficulties in reading and writing cannot be included and this may impose a system-atic bias on the findings. Similarly, using modern techniques such as the internet for collecting the data will exclude those not familiar with this technology or those not having access to it.

The aim of the survey must be of importance to those being addressed. The respondents should feel motivated to contribute to the study and they will do so if the focus of the study is of concern to them. This has implications for the sample. Also, activities to motivate and establish a relationship between the investigator and the respondents will most likely improve the respondents' willingness to participate in the study. Thus patients, current or previous, will be more likely to respond to questions related to their health condition, whilst the public in general may feel less motivated to respond about their health.

Whether using interviews or questionnaires, the risk of systematic dropout is extensive, involving especially vulnerable people: those who are very sick, those with reading or writing problems, the illiterate, poor people and other disadvantaged groups. This means that when there is dropout, this has to be explored, as to whether it is systematic, meaning that a particular group has dropped out of the study. The response rate may be regarded as satisfactory, for instance 80%, yet the 20% that did not respond may be these vulnerable people. Thus the findings will be distorted; for example, in a study on patient satisfaction it was shown that the most fragile people were excluded, either deliberately not given the form or not able to respond, or they died; thus the results reflected those in best condition and perhaps more likely to answer positively (Ehnfors & Smedby 1993). Dropout is unavoidable; therefore the investigator should carefully monitor the respondents and non-respondents in those variables that are likely to affect the variable under study (Hellström & Hallberg 2001). For instance, this can be age, gender, capacity for daily living, social network etc. In a study of patient satisfaction, factors such as length of hospital stay or disease severity may affect the patient's view of the hospital stay. It is more informative to be able to tell which respondents the study failed to include than it is to tell the percentage of response rate only (Table 17.1).

Formulating the aim and a hypothetical model

A survey requires an aim and the development of a hypothetical model of factors that may need to be included and/or controlled for to be able to draw trustworthy conclusion from the findings. This can be done by drawing a model describing the variable under study and areas and variables that are likely to affect it (Lyberg et al 1997). The

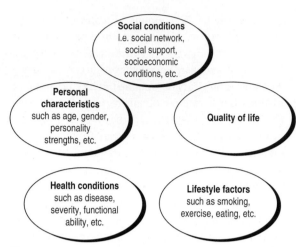

Figure 17.1 – *Example of how to explore possible domains and variables that may have an impact on the variable under study and variables that should be covered in the schedule.*

investigator may, for instance, want to explore quality of life in people with diabetes mellitus (Fig. 17.1). The level of quality of life may be affected by several other variables other than the disease and these could be factors on the background level, factors that are not easily manipulated: age, gender, stability in personality or physiological circumstances or other health problems. They can also be factors that may be open to manipulation: the social support available through the social network, lifestyle factors, education, economic situation, knowledge and understanding of the disease and how it can be

Table 17.1 – *Example of how to analyse and present respondents and non-respondents*

	Age			Total	Gender	
	75–79	*80–84*	*85+*		*Men*	*Women*
Population	3001	2563	1200	6764	2684	4080
%					39.7	68.3
Target sample, 30%	900	769	360	2029	805	1224
Response rate	684	446	144	1274	592	632
%	76.0	58.0	40.0	62.8	73.5	51.6

Comments: In addition, if possible other variables can be reported, for example level of ADL impairment, socio-economic variables.

controlled (Fig. 17.1). Thus, a survey needs to include other variables in addition to the variable at the centre of the investigator's interest. By analysing the variable, in this case quality of life, in relation to these other variables, the investigator will be able to draw more valid conclusions about the relationship between diabetes mellitus and quality of life. Such knowledge may be useful in setting up an intervention to improve their quality of life, targeting the factors that perhaps play the dominant role in low quality of life.

It goes without saying that a survey, especially using self-administered questionnaires, cannot be too long since that may negatively affect the respondents' motivation to respond. Thus, the number of variables included should be restricted. However, this makes development of the tentative or hypothetical model even more important. Once the model is developed, priority can be given to the variables and those judged to be most important are selected for inclusion. Thus when outlining the content of a survey study, whether intended to be performed in a personal interview or as a self-administered questionnaire, thorough planning is required. The literature review (see Chapter 8) preceding every study provides the investigator with the information needed to develop the hypothetical model in addition to clinical or personal experience.

Selecting the areas, questions and standardised measures to be included

Following development of the hypothetical model, the investigator has to decide how to measure the different areas that are to be included (Baker 1994). Here the investigator can choose between already developed and tested measures or questions developed for this particular study. The measures included can be those directly or indirectly assessing a phenomenon or a concept. Directly assessed aspects include a person's ability to manage daily living, using questions like: 'Can you dress by yourself?' Those indirectly assessing a

phenomenon such as quality of life are made up of a set of questions that may be added to each other in a certain way and likely to tap the concept of quality of life. The respondent may have to respond to several questions that together cover quality of life. In the example of 'Can you dress by yourself?' the respondent's own view of their ability to dress independently is given, whereas in the other example it is not the person's own view of their quality of life that is given but rather the level of quality of life as measured using a specific scale and defined concept. It is preferable to use already tested measures or questions developed and tested for their reliability and validity (Streiner & Norman 2003). The starting point for decisions should be the model that is likely to include single items and concepts, more or less well developed. Gender and age are examples of easily formulated questions whilst social network, social support, socio-economic conditions, personal strengths and quality of life are concepts that may be defined and assessed in different ways. Thus, the investigator has to explore these concepts and the way they have been defined, and on what basis different measures have been developed so that the choices made are in concordance with the model set-up. Figure 17.2 provides an example of layout and instructions for questions about health.

Pilot study

Before starting data collection a pilot study should be carried out. In a survey study, this can preferably be carried out in two steps. In the first step the interview schedule or the questionnaire can be tested, whilst in the second step the feasibility of the study as a whole can be tested.

Testing the interview schedule or the questionnaire can be done, for instance, by giving it to a smaller group (10–15 people) with the same characteristics as the target sample are supposed to have. These people should be asked to respond to all questions, marking those that may be difficult or ambiguous. They should also be asked to comment on readability, layout and clarity and whether they

Questions about how you view your health, how you feel and function in your daily life.
These questions cover how you view your health. Respond to the questions by putting an X in the box you believe fits you best.

1. In general, how would you say your health is nowadays?

☐ Excellent
☐ Very good
☐ Good
☐ Fair
☐ Poor

2. Compared to a year ago, how would you judge your general health condition nowadays?

☐ Much better than a year ago
☐ Somewhat better than a year ago
☐ About the same as a year ago
☐ Somewhat worse than a year ago
☐ Much worse than a year ago

Figure 17.2 – *Example of layout and instructions for the questions.*

regard the questionnaire as being too extensive, time-consuming or if they miss some questions that they would have expected to be included. If possible the pilot group could, after having responded, discuss the content and the way the schedule or questionnaire is put together. Thereafter adjustments can be made.

However, this pilot work gives information only about the feasibility of the questionnaire/schedule put together. It does not give any information about the feasibility of the survey study as a whole. Such information is obtained by actually doing the study exactly as it is planned to be carried out. All the steps from approaching the respondents, interviewing them or having them respond to the self-administered questionnaire, loading data into the computer, analysing the data and reviewing the results should be carried out. Through such a pilot study each step of the research process can be evaluated and adjusted to improve the quality of the study. It may seem to be a waste of time to analyse the data. However, by doing so the investigator can

review the questions included as regards the information they provide. Some of the questions perhaps provide no variation at all and are thus of no interest. Other questions may seemingly have been misunderstood and need to be adjusted. Thus, doing a pilot study includes doing each step of the process in the manner in which it is planned to be done, including the analysis. The size of a sample for a pilot study should be kept small, and depending on how easy/difficult it is to include respondents and whether it is interviews or self-administered questionnaires, something like 20–50 respondents may be included.

Informed consent

On the first page of the questionnaire there should be a brief description of the aim of the study, the context of the questionnaire and explanation of what the respondents are asked to do. This introduction should also contain information about how data will be treated and presented, and ensure the confidentiality of the respondents. Further, the respondents should be informed about ethical permission in accordance with the law of the country and they should explicitly be asked to participate. If they do not want to participate they should be informed about what to do with the questionnaire. A prepaid envelope should be enclosed if it is a posted questionnaire. The same type of information should be given in cases where data are collected in face-to-face interviews. It is commonly considered that informed consent has been obtained when the respondent returns the questionnaire, while in the face-to-face interview they may be asked to sign a consent form depending on the decision of the research ethics board.

Anonymity

Whether the survey study is going to be carried out anonymously or if identification is needed depends on whether the investigator wants to return to that specific person and/or link data from one data collection to a subsequent data collection, a longitudinal design. In any case some kind of identification is needed if a postal questionnaire is carried out, where reminders are going to be sent to those not responding. It may also be useful to keep a list of the sample meant to be included and through that list to keep track of respondents and non-respondents. By doing so, the investigator can analyse the dropout more thoroughly compared with no list was compiled of the target sample.

Technical aid

When a self-administered questionnaire is used it is of the utmost importance that the layout is done properly, not only so that it is easy for respondents to read and understand, but also for the next step, which is to transfer the data to a computer for statistical analysis.

There are various electronic systems available in which the interview schedule or the questionnaire can be created right from the beginning. When using such a technique, the data file is often created at the same time. Thus when the interviews or self-administered questionnaires have been returned, the responses can be scanned into the data file. This technique also commonly allows the form to be made available in a handheld computer or on the internet.

Sample issues

As in all other research, developing the sampling frame is a key issue so that it is a true representation of the population about which conclusions are meant to be drawn (Fowler 1993). It is as unethical to carry out a study with too small a sample as it is to have too large a sample. Thus the first step is to identify the population that the study is concerned with. In this process it is important to keep in mind that the phenomenon under study should exist in this population. It is a waste of people's time and research resources to go for a population that is broader than needed. For instance, if the study is about musculoskeletal pain in the population it may be of little interest to include very young people unlikely to have such pain. Furthermore, the interpretation of pain may be different in young people versus old or very old people, making the results not comparable. Also, it may not be possible or necessary to include all people having a certain characteristic or experiencing a certain phenomenon. Thus a representative sample is taken from the population about which conclusions are supposed to be drawn.

The ideal way to this is by drawing, at random, a sample from the population in mind (Fowler 1993). This sample must be drawn in a manner so that it is free from bias and everyone in the population has the same chance of being included in the study. However, there are other ways as well, depending on whether knowledge is wanted about certain questions, for instance, young people, men versus women, independent versus dependent. In such cases the population is organised in strata and the sample is drawn from each strata to a predetermined number, which is in proportion to the actual size of that particular group in the population. Over-sampling can also be decided on in a particular stratum to ensure that the group will be large enough to analyse. Also, sampling can be done in clusters, which means that a sample unit is a group of people instead of individuals. Calculating the size of the sample is as important in a survey study as it is in all other designs. This should be done on the basis that conclusions can be drawn satisfactorily to conclude that the findings have external validity (Kazdin 1998). It is the study variable in focus that should be the basis for this estimation. It is also important to bear in mind that if subgroup analysis is going be done, the estimation of the sample size needed should take that into consideration. Also, the likelihood of dropout should be taken into consideration. Thus if only 70% are estimated to respond, the target sample should be increased so that the final sample is large enough.

Another issue to reflect upon is how to obtain the sample and the possible distortion/bias that may affect the results depending on how the sample is obtained. The ideal sample is one that is truly representative of the population in mind.

Thus, collecting the sample in a waiting room or from a waiting list may be biased, depending on the definition of the population.

Analysis and presentation

Since this chapter is concerned with structured questions, statistical analysis is the appropriate manner to analyse and present the data. The level of data is nominal or ordinal in most cases and not likely to be normally distributed, and thus non-parametric statistics are used (Jakobsson 2004, Siegel & Castellan 1988).

The statistical analysis to be performed is driven by the aim and what the final sample allows in terms of analysis. A logical manner to present the findings is to start with descriptive data and continue with comparison, correlations and regression analysis if done (Fink & Kosecoff 1988).

A specific problem, especially prevalent in postal questionnaires, is the internal dropout, meaning that a respondent may have left several questions without a response. This is a specific threat to the reliability of the findings and should therefore be acted upon. This can be done by excluding individuals with a high level of internal dropout. In any case it should be declared along with the presentation of the results.

EXERCISES

1. Discuss and define the term survey in relation to self-reports and give examples of suitable and unsuitable research questions for survey research.
2. Discuss pros and cons of collecting data with mailed questionnaires, emailed questionnaires, versus personal interviews in survey research. Give examples of studies suitable for these various data collection procedures.
3. Discuss and give examples of how the external and internal dropout can be prevented and/or kept under control in survey research.
4. Discuss and give examples of how to select and approach the sample for your survey; analyse and discuss what your sample may or may not be representative of.
5. Select an area of interest and formulate an aim for a study on that area. In the next step develop a tentative model of how to study this area using a survey and by deciding on the variable under study and variables that should be included because of their possible influence on the variable under study. Give examples of how to measure these variables.

References

Baker T L 1994 Doing Social Research, 2nd edn. McGraw-Hill, New York

Ehnfors M, Smedby B 1993 Patient satisfaction surveys subsequent to hospital care: Problems of sampling, non response and other losses. Quality Assurance in Health Care 5: 19–23

Fink A, Kosecoff J 1988 How to Conduct Surveys. A Step by Step Guide. Sage, Beverly Hills, CA

Fowler F 1993 Survey Research Methods. Sage, Newbury Park, CA

Hellström Y, Hallberg I R 2001 Perspectives of elderly people receiving home help on health, care and quality of life. Health Social Care Community 9: 61–71

Herzog A R, Kulka R A 1989 Telephone and mail surveys with older populations: A methodological overview. In: Lawton M P, Herzog A R (eds) Special Research Methods for Gerontology. Bayword Publishing, New York

Jakobsson U 2004 Statistical presentation and analysis of ordinal data in nursing research. Scandinavian Journal of Caring Sciences 18: 437–440

Kazdin A E 1998 Research Design in Clinical Psychology, 3rd edn. Allyn and Bacon, Boston

Lyberg L, Biemer P, Collins M, et al 1997 Survey Measurement and Process Quality. John Wiley & Sons, New York

Polit D F, Hungler B P 1999 Nursing Research Principles and Methods, 6th edn. Lippincott, Philadelphia
Siegel S, Castellan N J Jr 1988 Nonparametric Statistics for Behavioural Sciences. McGraw Hill, New York
Streiner D L, Norman G R 2003 Health Measurement Scales. A Practical Guide to Their Development and Use, 3rd edn. Oxford University Press, Oxford

Werntoft E, Hallberg I R, Elmståhl S, et al 2006 Older people's views of how to finance health care costs. Journal of Ageing and Society 20. 1–18

Chapter 18

Experiments

Graeme Smith

- Introduction
- Clinical trials
- Randomised controlled trials
- Strengths and weaknesses of RCTs
- Other experimental approaches
- Ethical issues
- Hawthorne effect
- Conclusion

Introduction

An experiment can be defined as a set of actions and observations, performed to verify or falsify an hypothesis or research a causal relationship between phenomena. The essence of experimental design is the relationship between cause and effect and the experiment is a cornerstone in empirical approach to knowledge in many areas of research. In this chapter, the meaning and purpose of experimental research design in nursing will be explored with particular emphasis on the randomised controlled trial. Additionally, issues surrounding experimental design in nursing research will be used to illustrate/highlight issues in clinical practice.

In nursing research there are three requirements for a true experiment: intervention, control and randomisation. The choice of experimental design by the nurse researcher may be influenced by many factors including:

- research hypothesis;
- research aims;
- number of variables to be examined;
- degree of control required;
- resources available;
- ethical considerations.

Clinical trials

In general, clinical trials are any planned therapeutic or preventive studies involving patients comparing concurrently one intervention (drug, device or procedure) to another intervention, placebo or no intervention to determine their efficacy and safety.

In the health care setting experiments are usually referred to as clinical trials. These are a special type of experiment as they involve people. There are several types of clinical trial commonly used to evaluate new drugs, medical devices and other interventions, including psychological or complementary therapies for patients in strictly scientific controlled settings. Clinical trials are required by regulatory authorities to approve new treatments and, as such, are designed to assess the efficacy and safety of interventions.

Traditionally, clinical trials have used physiological or biomedical outcomes. However, these outcomes may not be relevant in certain clinical situations. In health care, clinical trials have been categorised as either explanatory or pragmatic (Roland & Togerson 1998). In explanatory trials a single main measure of clinical outcome may be appropriate. For example, if two antihypertensive drugs are compared for effect on high blood pressure then hypertensive control would be the main outcome. In pragmatic trials a single outcome measure may be insufficient to weigh up the risks and benefits of giving a specific intervention. The Cochrane Collaboration believed that several outcomes could be used in their examination of treatments for back pain and recommended that outcomes such as pain, functional status, ability to work and satisfaction with treatment were important in this patient group (Van Tulder et al 1997).

Randomised controlled trials

The first reported randomised controlled trial (RCT) took place in the United Kingdom in 1747. Since the early 1600s, many people had felt that citrus fruits might potentially reduce the incidence of scurvy during long ocean voyages. James Lind studied sailors with scurvy and evaluated six potential treatments, one of which involved using citrus fruits. The two sailors who received the citrus treatment got better, as Lind reported (www.jameslindlibrary.org):

The consequence was that the most sudden and visible good effects were perceived from the use of the oranges and lemons; one of those who had taken them, being at the end of six days fit for duty ... The other was the best recovered of any in his condition; and being now deemed pretty well, was appointed nurse to the rest of the sick.

However, it was not until 1795 that Lind's findings were actually used by the Royal Navy (McKibbon et al 1999).

Introduction to randomisation

The RCT is one of the simplest, most powerful and revolutionary tools of research (Jaded 1998). The process of assignment in experimental research design is vitally important. In an ideal world, representative, randomly selected samples of patients would be assigned in equal numbers to both the experimental and control groups. This process of allocation is of vital importance, as any partiality may confound the study and devalue the usefulness of the findings. Routinely, in an RCT a proposed new treatment option is evaluated against the best standard treatment currently available. Patients have a 50:50 chance of receiving either the standard treatment or the experimental arm.

To avoid the potential of selection bias it is important that the process of random allocation should be concealed from the individual recruiting for a study. Selection bias relates to potential biases that may be introduced into a study by the selection of different types of people into treatment and comparison groups. As a result, the outcome differences may potentially be explained as a result of pre-existing differences between the groups, as opposed to the treatment itself. Nelson et al (2006) suggested blinded or masked allocation methods to minimise selection bias. These methods include the generation of random number sequences, remote telephone randomisation and randomisation via sealed envelopes. Failure to adequately mask allocation increases the possibility of inflated estimated effectiveness of experimental interventions. Proper randomisation hinges on adequate allocation concealment (Schulz & Grimes 2002).

The randomised control trial is rooted in 'positivist' science. It is concerned with events that can be observed, requires a stable environment, should be quantifiable and aims to establish causal relationships (Proctor 1998). The RCT is recognised as the principal method for obtaining a reliable assessment of treatment effects (Richardson 2000).

Cooke et al (2005) employed an RCT design to examine the effect of music on preoperative anxiety in day surgery. One hundred and eighty subjects were randomly allocated to an intervention, placebo or control group in a study which supported the use of music as an independent nursing intervention for preoperative anxiety in surgical patients. Chan et al (2005) designed an RCT to evaluate the effectiveness of an osteoporosis education programme for women in Hong Kong. Pre-, post- and follow-up education outcome measures compared attitudes and consumption frequency before and after the education programme. Using an RCT they concluded that an educational programme can act as simple but effective nursing intervention to promote women's attitudinal and behavioural intentions towards osteoporosis prevention.

Randomised controlled trials are designed to use large numbers of subjects to test the effect of a treatment or an intervention and to compare the results with a control group who have not received the treatment or intervention. Randomised controlled trials have been used in medical science since the 1940s and they now form the basis for strength of evidence in clinical guidelines (National Institute for Health and Clinical Excellence 2007) often viewed as a 'gold standard' approach. These types of clinical trials (e.g. drug trials) are usually conducted in ideal circumstances and subjects are selected according to a narrow set of inclusion/exclusion criteria. They are a popular type of experiment for testing the effectiveness and cost efficiency of treatments and interventions in health care.

Randomised controlled trials are designed specifically to minimise selection bias. However, the researcher should also be aware of other potential forms of bias which may lead to systematic errors in an experiment. These include performance bias and attrition bias.

Performance bias relates to the experimental intervention, or exposure to other factors apart from the intervention of interest. For example, in a study examining the impact of massage therapy in the management of postoperative pain, patients who received psychological support from the nurse researcher in addition to their massage therapy may fare better than others in the study. This improvement may be related to the effect of the additional support rather than the massage therapy and, as such, would introduce bias into the study. Attrition bias relates to withdrawals or dropouts of participants from a study. The way the researcher deals with withdrawals or dropouts from a study has the potential to bias the results of an RCT, as the withdrawal may be related to the intervention or outcome.

Larson et al (2005) used a longitudinal, randomised controlled trial to examine the impact of a nurse-led support and education programme for 100 spouses of stroke victims. Participants were randomly assigned to either an intervention or control group for a 12-month period. The intervention group met six times for support during six months, which had a positive effect on their well-being.

Intervention

In the absence of an intervention, there is no experiment. The researcher must introduce an intervention to produce an outcome or effect. In nursing research, the term 'treatment' may be used instead of 'intervention'. In conducting an experimental study, the nurse researcher attempts to make things happen. Parahoo (1997) stated that many nurse researchers do not state their hypotheses or questions in studies. This, he argued, does not facilitate the task of the reader, who has to piece together the information in the paper, including the results, to ascertain the researcher's hypotheses, questions or objectives.

Chang et al (2002) used an RCT to investigate the effects of massage on pain reaction and anxiety during labour. The experimental group received massage intervention whereas the control group did not. The nurse-rated present behavioural intensity as a measure of labour pain and anxiety was measured with the visual analogue scale for anxiety. The intensity of pain and anxiety between the two groups was compared in the latent phase (cervix dilated 3–4 cm), active phase (5–7 cm) and transitional phase (8–10 cm). In both groups, there was a relatively steady increase in pain intensity and anxiety level as labour progressed. Chang et al demonstrated that the experimental group had significantly lower pain reactions in the latent, active and transitional phases. Anxiety levels were only significantly different between the two groups in the latent phase. Twenty-six of the 30 (87%) experimental group subjects reported that massage was helpful, providing pain relief and psychological support during labour.

Control

The researcher should attempt to control extraneous variables in order to test whether it is the manipulation of the independent variable that actually causes any change in the dependent variable. This high degree of control is a key feature of experimental research design. Some control can be imposed by the researcher upon a study by manipulating the independent variable, using a control group, and by random allocation of patients. These strategies increase the amount of control and, as such, enhance the internal validity of the research. Failure to control extraneous variables may threaten the internal validity of an experiment.

Examples of this are the Hawthorne effect and placebo effect, which are discussed later in this chapter.

Experimental/intervention group

The researcher should devise strategies to control extraneous variables to ensure that the intervention (treatment) is the only variable responsible for outcome in the study. Extraneous variables may influence the outcome of an experiment. For example, a nurse researcher may wish to use a randomised controlled trial to measure the impact of stress management techniques in patients with a chronic illness who display high levels of anxiety (Smith et al 2002). To confirm that stress management therapy did have a therapeutic impact, the researcher could compare the patients with a group of patients who did not receive relaxation therapy. The group of patients who received relaxation therapy is called the experimental/intervention group and the group to which comparison is made is called the control group. Patients should have a 50:50 chance of receiving either the standard treatment or the intervention.

Control group

Using an RCT, the researcher attempts to ensure that the intervention/treatment is the only variable that influences the outcome. As such, every effort must be made to control extraneous variables. In the above example, the nurse researcher wants to examine the 'measurement of stress management techniques in a group of anxious patients with a chronic illness'.

In such an experiment the researcher, using a validated measurement scale, may find that the anxiety score drops after a course of stress management. However, the researcher could not be certain that over time symptoms of anxiety may improve for a variety of reasons, e.g. life events or drug therapy. Therefore, the use of nurse-led stress management techniques may not have influenced the reduction in anxiety scores. To identify the effect of nurse-led stress management techniques and to ascertain whether these techniques were the only contributing factor, the nurse researcher could establish a control group. A control group of patients receiving no intervention/treatment could be compared with patients who received specific stress management techniques.

An additional problem for the nurse researcher relates to the fact that patients being examined in the health care setting may already be receiving some form of treatment. In this instance the nurse may choose to compare the patients receiving stress management with another group of patients receiving conventional treatment.

In the highlighted example, the group that receives the intervention (stress management) is the experimental group. The comparative group that receives no treatment/conventional treatment is the control group.

It should be the nurse researcher's goal to ensure that the two groups are as similar as possible. Characteristics such as sex, age, gender and presentation of anxiety should all be considered, as they could all potentially influence recovery.

Once an appropriate control group is established, the researcher can be more confident that the results will not be influenced by these characteristics and that they have exerted control over extraneous variables.

Placebo effect and blind techniques

The placebo effect is well recognised in health care research. The terms 'placebo' and 'placebo effect' are used interchangeably; however, it is important to distinguish between them.

Placebo is defined as a beneficial physiological or psychological change associated with the use of medications, sham procedures, or in response to therapeutic encounters. The placebo effect is a favourable response to an intervention, regardless of whether it is the real thing or a placebo, attributable to the expectation of an effect, i.e. the power of suggestion. The effects of many health care interventions are attributable to a combination of both placebo and 'active' (non-placebo) effects.

In clinical trials, experimental treatments are often compared with placebos to assess the treatment's effectiveness. This is usually conducted to compare its effects with those of a real drug or other intervention, but sometimes for the psychological benefit to the patient through a belief that he/she is receiving treatment. The placebo response may be responsible for a large part of the effect of non-inert substances. Placebos are used in clinical trials to blind individuals to their treatment allocation. In experimental research, placebos should be indistinguishable from the active intervention to ensure adequate blinding. In comparison to many nursing research projects, placebo controls are not difficult to establish in pharmaceutical trials. A review of the placebo effect in nursing care revealed that it occurs in up to 90% of nursing interventions (Kwekkeboom 1997). Chan and Thompson (2006) reviewed placebo, placebo effects and their measurement and application to nursing. They concluded that placebo effects are difficult to measure and control and the use of a credible placebo is sometimes impractical in clinical nursing research. These difficulties were illustrated by Griggs and Jensen (2006), who examined the effectiveness of acupuncture for migraine in 13 randomised controlled studies and identified that headache conditions, such as migraine, are sensitive to the placebo effect and that the use of sham therapies in clinical trials of acupuncture may be unnecessary as almost all produce this effect.

Single-blind and double-blind techniques

If a researcher is aware of whether an intervention is being given to the experimental or control group in an experiment, this may potentially introduce bias into an experiment. Outcome data in a study should always be collected in the same way, with the same rigour, for all study groups. To make this possible, health professionals and participants should be unaware of the intervention being received. The researcher may also be biased in favour of the treatment they are testing. The halo effect is the tendency for researchers to be influenced by one characteristic in judging other, unrelated characteristics.

Additionally, patients should also be unaware which group they have been randomly allocated as they potentially may have a preference for a particular drug or treatment which may influence their assessment of the intervention. To reduce the potential of bias it is possible to apply single-blind or double-blind techniques. With single-blind techniques the subject is unaware of which treatment is being received, but the investigator has this information. In unusual cases, the investigator and not the subject may be kept blind to the identity of the treatment. Double-blind technique is an experimental procedure in which neither the subjects of the experiment nor the persons administering the experiment know the critical aspects of the experiment; a double-blind procedure guards against experimenter bias, measurement bias and placebo effects.

The presence of these techniques of research control can potentially lead to problems in nursing research. There are situations where too much control can introduce bias. If a nurse researcher tightly controls key variables in a study, it is possible that the true nature of those variables may become concealed (Polit & Hungler 1995).

Cluster randomisation

Instead of randomising individuals to experimental and control groups, researchers are increasingly randomising in clusters. In cluster randomised trials (CRTs) clusters of people, or intact social units, rather than individuals, are randomised to intervention and control groups, and outcomes are measured on individuals within those clusters (Edwards et al 1999). CRTs are also known as group randomised trials and are becoming increasingly important in health technology assessment.

The Zelen design

In standard RCTs individuals who meet study criteria are randomised to experimental or control groups once they have consented to participate. This may lead to experimental bias as patients may not receive their preferred treatment and may then comply poorly with treatment received. With the Zelen design, individuals are randomised before they have given consent or are even aware of the study. Those randomised to standard treatment are not informed of their assignment. Those randomised to active treatment are informed of the study and asked to give informed consent

(Torgerson & Roland 1998). The Zelen design provides a very pragmatic study in which all subjects are used. However, it is an open approach and lacks blinding. Homer (2002) provides a comprehensive overview of the advantages and disadvantages of the Zelen design in nursing.

Strengths and weaknesses of RCTs

The main strength of experimental design is its power in establishing causality. In the study of inanimate objects in a laboratory, experimental design methods are very powerful. This very rigid approach to experimental research may be at the expense of or undervalue health, nursing or psychological studies, which are often difficult or impossible to double-blind. In nursing research it is rarely possible to reduce patient care/intervention into singular causal relationships. Nurse researchers often wish to study the effects of more than one variable on a range of other variables.

Therefore, in the context of nursing research when dealing with human subjects, these designs may have some weaknesses.

Other experimental approaches
Quasi-experimental design

In nursing research, for many reasons, practical and ethical, it may be difficult to undertake RCTs. In the clinical environment it may not be feasible to allocate patients randomly to a particular treatment or intervention because of clinical, organisational or ethical considerations. The structure of the quasi-experimental design appears very similar to true experimentation. However, it lacks the characteristic of control or randomisation.

In single group design only one group is used. The independent variable is manipulated and the researcher measures changes in the dependent variable. The main disadvantage of post-test only single group design relates to the lack of measurement of the dependent variable prior to manipulation. Without such a measure it is impossible to detect changes and to infer any causal effect.

One of the most widely used experimental designs by nurse researchers is the single group pre-test–post-test. It has a distinct advantage over post-test design as it includes a measurement of the dependent variable before and after the intervention, which allows changes to be identified. In pre-test–post-test design the initial measure of the dependent variable is termed the baseline measure. The post-test measure, which captures the outcome of the intervention, is termed the outcome measure.

Example of pre-test–post-test experimental design

MacLellan (2004) conducted a pre-test–post-test experiment to evaluate a nurse-led intervention to improve pain management following surgery. Intervention (independent variable) included education for nurses in the form of short pain courses, introduction of regular pain assessment and profiling of pain at hospital level. The dependent variable (pain) was recorded using a visual analogue scale at baseline and then 3-hourly, 8 a.m. to 8 p.m., from the day of surgery for two days post-surgery by patients, and changes over time were determined.

Both the post-test and pre-test–post-test single group experimental design provide the researcher with a snapshot measurement of the dependent variable. The extent to which any changes can be attributed to the independent variable is often questionable as other factors, such as subject variables, natural changes, pre-test sensitisation, as well as researcher expectancy, may account for changes.

Example of a non-equivalent control group pre-test–post-test design

Choi et al (2005) using a quasi-experimental design with a non-equivalent control group, demonstrated that t'ai chi programmes can safely improve physical strength and reduce the fall risk for older adults.

Cohort design

One variant of non-equivalent control design is the cohort design. In cohort design experimentation, the chosen control group is another group with a similar characteristic.

For example, if we wished to examine the effects of a new curriculum on nursing students, a previous group of students from the old curriculum could be used to compare with the new group of students on the new curriculum. The strength of this design depends on the extent to which the groups of students are similar in key characteristics. In this case characters such as age, gender, comparable educational entry level and previous experience would be relevant.

Quasi-experimental designs are illustrated in Table 18.1.

Ethical issues

Parahoo (2006) noted ethical concerns that surround the use of experimental methods in nursing research. Nurses act in a range of roles in research and as the United Kingdom Nursing and Midwifery Council states, nurses must 'act to identify and minimise the risk to patients and clients'. In most

Table 18.1 – *Quasi-experimental designs*

One group	No pre-test	→ Intervention	→ Post-test
One group	Pre-test	→ Intervention	→ Post-test
Two groups			
Experimental (non-random)	Pre-test	→ Intervention	→ Post-test
Comparison group	Pre-test	→ Intervention	→ Post-test

respects nurse researchers are in a similar position to other health professionals when it comes to ethics of research. For example, this may relate to the morality of withholding a potentially beneficial experimental treatment from a subject in a control group. Patients should have a clear understanding of the research they are participating in (informed consent) if they have agreed to participate in a blind study. It begs the question 'Is it ethical to withhold all treatment from the control group?' The nurse researcher may also be influenced by knowing which patients/individuals are in the control or experimental group.

Sometimes in experimental practice it may be possible to manipulate a variable; however, to do so would be unethical. For example, it would be unethical to ask an experimental group to take up smoking to examine the physiological effects it would have on the respiratory system.

For these pragmatic, ethical and technical reasons some nursing/health research problems cannot be addressed through RCT design.

Hawthorne effect

Another concern with RCT design is the contamination of results through the researcher's or subject's awareness of the nature of the study. This relates to a phenomenon known as the 'Hawthorne effect'. The Hawthorne effect was identified by a research study in the 1920s, which found that factory output increased when lighting was improved, but also that when lighting was decreased to the original levels, productivity increased still further. The study showed that personal factors were important influences in the factory – people, unlike machines, behave differently when they are being watched.

The Hawthorne effect can be overcome in randomised controlled trials by utilising a double-blind approach. This involves both the researcher and the subject being unaware which subjects have been in the experimental and control group during the measurement of the intervention. This raises another ethical issue related to the level of information provided during informed consent.

A major limitation of using an RCT design in health/nursing relates to the fact that many variables which are measured in health care research cannot be manipulated, for example social class, blood type, genetic make-up.

Conclusion

In this chapter, the meaning and purpose of using a randomised controlled trial approach to experimental design in nursing research has been explored. The main characteristics of an experiment – intervention, control and randomisation – have been identified. Issues related to the use of randomised controlled trials have been highlighted. The main differences between true experiment and quasi-experimental design have been emphasised.

The strengths and weaknesses of experimental approaches have been outlined with examples from recent nursing literature. In particular, emphasis has been given to issues surrounding the use of RCTs in nursing research.

Despite the fact that the RCT is not as popular in nursing research as other designs, such as the case study, it has a very important role to play in the current climate of evidence-based care.

References

Chan M F, Ko C Y, Day M C 2005 The effectiveness of an osteoporosis prevention education programme for women in Hong Kong: a randomized controlled trial. Journal of Clinical Nursing 14: 1112–1123

Chan W H C, Thompson D R 2006 The use of placebo in clinical nursing research. Journal of Clinical Nursing 15: 521–524

Chang M Y, Wang S Y, Chen C H 2002 Effects of massage on pain and anxiety during labour: a randomized controlled trial in Taiwan. Journal of Advanced Nursing 38: 68–73

Choi J H, Moon J S, Song R 2005 Effects of Sun-style Tai Chi exercise on physical fitness and fall prevention in fall-prone older adults. Journal of Advanced Nursing 51: 150–157

Cooke M, Chaboyer W, Schulter P, Hiratos M 2005 The effect of music on preoperative anxiety in day surgery. Journal of Advanced Nursing 52: 47–55

Edwards S L J, Braunholtz D A, Lilford R J, Stevens A J 1999 Ethical issues in the design and conduct of cluster randomised controlled trials. BMJ 318: 1407–1409

Griggs C, Jensen J 2006 Effectiveness of acupuncture for migraine: critical literature review. Journal of Advanced Nursing 54: 491–501

Homer C S E 2002 Using the Zelen design in randomized controlled trials: debates and controversies. Journal of Advanced Nursing 38: 200–207

Jaded A R 1998 Randomised Controlled Trials. BMJ Books, London

Kwekkeboom K L 1997 The placebo effect in symptom management. Oncology Nursing Forum 24: 1393–1399

Larson J, Franzin-Dahlin A, Billing E, et al 2005 The impact of nurse-led support and education for spouses of stroke patients: a randomized controlled trial. Journal of Clinical Nursing 14: 995–1003

McKibbon A, Eady A, Marks S 1999 PDQ Evidence-based Principles and Practice. B C Decker, Hamilton

MacLellan K 2004 Postoperative pain: strategy for improving patient experiences. Journal of Advanced Nursing 46: 179–185

National Institute for Health and Clinical Excellence (NICE) 2007 www.nice.org.uk

Nelson A, Dumville J, Togerson J 2006 Experimental Research. In: Gerrish K, Lacey A (eds) The Research Process in Nursing, 5th edn. Blackwell Scientific, Oxford

Parahoo K 1997 Nursing Research: Principles, Process, and Issues. Macmillan, London

Parahoo K 2006 Nursing Research: Principles, Process, and Issues, 2nd edn. Macmillan, London

Polit D F, Hungler B P 1995 Nursing Research: Principles and Methods, 5th edn. Lippincott, Philadelphia

Proctor S 1998 Linking philosophy and method in the research process: the case for realism. Nurse Researcher 5: 73–90

Richardson J 2000 The use of randomized control trials in complementary therapies: exploring the issues. Journal of Advanced Nursing 32: 398–406

Roland M, Togerson D J 1998 Understanding controlled trials. What are pragmatic trials? BMJ 316: 285

Schulz K F, Grimes D A 2002 Allocation concealment in randomised trials: defending against deciphering. Lancet 359: 614–618

Smith G D, Watson R, Roger D, et al 2002 Impact of a nurse-led counselling service on quality of life in patients with inflammatory bowel disease. Journal of Advanced Nursing 38: 152–160

Torgerson D J, Roland M 1998 What is Zelen's design? BMJ 316: 606

Van Tulder M W, Assendelft W W, Koes B W, Bouter L M and the Cochrane Back Pain Editorial Board 1997 Method guidelines for systematic reviews in the Cochrane Back Review Group for Spine Disorders. Spine 20: 2323–2330

Chapter 19

Single-case Studies

Rob Newell

Introduction – what are single-case experiments?

Single-case experiments are a particular example of experimental design. Strictly speaking, they are most often actually quasi-experimental, since they usually lack randomisation, and are therefore often referred to as single-case experimental designs (SCEDs). Their key distinguishing feature is that aspects of experimental control are applied to a single individual.

The researcher using single-case experimental methods applies the same ideas about control of variability as in traditional group experiments, attempting to control for bias which results both from subjects and from design. Thus, the single-case experiment is an attempt to examine cause–effect relationships in a single individual with the same amount of methodological rigour as in group experiments.

From the above, it should be immediately apparent that the SCED is a quantitative approach to research. Indeed, quantification is a defining characteristic of the approach. It is the crucial distinction between the SCED and the traditional case study.

Similarly, the randomised controlled trial (RCT) is itself problematic. RCTs are the gold standard in terms of the investigation of cause and effect because of their control of bias, but they have drawbacks. They cannot be swiftly mounted, since they require considerable planning and generally take a long time to complete. They typically require large numbers of participants before meaningful conclusions can be drawn. Finally, they are probabilistic, and so cannot offer definitive guidance to the clinician in a specific situation with a specific patient (Newell & Burnard 2006). Whilst none of these difficulties is insurmountable, the debate around the use of the RCT, and around evidence-based practice based on RCTs, has continued (Newell 2003), and is, if anything, more current today than when SCEDs first came to prominence.

What are single-case experiments for?

The SCED is firstly a way of investigating the effectiveness (or otherwise!) of our interventions with patients, using a credible research approach, during our everyday clinical practice (Newell 1992). In this sense, it can be useful in three main ways. First, we can monitor patient progress reliably. Second, we can monitor the effectiveness of a known treatment approach and, if necessary, assess our own competence in using it and identify training needs. Finally, we can start to develop innovative treatments, based on theory and clinical experience, applying them in novel situations with clients for whom no evidence base for intervention currently exists.

The SCED may also be an extension of this clinical use, where we can use experimental control to build up a systematic picture of a patient's characteristics or difficulties. This approach is rarely used in nursing, but is a mainstay of psychology, particularly where a patient presents with very unusual attributes. In such situations, group experiments would be almost impossible to mount, since sufficient numbers would simply not exist. This use of SCEDs is perhaps the most similar in intent to the traditional case study, which often seeks to document unusual cases, but once again, differs because of the inclusion of systematic measurement and control. One very accessible example from the psychology literature is *To See but Not to See* (Humphreys & Riddoch 1987), which uses a series of experimental approaches to arrive at a systematic description of the processes which underlie a particular case of visual agnosia.

Finally, SCEDs are a powerful experiential learning tool. It is surprising that, whilst both experiential learning and the need for adequate education in research have increased in importance and prominence in nursing, the two issues are rarely put together. This is, perhaps, because experience in research is often hard to come by, particularly for the novice. Yet research is most definitely a craft skill for nurses, in the same way that learning to give a bed bath, an injection or a flexible sigmoidoscopy are essentially nursing craft skills. Divorcing the theory from the craft leads to a view of these skills which is often inappropriate. SCEDs provide an antidote to an overly theoretical perception of the research process because they allow the novice actually to engage in research, rather than reviewing it. Whilst some qualitative projects also allow this, they do not have the power to explore cause/effect relationships, leaving SCEDs as the only viable option for the novice wishing to learn about the systematic research of treatment effectiveness through experiential learning.

What are the basic assumptions of single-case experiments?

The first basic assumption is that it is possible to examine cause and effect meaningfully in a single case. This assumption leads to the insistence on proper experimental control which we described earlier in this chapter. Thus, unlike in the case study, the treatment, the desired outcome and the assumed relationship between them are specified before the study begins, and then adhered to throughout. In experimental terms, this is the equivalent of saying that the independent variable and dependent variable are adequately operationalised and an hypothesis is stated. For the remainder of this chapter, we will use the treatment of a person with multiple sclerosis as a case example. The patient has identified two problems which are particularly affecting her life – fatigue and pain. For the moment, we will consider just pain. The dependent variable will be scores on the Multidimensional Pain

Inventory (MPI) (Kerns et al 1985); the independent variable will be relaxation exercises or no treatment; the hypothesis will be that the patient will report less pain when undertaking relaxation exercises than when having no treatment.

The second assumption of SCEDs is that the research design should be flexible in response to changing circumstances. This seems, of course, to contradict the first assumption, since this flexibility usually involves changing the nature of the independent variable (treatment). However, where treatment tactics are changed in response to varying clinical needs, these changes are explicitly acknowledged, and measurement is used to attempt to isolate the point at which treatment has changed, and maintain the integrity of the cause/effect chain. The general point, however, is that SCEDs are patient centred.

The third important assumption of SCEDs is the notion of generalisability. SCEDs are criticised for having poor external validity. One aspect of this is that it is argued that individual cases are unique and that this uniqueness prevents us from drawing any conclusions about the general effectiveness of a treatment for patients with similar problems. Proponents of SCEDs have sought to overcome this objection by invoking the idea of lawfulness. This idea was borrowed from natural sciences, principally by behaviourists in the 1940s and 1950s who sought to identify governing principles or laws of human behaviour which were similar in applicability to laws in the natural sciences, which govern such issues as the diffusion of gases or the rate of cooling of a liquid. The argument is that if human behaviour is lawful, a relationship which holds true in a single person will hold true for all other persons. Naturally, the greater the similarity between the person in whom the relationship was demonstrated and others, the better the law will hold, but this is regarded as being a matter of the test conditions under which the relationship was shown to exist, rather than a breach of the law supposedly governing that relationship.

How are single-case experiments designed?

Just as different group experimental designs seek to reduce different sources of bias, so do different single-case experimental designs. There are two different classes of SCED: AB designs and multiple baseline designs. Broadly speaking, these two classes of SCED correspond to repeated measures and independent groups designs in traditional group experimental designs (Newell & Burnard 2006). As we noted earlier in this chapter, SCEDs attempt to establish good internal validity. Their various designs represent different ways of dealing with threats to that internal validity. For the rest of this section, we will follow the patient with multiple sclerosis through a number of different design approaches which address threats to external validity while remaining flexible in response to her individual needs and allowing the nurse to try different interventions to meet these. The actual scores, however, are for illustrative purposes only, and should not be taken as endorsements of any particular treatment approach.

Case example: pain and fatigue in multiple sclerosis – 1: The AB design and its variants

In all AB designs, the A phase represents baseline measurement (a period of no intervention), whilst the B phase represents the introduction of an intervention.

The AB design

In this approach, the simplest way of systematically examining treatment outcomes, a period of baseline measurement is followed by introduction of the treatment, and is really little different from what goes on in clinical practice. We observe patient problems and respond. The crucial distinction, from a research point of view, is that both the observation and the response are quantified. As we can see from Figure 19.1, the patient has

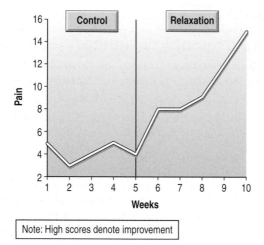

Figure 19.1 – *The AB design.*

measured her perception of pain on a regular basis, both before the introduction of relaxation exercises and during a period when these exercises have been practised on a regular basis. From the graphs, we infer that improvement has occurred.

The ABA design

Tempting as it is to infer improvement from the graph in Figure 19.1, this inference is oversimple, since the AB design, like the before–after design in group experimental designs, is vulnerable to maturation effects (physical or psychological changes as a result of time) and extraneous environmental effects over time. These effects confound our ability to attribute causation to the independent variable in both SCEDs and repeated measures group designs, and have led in the past to inflated estimates of treatment effectiveness. In the case of the multiple sclerosis patient, the improvement in pain might have been caused by a change in medication or the fact that multiple sclerosis is variable in its course, rather than as a result of relaxation exercises. However, it is relatively simple to test these propositions by the introduction of a further A phase – a return to baseline, during which relaxation is not practised (Fig. 19.2). One shortcoming here is that, for some interventions, return to baseline is not possible. For example, if we offer information, it is, by and large, not possible to ask a person to forget consciously that information. However, if an intervention requires continuing input (as is often the case in long-term illness, for example), then a return to baseline is a powerful way of increasing our confidence in the internal validity of the study.

The ABAB design

In the above example, the patient's improvement has not been maintained following return to

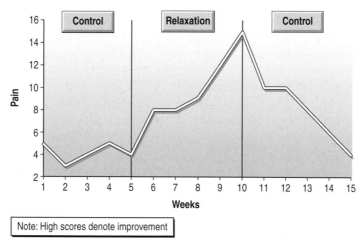

Figure 19.2 – *The ABA design.*

baseline. It is sometimes argued that it is unethical to use return to baseline for this reason, but this argument is difficult to sustain, since it is important that clinicians know whether a treatment is in fact the cause of changes in the patient's status. If it is not, and the patient continues to undertake the intervention, that is a waste of their time and effort, and therefore is itself unethical. However, if the patient does not maintain gains during the return to baseline, this is evidence for the effectiveness of the intervention, and it would, in this case, be unethical to leave the patient at the return to baseline phase. In SCEDs, the design modification reflects what we would probably do in clinical practice – we reintroduce the treatment phase, resulting in an ABAB design (Fig. 19.3).

Apart for the ethical reason for introduction of a further B phase, there is a compelling methodological advantage in doing so, in that the number of potential phases to be compared is increased. In the example in Figure 19.3, we can draw comparisons between the following phases: A1 and B1, A2 and B2, A1 and B2, A1 and A2. Obviously, the more differences we see between A and B phases, the more confident we can be that treatment

has changed the patient's health status. Moreover, whilst similarity between the two baseline phases (A1 and A2) would likewise increase such confidence, differences between them would tend to decrease it, since it would suggest that the baseline was unstable. This instability might be making an important contribution to apparent differences between the treatment phases.

Extending AB designs

In treatment situations, we may often have several competing treatment approaches, all of which are potentially useful in addressing particular patient problems. For example, relaxation is just one way of addressing the problem of chronic pain. One treatment, which does not rely on relaxation but instead involves deliberately entering situations where pain may occur, has been developed from the fear-avoidance model of pain perception proposed in the 1980s by Lethem and co-workers (Lethem et al 1983) and tested by Rose and colleagues (Rose et al 1992). In this approach, the patient reintroduces in a graded way activities which they fear may cause pain. Of course, there are also pharmacological approaches, such as the

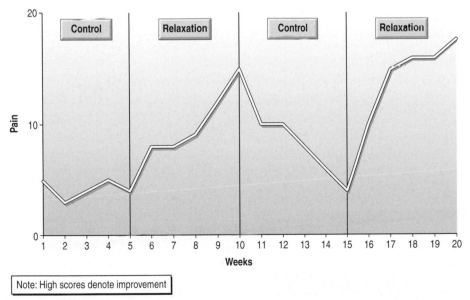

Figure 19.3 - *The ABAB design.*

appropriate, regular use of analgesia. As nurses, we may wish to offer the patient any or all of these alternatives.

We can extend the AB design to allow us to do so, by introducing additional treatment phases, each of which is distinguished from the others by a different letter. We can, thus, speak of ABAC designs, and so on, with each different letter representing a different treatment. In the clinical example above, we would have: A (baseline); B (relaxation); A (baseline); C (reintroduction of activities); A (baseline); D (medication management). Finally, as in group experiments, each condition does not necessarily consist of a single treatment. We could, for example, describe a combination of treatments as a single treatment condition. Clinically this would often represent an attempt to help a patient by combining the most promising interventions. So, in the example above,

we could add a further return to baseline, then a further treatment phase: E (reintroduction of activities + medication management). Naturally, each of these different treatment phases is a different level of the independent variable.

In clinical practice we often do much the same thing, but there is a tendency to omit the baseline phases. This is discussed further when we talk about disadvantages of SCEDs later in this chapter. However, in the SCED, the importance of always interposing baseline phases between treatment phases is considerable, since it allows us to compare each treatment independently with a baseline. In the absence of such baselines, we would not be able to tell, for example, whether any apparent superiority of treatment C is, in fact, contributed to by a carry-over from the effectiveness of treatment B. This point is clarified in Figure 19.4, which

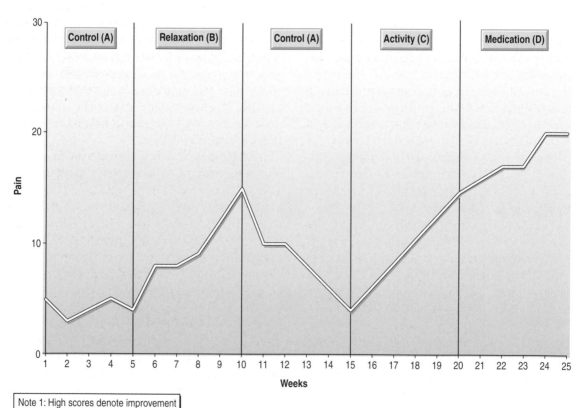

Note 1: High scores denote improvement
Note 2: Final A phase omitted

Figure 19.4 – *The ABACAD design.*

shows an ABACAD design, but with the third A phase omitted (ABACD). In this situation, we do not know whether the patient's pain would have returned to baseline between C and D. In the absence of such a return to baseline, we have no evidence for inferring that the continuing improvement at D (medication management) is anything more than a carry-over from the effectiveness of reintroduction of activities at C.

Case example: pain and fatigue in multiple sclerosis – 2: The multiple baseline design

Although the AB design is capable of almost infinite modification, all these designs share a single assumption: that difference in the patient's health status can be inferred from differences between the sequential baseline and treatment phases. By contrast, multiple baseline designs infer causation by observing comparisons between scores on treated and untreated problems at the same time. The rationale for this inference is based on the notion that if a treatment is specific to a particular problem, it will not affect other problems. Therefore, if the treated problem improved, but others do not, it is likely that the improvement was caused by the treatment. By contrast, if all problems have improved, it is likely that the improvement was caused by some extraneous effect, such as maturation.

For example, if I were to exercise my arm muscles and, as a result, my biceps circumference increases, I could reasonably attribute this increase to the exercise regime. However, if my thigh circumference increased at the same rate at the same time, I would be much less confident that arm exercises had truly caused the increase in biceps circumference. This example also, of course, points to the shortcoming of multiple baseline designs, which is that, to be useful as a source of comparison, the untreated problem must genuinely be unlikely to be affected by the treatment. To return to our exercise example, suppose we chose sleep as the untreated problem. Since exercise reliably improves sleep, it would be quite reasonable for my sleep to improve, even though I had not thought I was directly targeting it with exercise. Accordingly, improvement in both physique and sleep would not refute the suggestion that exercise had been responsible for the change in physique. As a general rule, the more a treatment is specific to a particular difficulty, the more we can use untreated difficulties as controls.

In discussing AB designs, we noted that, in some cases, it was not possible to return to baseline. Typically, this would be the case in treatments which when applied, do not need to be repeated by the patient for their effect to continue. Many drug treatments are of this form, but so are a number of psychological, social and educational interventions. Imagine, for example, trying to return to baseline after having learnt to read the word 'baseline'. In the absence of some gross memory disturbance, you do not need to continue consciously rehearsing this activity to be able read 'baseline' next time you encounter it, and the absence of an ability to return to baseline deprives us of a potentially powerful source of causal inference. In such situations, the multiple baseline design is a viable alternative, since it does not rely on sequential phases in order to draw causal inferences.

In the example below, the patient is given a relaxation exercise for pain and a programme of graded exercise for fatigue (which she rates on the Chalder fatigue scale (Chalder et al 1993)). Of course, it is quite likely that relaxation itself might reduce fatigue and we might, therefore, feel that the independence between the two conditions is insufficient to allow adequate confidence in any apparent effect of exercise on fatigue. However, exercise is known to affect fatigue considerably, whilst the evidence of relaxation is relatively weak. For this reason, relaxation was introduced as the first condition, so as to minimise any carry-over effect. Moreover, the overall extent of the difference between conditions is important in attributing causation to the relevant independent variable. Finally, in the instance shown in Figure 19.5, the researcher introduced a return to baseline for

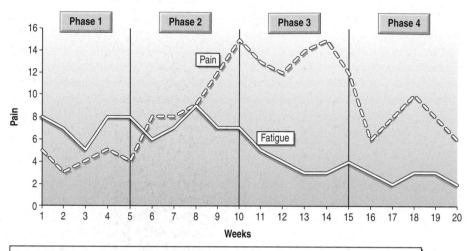

Note 1: Phase 1 = Control all conditions; Phase 2 = Relaxation for pain, control for fatigue; Phase 3 = Relaxation for pain, exercise for fatigue; Phase 4 = Control for pain, exercise for fatigue
Note 2: High scores on pain scale denote improvement; low scores on fatigue scale denote improvement

Figure 19.5 – *The multiple baseline design.*

the relaxation/pain condition, precisely to separate further the effects of the two independent variables. Although this is unusual in multiple baseline designs, it should be noted that the return to baseline is not to allow comparison between the sequential treatment and control phases for pain, but between the no treatment phase for pain and the exercise treatment phase for fatigue at the same time point. It is also possible to combine elements of multiple baseline and AB approaches in order to allow further possible data comparison points, some between different problems and some between treatment and no treatment phases for the same problem.

How are single–case experiments analysed?

From their inception, SCEDs have always relied primarily on visual inspection of data as the main form of analysis (Kazdin 1982 and 1984, Parsonson & Baer 1992). This arose for several reasons. SCEDs were intended as an aid for people in clinical practice and it was argued that any improvements in a patient's condition which were sufficiently large

to be important to them would be obvious from visual inspection.

As well as being important for patients, visible differences in scores are also easy to analyse. Once again, this issue has its roots in clinical practice, since clinicians are not necessarily skilled in statistical analysis, and even if they possess these skills, may find it impractical to undertake such analyses during the course of busy clinical practice. A further, related factor which has inhibited the use of statistics to analyse SCEDs in clinical practice is the fact that the statistical tests with which most people are familiar are often inappropriate.

Nevertheless, in the absence of statistical approaches, the visual inspection of SCED data can be relatively sophisticated. Thus, the researcher can compare not only raw scores between conditions, but also mean scores, differences between the final score in one condition and the next, differences in trends across conditions and differences in latency of onset of change across conditions, as well as combinations of these approaches.

Regardless of the degree of sophistication of visual inspection, however, there remain convincing counter arguments to relying on such an approach to the analysis of SCEDs. Many of these are summarised in Kazdin (1984), but they are essentially of two kinds, methodological and therapeutic. Methodologically, it turns out that our analysis of visually presented data is often biased (House 1980). Thus, Wampold and Furlong (1981) found systematic bias in the way visually presented clinical data were interpreted: there is a tendency to overlook or underestimate small changes but to overestimate large ones.

In therapeutic terms, the weakness of visual inspection comes from the difficulty in defining what level of improvement is likely to be important in different circumstances. Whilst we may intuitively think that only large, obvious changes are likely to be important to patients, this is not necessarily the case. For example, in long-term conditions, a small change in someone's status may be extremely important to them. Similarly, in such conditions, change may take a long time and our snapshot may not recognise that the small changes we see are part of a general upward trajectory which will eventually lead to large, important changes. Also, the examination and detection of small changes may help us to tailor treatment to patient needs. Finally, by their very nature, SCEDs are often used to investigate innovative interventions in unusual cases. In these situations, it may be very useful to detect small changes. If we are developing a novel treatment, it may be that it is not, initially, very powerful, but that with modification, the changes it has produced may be increased, leading to an intervention that is powerful and meaningful in terms of clinical change.

Although statistical analysis may be important, there are difficulties in applying standard statistics to SCEDs. This is principally because standard approaches of the kind used in group experiments are poor at dealing with autocorrelation (the situation where a given value of measurement is a function of the previous value of that measurement) (Gorman & Allison 1997), a characteristic of the data that is particularly frequent in SCEDs (Huitema 1986). It is, in theory, perfectly permissible to use standard statistics if it can be demonstrated

that autocorrelation is not present (Kazdin 1984), for example by the use of correlational testing. In practice, however, the simple lack of significance in correlational testing is not necessarily sufficient to establish that autocorrelation does not exist (Busk & Marascuilo 1992).

However, a number of alternative statistical approaches have been designed for use with SCEDs. Of these, time series analysis is arguably the most powerful, but, from a clinical viewpoint, suffers from two important shortcomings. First, time series is a conceptually complex general approach to data analysis, rather than a simple test. Second, its application requires a large number of data points which, in turn require frequent measurements of the targeted behaviour. This frequent measurement may itself place a high burden on patient and clinician, but, equally importantly, target behaviours which are of high frequency may be hard or impossible to identify for a given patient problem.

By contrast with this complex approach to analysis, one of the earliest and simplest techniques developed for analysis of single-case experiments is the split middle technique, recommended by Kazdin (1984). This is a logical extension of visual inspection, in which trends are plotted and compared statistically. Specifically, the researcher extrapolates a trend line from the data points of one condition into the next, then examines how many data points from this next condition fall above and below the extrapolated trend line, and compares this number with that which would be expected by chance using a binomial test.

More recently, there has been considerable discussion of the use of non-parametric tests intended for group experimental designs. Edgington (1992) recommended the use of such tests, which do not have the same assumptions about autocorrelation as parametric tests, for ordinal and nominal level data. Essentially, in such approaches, each value is regarded as a separate case for calculation purposes. Edgington recommends use of Mann–Whitney U and Kruskall–Wallis for ordinal level data and Fisher's exact test and chi square for nominal level data (for two or three or more conditions, respectively). However, there is no reason why tests for ordinal level data could not be applied to interval level data also, provided one is prepared to accept the loss of statistical power inherent in such an approach.

Conclusion

There are numerous advantages to the use of single-case experimental designs in clinical practice. It has been argued that SCEDs are client-centred, allow monitoring of clinical practice, facilitate the description of unusual patient characteristics and responses to treatment, assist in the development

of novel interventions, and are practical enough to be employed as part of everyday practice. It is, perhaps, the last of these advantages which makes SCEDs potentially so useful to practitioners. Using SCEDs, it is not necessary to have dedicated time for research in order to undertake rigorous analysis of one's clinical practice or to be involved in the process of research. On the contrary, rather than something different from clinical practice, SCEDs allow research to become united with it. For clinicians, this raises awareness of research as a legitimate practice activity, whilst for teachers, it offers an accessible route by which to teach practitioners and students this all important clinical skill.

EXERCISES

1. Consider a patient from your current practice and identify one of her difficulties: operationalise an independent and dependent variable and state an hypothesis.
2. Identify an appropriate way of measuring changes in the dependent variable.
3. Consider how you will design the study. Will it be AB, ABA or a variant, or will it be multiple baseline?
4. Decide on how you will enlist the patient's support in:

   (a) participation in the measurement of treatment
   (b) participation in the withholding of treatment during baseline(s).

5. Devise an approach to analysis of the data. What support (if any) do you need from others?

References

Busk P L, Marascuilo L A 1992 Statistical analysis in single-case research: issues, procedures and recommendations with applications to multiple behaviors. In: Kratchowill T R, Levin J R (eds) Single Case Research and Analysis. Lawrence Erlbaum, Hillsdale, NJ

Chalder T, Berelowitz C, Pawlikowska T 1993 Development of a fatigue scale. Journal of Psychosomatic Research. 37: 147–154

Edgington E S 1992 Nonparametric tests for single case experiments. In: Kratchowill T R, Levin J R (eds) Single Case Research and Analysis. Lawrence Erlbaum, Hillsdale, NJ

Gorman B S, Allison D B 1997 Statistical alternatives for single case designs. In: Franklin R D, Allison D B, Gorman B S (eds) Design and Analysis of Single Case Research. Lawrence Erlbaum, Mahwah, NJ

House A E 1980 Detecting bias in observational data. Behavioral Assessment. 2: 29–31

Huitema B E 1986 Autocorrelation in behavioral research: Wherefore art thou? In: Poling A, Fuqua R W (eds) Research Methods in Applied Behavior Analysis: Issues and Advances. Plenum, New York: 187–208

Humphreys G W, Riddoch M J 1987 To See but Not to See: A Case Study of Visual Agnosia. Lawrence Erlbaum, London

Kazdin A E 1982 Single Case Research Designs. Oxford University Press, New York

Kazdin A E 1984 Statistical Analyses for Single-case Experimental Designs. In: Barlow D H, Hersen M Single Case Experimental Designs. Pergamon, New York

Kerns R D, Turk D C, Rudy T E 1985 The West Haven–Yale Multidimensional Pain Inventory (WHYMPI). Pain. 23: 345–356

Lethem J, Slade P D, Troup J D G, et al 1983 Outline of a fear-avoidance model of exaggerated pain perception – I. Behaviour Research and Therapy. 21(4): 401–408

Newell R J 1992 The single case experiment: a research method for everyday use. Nursing Practice. 6: 24–27

Newell R 2003 Using evidence to inform practice. In: Hannigan B, Coffey M (eds) The Handbook of Community Mental Health Nursing. Routledge, London

Newell R, Burnard P 2006 Vital Notes for Nurses: Research for Evidence-based Practice. Blackwell, Oxford

Parsonson B S, Baer D M 1992 The visual analysis of data, and current research into the stimuli controlling it. In: Kratchowill T R,

Levin J R (eds) Single Case Research and Analysis. Lawrence Erlbaum, Hillsdale, NJ

Rose M J, Klenerman L, Atchison L, et al 1992 An application of the fear avoidance model to three chronic pain problems. Behaviour Research and Therapy. 30: 359–365

Wampold B E, Furlong M J 1981 The heuristics of visual inspection. Behavioral Assessment. 3: 79–92

Chapter 20

Action Research

Heather Waterman and Kevin Hope

- Introduction: history, definitions and typologies
- Characteristics of action research
- The practicalities of carrying out action research
- Example of action research
- Conclusion

Introduction: history, definitions and typologies

There is a complex history to the development of action research (Hart & Bond 1995). No single model can encapsulate the variety of thinking about action research (Elden & Chisholm 1993) and, recognising this diversity, Reason and Bradbury (2001) describe it as a 'family' of approaches to research made up of participative, experiential and action-oriented methods.

There are multiple definitions of action research depending on where the author sees action research to be located philosophically. The minority view locates action research within the constructivist interpretivist domain, seeing it as a method for gaining access to subjects' understandings of their situations. A stronger case is made for locating action research within the domain of critical theory (Carr & Kemmis 1986), recognising its potential as a method for addressing ideological and power-related issues in the social situation as well as providing an impulse for action. Finally, a relatively recent addition sees it located within a participatory paradigm (Heron & Reason 1997) which places emphasis on the experiential knowledge of participants and the collaborative aspects of the method.

For some, this confusion is a source of irritation ranging from a straightforward expression of dissatisfaction with the situation ('terminological anarchism' according to Kalleberg (1990)) to a concern that the term might be over-applied in practice leading to a dilution in meaning (Hart & Bond 1995).

Waterman et al (2001, p. 11) define action research as:

... a period of inquiry, which describes, interprets and explains social situations while executing a change intervention aimed at improvement and involvement. It is problem-focused, context specific and future oriented. Action research is a group activity with an explicit critical value base and is founded on a partnership between action researchers and participants, all of whom are involved in the change process. The participatory process is educative and empowering, involving a dynamic approach in which problem identification, planning, action and evaluation are interlinked. Knowledge may be advanced through reflection and research, and qualitative and quantitative research methods may be employed to collect data. Different types of knowledge may be produced by action research, including practical and prepositional. Theory may be generated and refined, and its general application explored through the cycles of the action research process.

Because of the systematic methodology used, this definition encapsulates many of the facets that other authors refer to and is offered as a comprehensive and inclusive definition.

To make sense of the range, authors have identified typologies of action research (Table 20.1). These are offered as 'ideal types' (Hart & Bond 1995) which are not intended to be as prescriptive, but attempt to clarify and simplify the complex processes involved.

Holter and Schwartz-Barcott (1993) identify three approaches: the technical-collaborative approach is where particular interventions are tested based on pre-specified theoretical frameworks; the mutual collaboration approach is when 'the researcher and practitioners come together to identify potential problems, their underlying causes and possible interventions' (p. 301) and plan change based on understanding of their practice; the enhancement approach aims to increase the closeness between actual problems and theory used to explain these and raise 'collective consciousness' to assist practitioners to identify and articulate problems (via critical reflection).

There are problems in trying to group action research in this way. Hart and Bond (1995) suggest that the type of action research engaged in might vary over the life course of a project and vary between or in different cycles. Additionally, a typology implies that action researchers will, at any time, be able to locate themselves within a given frame of reference and ignores complexities of the method. It seems more appropriate, therefore, to avoid falling into the trap of over-categorisation and focus on characteristics of action research. These are outlined in Box 20.1 and considered individually.

Characteristics of action research
Involves collaboration and participation

Action research is a collaborative process between action researchers and participants or co-researchers. Co-researchers participate in all aspects of the action research; the emphasis is on researching 'with' rather than 'on' people. Participation has been described variously as a 'defining characteristic' (Rolfe 1996), 'distinctive' (Elden & Chisholm 1993, Waterman et al

Table 20.1 – *Types of action research*

Lewin (1948)	Kingsley (1985)	Holter and Schwartz-Barcott (1993)	Hart and Bond (1995)
Experimental	Management model	Technical-collaborative	Experimental
Empirical	Autonomy model	Mutual collaborative	Organisational
Diagnostic	Underclass model	Enhancement	Professional
Participative			Empowering

Box 20.1 – *Characteristics of action research*

- Action research involves participation/collaboration
- Action research has a political, emancipatory and developmental role
- Action research involves change and improvement
- Action research focuses on the practical and is context specific
- Action research is cyclical
- Action research generates theory
- Action research involves reflection and reflexivity

2001), 'essential' (Wallis 1998) or constitutes a minimal requirement or central position (Carr & Kemmis 1986, Holter & Schwartz-Barcott 1993). Brydon-Miller et al (2003) suggest that a shared commitment to democratic change is one of the unifying beliefs of action researchers. Arguably, participation is the key functional element through which democracy is achieved.

Holter and Schwartz-Barcott (1993) point out that participation can be continuous or periodic while Reed (2004) highlights some of the difficulties in achieving and maintaining collaboration. For others, the issue is about how participation and collaboration change over the course of a study with ownership of change shifting towards participants (Wallis 1998); collaboration is not a fixed concept.

Has a political, emancipatory and developmental role

There appears to be consensus that action research is about empowering others because there is analysis of power and its distribution within a given social setting. However, there is variation as to expectations regarding the nature and degree of this, with changes at a structural or organisational level seen by some as a primary aim whereas others tend to focus on the impact on the individual.

An example of the organisational perspective in nursing is demonstrated by Robinson (1995).

His starting point is a critical examination of the manner in which power is played out, often in ways unnoticed in daily work, which reinforces inequalities. In contrast, we can turn attention to Lewin's (1948) original view that raising self-esteem of participants is a goal and Elden and Chisholm's (1993) position that change should be a self-generating and self-maintaining process. Arguably, change that has an impact on power differentials within a given environment both requires and determines increased self-confidence and esteem of participants.

Is about change and improvement

Important aims of action research are to change and improve. Some argue that change is a prerequisite of action research. For example, Elden and Chisholm (1993) are dogmatic about this, indicating that change-based data is one of five elements that need to be evident for any research to be classified as action research. Others argue that change is not always achievable (Webb 1989) nor indeed an indicator of the success of a project (Waterman et al 1995). Van Mannen (1990) challenges the change assumption and suggests that 'maybe more significantly action research must learn to deal with what we should have done' (p. 154). The intention to change or improve needs to be present.

Webb (1989) suggests that action research builds on existing motivation in a working environment and brings with it the authority to change. In addition, nurses operate in a professional context within guidelines and parameters laid down by professional bodies. Rules, regulations, guidelines and codes of practice can serve as orientating or motivational forces which point action research groups in the right direction or which can serve as supportive evidence for defending the route being taken.

Focuses on the practical and is context specific

For nursing, the focus on practice is an attraction of the approach and is reflected in Holter and Schwartz-Barcott's (1993) assertion that the solution of practical problems is one of its central characteristics. A closely related characteristic is the view that action research is context specific (e.g. Hart 1996, Hart & Bond 1995, Hendry & Farley 1996, Lathlean 1994). For Lyon (1998) contextual awareness means that change is more likely to occur because judgement about options available is made with reference to salient aspects including relevant contextual factors. Conversely, critics maintain that, due to its specificity, the generalisability of the research is low and that the subjective influence of participants contaminates the research environment.

Action research is cyclical

The notion of a cycle including planning, acting, observing and reflection was first articulated by Lewin, the central principle being that the floor of subsequent cycles is determined by the ceiling of previous ones. For Hart and Bond (1995), the cycle is seen as a means of interlinking research, action and evaluation. In reality several cycles of activity may occur simultaneously which could influence the direction of the major change. Heron (1996) suggests that this 'research cycling' can be conceptualised as having a pruning effect. As a consequence, needless vagueness and ambiguity is reduced but amplification and deepening of the research focus is enhanced. He sees the cycle as having a positive influence on the subsequent validity of a piece of action research.

Theory generation

Another recognisable characteristic is that action research should generate theory (Holter & Schwartz-Barcott 1993, Susman & Evered 1978). This aspect is seen as something that differentiates action research from other forms of change strategies, audit and evidence-based practice (Holter & Schwartz-Barcott 1993, Wallis 1998, Waterman 1996).

Rolfe (1996) argues that the outcome of action research is a highly personal form of knowledge which he terms 'grounded practice'. For Rolfe (1996):

The researcher-practitioner evaluates a situation, develops a theory to account for that situation,

tests the theory by constructing and implementing a clinical intervention, evaluates the new, transformed situation, modifies the theory accordingly and so on... (Rolfe 1996, p. 1317)

He points out that such theory is particular to the clinical setting being studied and, as such, cannot be separated from, or generalised beyond, that setting.

Greenwood (1994) aligns with the perspective that there are generalisable aspects suggesting what should happen in a given situation, all things being equal. Greenwood (1994) appears to be arguing that there is the possibility of generating theory about how change is or is not brought about.

Involves reflection and reflexivity

Robinson (1995) argues that action research is 'essentially an interactive reflexive process' (p. 67) which, according to Koch and Harrington (1998), is characterised by 'ongoing self critique and self appraisal' (p. 887). There appears to be a potential for the terms reflection and reflexivity to be used interchangeably. With regard to the latter, Waterman (1994) has traced different interpretations ranging from a stated need to understand, reflect and analyse the effects that the researcher has on the research process to one which emphasises the nature of the context specificity of understanding. For Waterman (1994), subjectivity is an inescapable aspect of the research process and reflexivity is the means by which we acknowledge, monitor and understand it.

The practicalities of carrying out action research

Box 20.2 contains the key activities involved in undertaking an action research project.

Selecting participants

First, if you do not already have a group of core people who are keen to solve the problem, you need to plan who to involve. Even if there is a natural group, it is worth considering who else needs to

Box 20.2 – *Key activities in action research*

- Selecting participants
- Setting up the project
- Managing meetings
- Clarifying the problem
- Fact-finding or reconnaissance
- Gaining ethics approval
- Research
- Critical reflection
- Describing and explaining the problem
- Planning
- Action
- Evaluation
- Closure

be represented. Second, identify representatives of those who say there is a problem, are affected by the problem, manage the problem, and control finances in the problem area. You will probably involve health care and social professionals from hospitals and the community, managers, accountants, and health and social care users and carers. You need broad representation to ensure ownership and a willingness to solve the problem, and to explore the problem critically from all perspectives. This should lead to increasing understanding in participants, and creative and better solutions.

Setting up the project

The next step is to invite potential participants to an introductory meeting. This means that action researchers have to become skilled at identifying the best times to meet, be sensitive to when people are too busy, motivate and enthuse participants, work with managers to arrange off-duty meetings, locate meetings as near as possible to the work environment, and be resourceful by, for example, attaching action research meetings to the end of staff meetings. Once commitment to the project has been gained, people generally manage to attend. However, since there are so many other calls on their time, we have found it helps to speak to people face-to-face on the same day to encourage

attendance. Lack of attendance does compromise the project because developments and research will be delayed. To minimise these outcomes, it is important that the true cost of staff involvement is included in the project budget.

Managing meetings

One of the most daunting aspects of becoming an action researcher is running core group meetings. Group dynamics may be difficult to manage, especially if there are people who dominate or groups who do not contribute because they are unused to public speaking. The overall purpose and goal of the meeting should be agreed. Depending on the purpose of the meeting, you need to work out whether you need to be directive, whether questions need to be open or closed, how many participants will attend, how to devise ground rules with the group, how to draw people into discussions and how to move on to different subjects. Action researchers may find textbooks on how to moderate focus group interviews helpful (Morgan 1998, Stewart & Shamdasni 1990). The core group meetings differ from focus group interviews because they will also include: project management, research, reflection, planning, monitoring and evaluation.

Clarifying the problem and activities

One of the first activities of the group is to clarify and negotiate the problem (Kemmis & McTaggart 1988, Winter & Munn-Giddings 2001). This process may take longer than expected for it may only be clearly stipulated after research and reflection. For example, someone may have a problem with introducing clinical supervision for community specialist nurses. When the problem is phrased like this, it tends to concentrate activities on one particular issue, i.e. 'clinical supervision', which may not be the most appropriate activity on which to work. If instead, the problem behind the solution is linked to an action (Elliott 1991), for example 'how to make community specialist nurses feel more supported and confident', a range of possible avenues for action can be visualised.

Next, the group must decide in general terms its objectives for the first phase. Thought needs to be given to whether the objectives are going to be achieved concurrently or sequentially. We have found it best to carry out activities in parallel. Although this may add to the complexity of the task, it allows for a broad, gradual and increasing understanding of the problem. As previously mentioned, action research aims to be democratic and, therefore, participants are invited to be co-researchers playing a proactive role in the action research as much as possible given their other commitments. All research projects including action research need adequate funding. However, too often in the past action researchers have underestimated this element and subsequently their work is compromised and open to criticism. In general in the UK, we would discourage action research that has not received any funding, either financial or in kind. McNiff et al (1996) offer a useful budget checklist for action research including: source of funding, contingency funds, stationery and printing, technology and staff time.

Fact–finding or reconnaissance

The first phase of action research consists of fact-finding (Lewin 1948) or initial reconnoitre (Kemmis & McTaggart 1988) of the problem. Action research textbooks (Atweh et al 1998, Kemmis & McTaggart 1988, McNiff et al 1996, Stringer 1996, Winter & Munn-Giddings 2001), offer frameworks for this phase but essentially it requires the group to undertake a full analysis of the problem prior to changing practice. The group may gather published information from research, historical, legal, ethics and policy documents and visit other places that have already advanced their practice in the area of the problem.

Ethics

Principles of informed consent, protection from harm and maintenance of privacy are as important in action research as in other research approaches and approval from a research ethics committee is required (Winter & Munn-Giddings 2001). Action research applications can appear vague because detail of later phases is dependent on the former. We have found that if an application is submitted after initial fact-finding before any formal data collection commences, then approval can be secured. Amendments can be submitted to the ethics committee as it becomes clearer what will be carried out in each subsequent phase/cycle.

Research

The group may also choose to carry out research to investigate the nature and extent of the problem in their area (McNiff et al 1996). The research may be qualitative or quantitative depending upon the research questions posed. More than one piece of research may take place at a time; for example, observation of nursing care and interviews with patients may be carried out in parallel.

Critical reflection

Critical reflection is also undertaken by members of the core action research group. Sometimes critical reflection can also be facilitated amongst a wider group of staff in focus group interviews. Kemmis and Wilkinson (1998) argue that critical reflection is a process by which people challenge and reconstruct 'irrational, unproductive, (or inefficient), unjust and/or unsatisfying (alienating) ways of interpreting and describing their world (language/discourses), ways of working (work), and ways of relating to others' (p. 24). Critical reflection requires a critical stance that asks us to delve beneath the mundane and routine to consider the influential ideologies in our lives and whose purposes these beliefs serve. Critical reflection enables participants to listen and learn from perspectives different to their own, and to verbalise and evolve their values. Critical reflection is educative and gives rise to options or choices for action and thereby is empowering for those concerned. Critical reflection also involves 'unpacking' concepts and related actions;

for example, what do we really mean when we use the expression 'user involvement'? How do we put it into practice and does it fulfil our expectations? Does everyone have the same understanding or is it used differently by different groups of professionals? How does it help us to put our values into practice? Are there any contradictions between what we say we do and what happens in practice?

As discussed, the first phase of action research consists of several elements which may take months to complete. Therefore, action researchers report a tension between a need for change or improvement and the desire for research, reading and reflection before implementing changes. In nursing action research, it is not uncommon to hear about changes occurring before the first phase is finished. Changes that occur prematurely are useful reflections of 'taken for granted' assumptions about the problem and need not be detrimental to a project (Waterman et al 2005).

Describing and explaining

When the first phase is complete, the core action research group must attempt to summarise and explain the problem (Stringer 1996). They will do this amongst themselves or with reference to a wider group. They draw up a plan of action identifying their objectives and courses of action whilst explaining their reasoning behind changes or innovations. These descriptions and explanations make useful reference points when changes are monitored and evaluated later.

Planning

Several action objectives will be written and the group decides whether to implement them all or whether to take a few at a time and observe their effect before introducing others (Elliott 1991). If all objectives are implemented this will make evaluation more complex because it will be difficult to attribute the cause to a single change in practice. In this case, the evaluation would consider the changes as a whole. Evaluating one change at a time may not be an option in the health care environment because of time. Subtle changes in behaviour and relationships between participants will have occurred through critical reflection and will make it difficult to attribute cause from one action change alone.

The plan of action will be detailed and contain not only objectives geared towards changing behaviour and systems but further research and reflection. Objectives also need to be agreed on how actions are to be monitored, for example through regular meetings. Having carried out phase one, action researchers are in a good position to determine how best and why to make changes. Kemmis and McTaggart (1988) argue that action researchers should plan changes that cause least disturbance but have maximum effect. The core action research group devises action objectives; however, as McNiff et al (1996) indicate, these need to be agreed/approved via the usual decision-making structures of the organisation. The most influential people in getting changes accepted and actioned in the organisation may also know least about the project (McNiff et al 1996). In trying to gain organisational approval, changes may be prevented or diluted (Waterman et al 2001). Managerial and financial representation on the core action research group helps to mitigate this problem.

Action

The third phase is one of 'action' in which the plan is enacted. Kemmis and McTaggart (1988) highlight that changes to the plan occur as soon as it is implemented. This is because, for example, new policies are implemented or new people arrive. The core action research group therefore should expect to amend the plan at regular intervals. Flexibility keeps the project up-to-date and context relevant and therefore is viewed as a strength of action research.

Evaluation

The group will need to consider the indicators of success including the key behaviours, relationships or documentation that will have changed through the enactment of the plan (McNiff et al 1996) and decide whether they need to carry out descriptive qualitative and/or inferential research. Each member of the core group will participate in the evaluation as far as possible and appropriate. Listening to feedback on changes or innovations implemented will add to their understanding of the problem. Following the evaluation, the plan is revisited and the descriptions and explanations (theory) regarding the problem are altered accordingly. The whole cycle is rerun and so forth until funding is exhausted or until the core action research group takes a decision to terminate the project. Action research therefore avoids premature theoretical and practical closure, and challenges popular orthodoxies and taken-for-granted solutions.

Closure

A few months before the project finishes, members of the action research group will begin to discuss whether and how to 'wind down' the project. Typically, a great deal of energy and emotions are invested in action research, which some people may find difficult to end, and therefore members have to be sensitive to one another's needs at this time. We find that there tends to be a gradual slowdown of the project with meetings and new activities becoming less frequent until they stop. Presentations and publications are important means of disseminating, celebrating and demonstrating that the work is coming to an end.

Example of action research

Problems with symptom management, provision of services, and practical support and team working were the impetus to an action research project which developed and implemented a framework for palliative primary care services (Daniel & Linnane 2001). The participatory nature of action research was attractive because active involvement of primary team members and patients was desired in order to improve practice. All the professional staff of one general practice and all the palliative care patients that were well enough to participate were approached to take part. Phase 1 of the project mainly consisted of team building and value clarification. A range of data collection methods were employed that promoted critical reflection: field notes, questionnaire on staff views of palliative care, semi-structured interviews with staff on palliative care roles and with patients to determine their views on service provision, and review of patients' care pathways. From the findings of phase 1, it was decided to implement three pilot nurse-led palliative care clinics. For phase 2, patient feedback spurred more clinics, implementation of a key worker for each patient, more multidisciplinary meetings, use of a patient-held record system, education seminars, and an audit framework. Phase 2 was evaluated through staff and patient questionnaires and audit data. The findings suggest that team working was improved, the key worker role was the most useful change, patients supported the clinics, and the seminars were helpful. The audit identified that psychological care was the most frequently documented problem. A framework for multidisciplinary palliative care was articulated from the findings which may have relevance in other primary care settings.

Conclusion

For staff keen to advance health care within the context of their work environment, action research provides a helpful theoretical and practical framework. Action research is a participative and empowering process that promotes sustainable change.

EXERCISES

1. *Differentiating between action research and experimental research.* Read the chapter on experimental research (Chapter 18). Then draw up a list of characteristics that differentiate action research from experimental research. Next list those characteristics that action research has in common with experimental research.

ANSWER

Different characteristics:

In action research the researcher roles are blurred, the method is participatory and empowering, there is the intention at least to change the setting, complexity is embraced, reflexivity is important, critical reflection and learning are an important part of the process, and the process is flexible and may be unpredictable.

In experimental research, the researcher is distant and neutral, the setting is controlled, the focus is on a small number of variables, objectivity is important, emphasis is on measurement, outcome and causality are important, production of knowledge is a prime goal, and process is predetermined.

Similar characteristics:

Both approaches generate knowledge and need appropriate funding.

2. *Critical reflection.* Given the information provided in this chapter:

   a. Select a problem. This could be an area of work that causes bother, tensions, or conflicts. Or an area in which there are contradictory practices and/or policies.
   b. Describe three examples that illustrate the problem.
   c. Check you have described the problem and not a potential solution to a problem.
   d. If you think you have written about a solution, go one step back and think about what the problem is that the solution is supposed to be solving.
   e. Undertake critical reflection; ask yourself:

       - What attitudes and feelings are revealed in the behaviour exhibited by the professionals and clients?
       - What values are being exhibited in the examples?
       - Do the values match your personal values about nursing care?
       - Who has power in the relationships and how is this revealed?
       - Does the 'everyday' terminology applied tell you anything about how the problem is perceived, e.g. some primary care practitioners may refer to the term 'heart-sinkers' – what does that symbolise?
       - Could more constructive words be used to describe the issue?
       - What concepts lie behind the actions exhibited?
       - Are they executed as well as they might?
       - Does care occur differently in different contexts for the same issue?

References

Atweh B, Kemmis S, Weeks P 1998 Action Research in Practice: Partnerships for Social Justice in Education. Routledge, London

Brydon-Miller M, Greenwood D, Maguire P 2003 Why action research? Action Research 1: 9–28

Carr W, Kemmis S 1986 Becoming Critical: Education, Knowledge and Action Research. The Falmer Press, London

Daniel L, Linnane J 2001 Developing a framework for primary palliative care services. British Journal of Community Nursing 31(1): 238–247

Elden M, Chisholm F 1993 Emerging varieties of Action Research: Introduction to the special issue. Human Relations 46: 121–142

Elliott J 1991 Action Research for Educational Change. Open University Press, Milton Keynes

Greenwood J 1994 Action research: a few details, a caution and something new. Journal of Advanced Nursing 20: 13–18

Hart E 1996 Action research as a professionalizing strategy: issues and dilemmas. Journal of Advanced Nursing 23: 454–461

Hart E, Bond M 1995 Action Research and Health and Social Care: A Guide to Practice. Open University Press, Buckingham

Hendry C, Farley A H 1996 The nurse teacher as action researcher. Nurse Education today 16: 193–198

Heron J 1996 Co-operative Inquiry: Research into the Human Condition. Sage, London

Heron J, Reason P 1997 A participatory inquiry paradigm. Qualitative Inquiry 33: 276–294

Holter I M, Schwartz-Barcott D 1993 Action research: what is it? How has it been used and how can it be used in nursing? Journal of Advanced Nursing 18: 298–304

Kalleberg R 1990 The construct turn in sociology. Working paper. Institute for Social Research, Oslo, April

Kemmis S, McTaggart R 1988 The Action Research Planner, 3rd edn. Deakin University Press, Geelong

Kemmis S, Wilkinson M 1998 Participatory action research and the study of practice. In: Atweh B, Kemmis S, Weeks P (eds) Action Research in Practice: Partnerships for Social Justice in Education. Routledge, London: 21–36

Kingsley S 1985 Action research: method or ideology? Occasional Paper No 8. Association of Researchers in Voluntary Action and Community Involvement (ARVAC)

Koch T, Harrington A 1998 Reconceptualizing rigour: the case for reflexivity. Journal of Advanced Nursing 28: 882–890

Lathlean J 1994 Choosing an appropriate methodology. In: Buckledee G, McMahon R (eds) The Research Experience in Nursing. Chapman & Hall, London, 31–46

Lewin K 1948 Resolving Social Conflicts: Selected Papers on Group Dynamics. Harper and Brothers, New York

Lyon J 1998 Applying Hart and Bond's typology: implementing clinical supervision in an acute setting. Nurse Researcher 6: 29–56

McNiff J, Lomax P, Whitehead J 1996 You and Your Action Research Project. Routledge, London

Morgan D 1998 Planning Focus Groups: Focus Group Kit 2. Sage, London

Reason P, Bradbury H 2001 The Handbook of Action Research: Participative Inquiry and Practice. Sage, London

Reed J 2004 Using action research in nursing practice with older people: democratizing knowledge. Journal of Clinical Nursing 14: 594–600

Robinson A 1995 Transformative 'cultural shifts' in nursing: participatory action research and the project of possibility. Nursing Inquiry 2: 65–74

Rolfe G 1996 Going to extremes: action research, grounded practice and the theory–practice gap in nursing. Journal of Advanced Nursing 24: 1315–1320

Stewart D W, Shamdasani P N 1990 Focus Groups: Theory and Practice. Sage, London

Stringer E 1996 Action Research: A Handbook for Practitioners. Sage, Thousand Oaks, CA

Susman G I, Evered R D 1978 An assessment of the scientific merits of action research. Administrative Science Quarterly 23: 582–603

Wallis S 1998 Changing practice through action research. Nurse Researcher 6: 5–15

Waterman H 1994 Meaning of visual impairment: developing ophthalmic nursing care. PhD Dissertation, Victoria University of Manchester

Waterman H 1996 A comparison of action research with quality assurance. Nurse Researcher 3(3): 15–23

Waterman H, Webb C, Williams A 1995 Parallels and contradictions in the theory and practice of action research and nursing. Journal of Advanced Nursing 22: 779–784

Waterman H, Tillen D, Dickson R, et al 2001 Action research: a systematic review and assessment for guidance. Health Technology Assessment 5(23): 1–166

Waterman H, Harper R, MacDonald H, et al 2005 Advancing ophthalmic nursing practice through action research. Journal of Advanced Nursing 52: 281–290

Webb C 1989 Action research: philosophy, methods and personal experiences. Journal of Advanced Nursing 14: 403–410

Winter R, Munn-Giddings C 2001 A Handbook for Action Research in Health and Social Care. Routledge, London

van Mannen M 1990 Beyond assumptions: shifting the limits of action research. Theory Into Practice 24: 152–157

Chapter 21

Grounded Theory

John Cutcliffe

Introduction

One of the beauties of science, irrespective of the 'field', discipline or area, is the persistently evolving nature of knowledge. Moreover, it is not only the knowledge base that expands, deepens and becomes more dense it is also how we acquire, refine, test and refute this knowledge. Epistemological and methodological developments are just as much an advancement of the academe of science as are new discoveries of the behaviour of quarks (sub-atomic particles), the discovery of new interstellar bodies or, on a more human level, discoveries relating to the most effective preoperative care package and how nurses can inspire hope in people.

One such methodological discovery that has had a significant impact on nursing science is the creation (and subsequent development) of grounded theory (GT) methodology. There are, currently, at least two different perspectives on GT; furthermore, there has been a well-documented disproportionate emphasis on and resultant familiarity with Strauss and Corbin's (1990) version of GT (see, for example, Melia 1996). However, I accept Glaser's cogent 1992 (and subsequent) arguments that Glaserian GT is 'real' GT and I have no wish to skew the extant literature even further towards the Straussian version of GT. As a result, this chapter focuses on Glaserian GT. For those readers interested in Straussian GT (or what Glaser 1992 calls 'full conceptual description'), I refer you to Strauss and Corbin (1990) and Charmaz (1990).

An introduction to grounded theory methodology

In 1967, Glaser and Strauss published their text, *The Discovery of Grounded Theory: Strategies for Qualitative Research*. Since that time the method (Glaser describes grounded theory as both a method and a methodology; for simplicity, the chapter will refer to grounded theory as a method) has become well established in a wide range of disciplines (and the number continues to grow); the book is regarded as a seminal work and GT has a demonstrated international utility. One of the many striking features of the 1967 text was that, for the authors, it was regarded as only the beginning of the venture into the development of methods; it would be appropriate if not expected, that the method itself would evolve and develop. As a number of authors have noted, this led to a propagation of GTs and, more worryingly, many of these share little methodological similarity with the original method (Becker 1993, Benoliel 1996, Cutcliffe 2000, 2005, Melia 1996, Wilson & Hutchinson 1996). Accordingly, it is necessary to examine the key elements of GT that have been present since its genesis, as such examination ought to assist in its subsequent application and operationalisation.

Grounded theory: an overview

GT was developed, like other scientific advances that are prefaced by disenchantment with the prevailing orthodoxy, as a reaction to the then over zealous preoccupation with verification of theory. GT's basic and central theme is generating theory from data that are systematically obtained from social research; consequently, GT is an inductive process (Glaser & Strauss 1967). It is a method for inducing and developing theory that should provide clear enough categories and hypotheses to explain and aid understanding of the basic (psycho)social process being studied. The theory evolves continuously from the data during the process of the research in that, unlike many other methods, the researcher does not commence with existing literature but begins with an identified area of study. Then, as data are collected, the process of constant comparative analysis occurs (a central feature of GT) whereby each item or label of data is compared with every other item or label. Glaser and Strauss (1967, p. 32) stress that this strategy of comparative analysis within the induction of grounded theory puts a high emphasis on:

Theory as process, that is, theory as an ever-developing entity, not as a perfected product.

GT usually occurs when there is little or no research into the subject or area. Consequently, research questions in GT (if present at all) are markedly different to research questions postulated at the start of a deductive study. Indeed, Glaser (1978, 1992, 1995a, 1995b) repeatedly purports that a 'true' GT begins only with a 'general wonderment'. The key research question, Glaser predicates, will emerge as the key (psycho)social problem facing the population being studied. Though it should be noted that a more contemporary view outlines the difficulties that such an approach creates and how it may be prudent, for a number of reasons, to include a non-specific question (Cutcliffe 2005).

A crucial difference between GT and other approaches is its emphasis on theory generation and development (Glaser & Strauss 1967, Glaser 1998, 2001). It is a way of thinking about and conceptualising data, to induce theory that is grounded in the reality of the research participants (Smith & Biley 1997). As a result, the theory can be seen to originate from the 'ground level' from the (psycho)social world from where the data originate. As Stern (1985), who was among the first nurses to use GT in a nursing focused study suggests, GT scientists construct theory from the data rather than applying a theory constructed by someone else from another data source. As a result, a GT should therefore 'fit' the situation being researched. To sum up:

a well constructed grounded theory will meet its four most central criteria: fit, work, relevance, and modifiability. If a grounded theory is carefully induced from the substantive area its categories and their properties will fit the realities under study in the eyes of subjects, practitioners and researchers in the area. If a grounded theory works it will explain the major variations in behaviour in the area with respect to the processing of the main concerns of the subjects. If it fits and works the grounded theory has achieved relevance. The theory itself should not be written in stone or as a 'pet', it should be readily modifiable when new data present variations in emergent properties and categories' (Glaser 1992, p. 15).

Key features/elements of grounded theory

Generating theory

As stated above, a principal feature of GT is its emphasis on theory generation, not conceptual description, nor theory verification. That is not to say that description or verification have no place within GT; these processes, however, are subsumed within the overall process of theory generation. A generated GT then can be presented in many forms:

Grounded theory can be presented either as a well codified set of propositions or in a running theoretical discussion, using conceptual categories and their properties. (Glaser & Strauss 1967, p. 31)

GT produces two basic kinds of theory, substantive or formal theory. Grounded substantive theory is theory that has been developed for a substantive or empirical area of (psycho)social enquiry, for example client care. Grounded formal theory is theory that has been developed for a formal or conceptual area of (psycho)sociological enquiry, for example deviant behaviour. Glaser and Strauss (1967, p. 34) asserted that substantive theories are usually induced from the data and formulated first and then these substantive theories are followed by formal theories. Furthermore, they pointed out that it is the induced substantive theories that then enable new formal theories to be generated. As such:

Substantive theory in turn helps to generate new grounded formal theories and to reformulate previously established ones.

When referring to grounded substantive and grounded formal theory, Glaser and Strauss (1967, p. 32) indicated:

Both types of theory may be considered as middle-range.

Glaser and Strauss (1967) indicated that a GT will have theoretical elements that are generated by comparative analysis; these are conceptual categories and their properties, and hypotheses or generalised relations among the categories. Each of these elements is defined as:

- categories: a conceptual element of the theory that stands by itself (p. 36)
- property: a conceptual aspect or element of a category (p. 36)
- hypotheses: a suggested, not tested, relation among categories and their properties (p. 39).

As categories begin to emerge from the data, the researcher's attention is fixed on a category (Glaser 1992). This attention then helps the researcher discover emergent properties about the category. At this point in the theory generation though, such categories and their properties only conceptualise what the researcher can see (Glaser 1978), and the researcher needs the theoretical coding, which forms the connections between them which yield hypotheses. In turn, these hypotheses suggest how the incidents and categories may be related to each other (Glaser 1978).

However, Glaser and Strauss (1967) point out that these hypotheses have at first the status of suggested, not tested, relations amongst categories and their properties. The generation of such tentative hypotheses does not require an extensive compilation of evidence to establish proof, just evidence enough to establish a suggestion. In the early stages of the research, these hypotheses may seem unrelated, but through the ongoing processes of data collection, constant comparison, and the subsequent emergence of categories and properties, and their development in abstraction and interrelations, they begin to form an integrated central theoretical framework (Glaser & Strauss 1967).

Theoretical sampling

Glaser and Strauss (1967, p. 45) pointed out that theoretical sampling involves:

The process of data collection for generating theory whereby the analyst jointly collects, codes and analyses his data and decides what data to collect next and where to find them, in order to develop his theory as it emerges.

Whether the researcher is concerned with inducing a substantive or a formal GT, the process of data collection is thus guided and controlled by the emerging theory. Glaser (1978, p. 36) embellished this initial description when he added that theoretical sampling is concerned with eliciting initial codes from the data from the start of the data collection through constant comparative analysis, and then:

To use the codes to direct further data collection, from which the codes are further theoretically developed.

Glaser and Strauss posit that this method of sampling is a radical shift away from the methods used when attempting to generate theory, whereby the limits, scope and origins of the sample are predetermined. A 'GTist', however, still needs a starting point, and Glaser and Strauss described this starting point as the researcher beginning the research with a partial framework of local concepts, which designate a few principal or gross features of the structure and processes under study. They provide a useful example of such local concepts and principal/gross features. If I am going to study hospitals, then I am aware that there will be doctors, nurses, patients, wards, treatment rooms, admission and discharge procedures. However, the researcher will not have any *a priori* frameworks of how these concepts interact and relate.

Theoretical sampling also involves the researcher's sensitivity (Glaser & Strauss 1967, Glaser 1978, 1992). To enable the theory to emerge from the data, the researcher needs to be sufficiently theoretically sensitive to be open to the emergence of whichever codes emerge. Glaser (1992, p. 27) added that:

It is a personal attribute of the researcher who has the ability to give conceptual insight, understanding and meaning to his substantive data.

Glaser (1992) argued that theoretical sampling within GT can be simple and direct. Once the decisions regarding the collection of initial data have been made, plans for the collection of further data cannot be made in advance of the emerging theory. As the emerging theory points the way towards the next source of data, the researcher does not know which 'way' to go until he has collected, coded and analysed the initial data. Future sources of data are thus dictated by the answers given to earlier questions. Glaser (1992) suggests that this process allows researchers to reach the limits of their data and data collection resources, and thus reaches the relevant theory expediently. Similarly, a GTist using theoretical sampling is unable to cite the total number, the nature, or type of groups from which the data were collected until the research is completed (Glaser 1978).

A GTist selects a theoretical sample based on the criteria of theoretical purpose and relevance, not of structural circumstance (Glaser & Strauss 1967). Consequently, the basic criterion which governs the selection of comparison groups is their theoretical relevance for furthering the development of emerging categories. The researcher seeks out any groups or units which may enhance the understanding of the categories by generating, to the fullest extent, as many properties of the categories as is possible and that will enable categories to link with each other.

Importantly, Glaser and Strauss (1967) highlight how the properties of the categories are influenced by diverse conditions; as a result, the researcher needs to be clear on the basic types of groups to be compared to control the effect on the conceptual level of the theory. They indicate that if the researcher intends to induce a substantive theory that is applicable to one substantive group, then the researcher needs to sample groups of the same substantive type. For example, in my doctoral study I was concerned with inducing theory that might aid the understanding of certain processes within bereavement counselling; therefore, it was appropriate to restrict the sampled groups to bereavement counsellors and their clients.

A more general or wider substantive theory would thus be induced by sampling wider substantive groups. Returning to the above example, I could have widened the substantive groups to include groups who attempt to help clients with bereavement problems, but who are not necessarily bereavement counsellors, for example, palliative care nurses, CRUSE counsellors and pastors. If the researcher is concerned with inducing a formal theory, he or she will select dissimilar substantive groups from the larger class and thus increase the theory's scope. For example, if a researcher was concerned with examining if and how hope is inspired in any form of counselling then it would be appropriate to widen the theoretical sample to include many types of counselling (e.g. counselling for substance misuse problems, for post-traumatic disorder, for couples/marriage guidance, for general anxiety states etc.) Consequently, according to Glaser and Strauss (1967, p. 52):

The scope of the theory is further increased by comparing different types of groups within different larger groups.

A GTist using theoretical sampling begins the generation of a substantive theory by minimising the differences in the sample (Glaser & Strauss 1967). Such endeavours help establish the basic categories and properties. Once this initial work is completed, the researcher increases the variation between the sample units, in accordance with the type of theory he or she is inducing, in order to stimulate the generation and refinement of theoretical properties. The outcome of this is that the scope of the theory is broadened (Glaser 1978). Theoretical sampling ceases once the categories are saturated and the researcher has achieved category saturation when:

No additional data are being found whereby the sociologist can develop properties of the category. (Glaser & Strauss 1967, p. 61)

They qualify their remarks stating that as the researcher:

Sees similar instances over and over again, the researcher becomes empirically confident that he has saturated his categories.

It should be noted here that, as with any decision about 'completeness' of one's data, and bearing Popper's (1965) cogent argument in mind, this requires 'a leap of faith' on the part of the researcher (see Cutcliffe & McKenna 2002).

However, as Glaser and Strauss (1967) pointed out, GT can be seen as process, in that a GT is never complete. As it is applied and explained, the theory becomes an ever developing entity and can evolve continuously (Glaser 1992, 2001). A saturated GT, made up of saturated categories then represents the most complete theory possible for that substantive group (or formal) group at that particular moment in time.

Lastly, Glaser and Strauss (1967) pointed out that in the same way that GT methods can and should evolve over time, the processes of theoretical sampling should also evolve with time. It is unlikely, then, that a study carried out in the late 1990s will have precisely the same operationalisation of theoretical sampling as that described in Glaser and Strauss' original work.

Constant comparative method

Glaser and Strauss (1967) proposed that a central feature of the GT method is the constant comparative method of qualitative analysis. In replying to what Glaser felt was Strauss' deviation from this central feature, Glaser (1992, p. 40) strongly re-emphasised the need for the constant comparative method in GT theory:

We do mean comparing incident to incident and/ or to concepts as the analyst goes through his data. We look for patterns so that a pattern of many similar incidents can be given a conceptual name as a category.

In their original text, Glaser and Strauss (1967, p. 105) describe four stages to the process of constant comparative method (Box 21.1).

Box 21.1 – *The four stages of the constant comparative method*

1. Comparing incidents applicable to each category
2. Integrating categories and their properties
3. Delimiting the theory
4. Writing the theory

It is important to note that these stages have a degree of linearity in that after a time, each stage is transformed into the next; they are also cyclic, in that the earlier stages remain in operation simultaneously throughout the analysis until the analysis is complete (Glaser & Strauss 1967).

Comparing incidents applicable to each category

In this stage the researcher codes the data and then compares each of these coded incidents with one another. The researcher codes these incidents into as many categories of analysis as is possible in order to let the categories emerge from the data. Glaser and Strauss (1967, p. 106) submitted that there are various ways that the researcher can code the data, (e.g. making notes on the margins of the transcript, separate index cards for each code); however, whichever way the researcher chooses it is important that these codes indicate which emerging category(s) the code belongs to. Glaser and Strauss provide a useful defining rule in order to help the researcher with this procedure which states:

While coding an incident for a category, compare it with the previous incidents in the same and different groups coded in the same category.

Further coding and comparison will enable the researcher to determine the properties of the categories and aid the process of developing the full range of theoretical notions which may apply to the category. Glaser and Strauss (1967, p. 107) declare that during such repeated coding, the researcher should record or memo these theoretical notions in order to preserve their initial freshness. They add a second useful defining rule here, suggesting that the researcher:

Stop coding and record a memo on your ideas.

Later, Glaser (1978) reasoned that the use of such memos constituted a core stage of and could be regarded as the bedrock of the process of inducing a GT. Such was Glaser's (1978) strength of feeling on this matter that he argued if a researcher misses out theoretical memoing, then the researcher is not doing GT. Glaser (1978) regarded these memos as the writing up (and subsequent recording) of the researcher's theorising and ideas about codes and their relationships as they came to mind. Such coding enables ideas to be developed with complete freedom, and recorded into a memo fund that is highly sortable.

Integrating categories and their properties

In this stage, as coding continues, the constant comparative units change from comparing incident with incident, to comparing incidents with the categories of the properties (Glaser & Strauss 1967). As a result of these comparisons, the categories are developed, the properties of the category are refined and begin to become integrated, that is, they relate in many ways. Glaser (1978) pointed out that as a consequence of further comparison this deeper understanding of the properties results in a more unified whole.

Delimiting the theory

In this stage, the delimiting of the theory occurs at two levels, the theory and the categories (Glaser & Strauss 1967). The first of these, the delimiting of the theory, occurs as a result of the theory solidifying, in the sense that major modifications become fewer and fewer. Later modifications, indicated as a result of further comparison of incidents with properties, take the form of clarifying the logic, taking out non-relevant properties, and integrating details of properties into the major outline of inter-related categories. According to Glaser and Strauss (1967), the most important process involved in this delimiting of the theory is reduction. This enables the researcher to formulate the theory with a smaller set of higher level concepts and hence delimit the theory in its terminology and text (Glaser & Strauss 1967).

It is interesting to note that Glaser and Strauss (1967) suggested that discovering these underlying uniformities and reducing the terminology enables the researcher to widen the scope of the theory and generalise to a wider population. Also, the reduction of terminology and subsequent possibility to broaden the scope of the theory is brought about by further comparison including some comparison with literature. Hence at this stage in the theory reduction, Glaser and Strauss (1967) advocate sampling the relevant empirical literature. As a consequence of this delimiting of the theory, the analyst begins to achieve two major requirements of theory: (a) parsimony of variables and formulation, and (b) broadening of the scope or applicability of the theory (Glaser & Strauss 1967).

The second of these, the delimiting of the categories, occurs as a result of reducing the number of categories. Reduction in the number of categories is achieved by discovering underlying uniformities. The researcher examines the categories and their properties and begins to perceive links of various kinds and this allows the original list of categories to be cut down. A further factor which contributes to delimiting the theory is theoretical saturation (which was detailed in the preceding section, 'Theoretical sampling').

Writing the theory

If the researcher is convinced that the analytical framework forms a systematic substantive theory and considers that the theory is couched in a form that is accessible to others in the substantive area studied, then he or she can proceed to publish the work with a degree of confidence.

Theoretical sensitivity

Building on the initial discussion on theoretical sensitivity contained in Glaser and Strauss' (1967) original text, Glaser returned to this central aspect of GT with conspicuous regularity (see Glaser 1978, 1992, 1998, 2001, for example). Theoretical sensitivity is concerned with assisting the researcher in achieving a certain depth of analysis (Glaser 1978) and it features two processes which are pivotal to that end, namely, searching for and discovering the core variable and the need for all GT to have a temporal dimension or identified stages.

In explaining the importance of the core variable, Glaser (1978) posited that searching for patterns in the generation of theory revolves around a core category. (Interestingly, Glaser interchanges the expressions, core variable and core category.) Without an identified core variable, a GT is incomplete and limited in its application. In his 1978 work, he proceeded to list criteria for establishing the core variable and these are described in Box 21.2.

The second process crucial to theoretical sensitivity is that of GTs having a temporal dimension or stages (Glaser 1978, 1998, 2001). The core variable will have two or more clear emergent stages and these stages should differentiate and account for variations in the pattern of behaviour (Glaser 1978). Since, in Glaser's (1978) view, a process is something that occurs over time and involves change over time, the variations over time within the core variable can be explained by the stages. As Glaser (1978, pp. 98/99) stated:

Stages are perceivable because they sequence with one another within certain temporal limits.

And:

Stages have a time dimension. That is they have a perceivable beginning and end.

A GT then should, according to Glaser, contain these stages or temporal dimensions of the (psycho)social process being studied and they enable the changes over time to remain in the 'grasp' of the theoretical whole.

Box 21.2 – *Criteria for establishing a core variable (Glaser 1978, pp. 95–96)*

- It must be central, that is related to as many other categories and their properties as possible and more than other candidates for the core category. The criterion of centrality is a necessary condition to make it core.
- It must reoccur frequently in the data. By its frequent reoccurrence it comes to be seen as a stable pattern and becomes more and more related to other variables.
- By being more related to many other categories and reoccurring frequently, it takes more time to saturate the core category than other categories.
- It relates meaningfully and easily with other categories. These connections are not forced, rather their realisation comes quick and richly.
- It has clear and grabbing implication for formal theory.
- It has clear and considerable carry through in that it does not lead to dead ends in theory nor leave the analyst high and dry.
- It is completely variable in that its frequent relations to other categories make it highly variable in degree, dimension and type. It is readily modifiable through these dependent variations.
- It is also a dimension of the problem. Thus, it in part explains itself and its own variations.

Example of a (modified) grounded theory study

The example of a GT study is that undertaken by Cutcliffe, Stevenson, Jackson and Smith (2006) and published in the *International Journal of Nursing Studies*.

A modified grounded theory study of how psychiatric nurses work with suicidal people

Background. People with mental health problems continue to present a disproportionately high risk of suicide. Despite the relevance of suicide to psychiatric/mental health (P/MH) nurses, there is a documented paucity of research in this substantive area undertaken by or referring specifically to P/MH nurses; there is currently no extant theory to guide P/MH nursing care of the suicidal person.

Objectives. Accordingly, this paper reports on a study undertaken to determine if P/MH nurses provide meaningful caring responses to suicidal people, and if so how.

Design. The study used a modified grounded theory method and was conducted in keeping with the Glaserian tenets of grounded theory.

Settings. The study was conducted in two geographical locations within the United Kingdom, one in the North and the other in the Midlands; both locations contained large urban centres.

Participants. A total of 20 participants were selected across the locations by means of theoretical sampling. All the participants were over 18 years old, had made a serious attempt on their lives or felt they were on the cusp of so doing and had received 'crisis' care from the 'emergency' psychiatric services.

Methods. The study adhered to the principal features of Glaserian grounded theory, namely (a) theory generation, not theory verification; (b) theoretical sampling, (c) the constant comparative method of data analysis; and (d) theoretical sensitivity (searching for/discovering the core variable, one which identified the key pychosocial process and contains temporal dimensions and stages). Further, the authors ensured that the study was concerned with generating conceptual theory, not conceptual description.

Findings/Conclusion. The findings indicate that this key psychosocial problem is addressed through the core variable: 'Reconnecting the person with humanity'. This parsimonious theory describes and explains a three-stage healing process consisting of the sub-core variables: 'Reflecting an image of humanity', 'Guiding the individual back to humanity' and 'Learning to live'.

EXERCISES

1. Locate at least five research studies in the extant nursing literature which claim to be using a GT method: see if you can identify if the studies use a Glaserian or a Straussian GT method.
2. Compare the theoretical products (i.e. the findings, the theory) of a Glaserian and Straussian GT – what principal differences do you notice?
3. Given Glaser's comments regarding a GT having 'fit, grab', try and locate a GT undertaken in a substantive area you are interested/work in and consider for yourself, 'Does it have fit and grab for you? – if not, why not?'

References

Becker P H 1993 Common pitfalls in published grounded theory research. Qualitative Health Research 3: 254–260

Benoliel J Q 1996 Grounded theory and nursing knowledge. Qualitative Health Research 6: 406–428

Charmaz K 1990 'Discovering' chronic illness: Using grounded theory. Social Science and Medicine 30: 1161–1172

Cutcliffe J R 2000 Methodological issues in grounded theory. Journal of Advanced Nursing 31: 1476–1484

Cutcliffe J R 2005 Adapt or adopt: developing and transgressing the methodological boundaries of grounded theory. Journal of Advanced Nursing 51: 421 428

Cutcliffe J R, McKenna H P 2002 When do we know that we know?: Considering the truth of research findings and the craft of qualitative research. International Journal of Nursing Studies 39: 611–618

Cutcliffe J R, Stevenson C, Jackson S, et al 2006 A modified grounded theory study of how psychiatric nurses work with suicidal people. International Journal of Nursing Studies 43: 791–802

Glaser B G 1978 Theoretical Sensitivity: Advances in the Method ology of Grounded Theory. Sociology Press, Mill Valley, CA

Glaser B G 1992 Basics of Grounded Theory Analysis: Emerging Versus Forcing. Sociology Press, Mill Valley, CA

Glaser B G 1995a Grounded Theory 1984–1994, Vol 1. Sociology Press, Mill Valley, CA

Glaser B G 1995b Grounded Theory 1984–1994, Vol 2. Sociology Press, Mill Valley, CA

Glaser B G 1998 Doing Grounded Theory: Issues and Discussions. Sociology Press, Mill Valley, CA

Glaser B G 2001 The Grounded Theory perspective: Conceptualisation Contrasted with Description. Sociology Press, Mill Valley, CA

Glaser B G, Strauss A L 1967 The Discovery of Grounded Theory: Strategies for Qualitative Research. Aldine, Chicago

Melia K 1996 Re-discovering Glaser. Qualitative Health Research 6: 368–378

Popper K 1965 Conjectures and Refutations: The Growth of Scientific Knowledge. Harper and Row, New York

Smith K, Biley F 1997 Understanding grounded theory: principles and evaluation. Nurse Researcher 4: 17–31

Stern P 1985 Using grounded theory methods in nursing research. In: Leininger M (ed) Qualitative Research Methods in Nursing. Grune and Stratton, New York: pp. 78–95

Strauss A, Corbin J 1990 Basics of Qualitative Research. Techniques and Procedures for Developing Grounded Theory. Sage, London

Wilson H S, Hutchinson S A 1996 Methodologic mistakes in grounded theory. Nursing Research 45. 122–124

Chapter 22

Phenomenology

Tanya McCance and Sonja Mcilfatrick

Introduction

One of the main reasons for the increased popularity of phenomenology in nursing research is that it provides a research approach that is consistent with the art, philosophy and practice of nursing: 'understanding unique individuals and their meanings and interactions with others and the environment' (Lopez & Willis 2006, p.726). However, there is much debate about adopting this approach within nursing, particularly without an adequate grasp of the underlying philosophy (Barkway 2001, Crotty 1996, Paley 1998). Lopez and Willis (2006) argued that a failure to examine the philosophical basis of a research method can result in research that is ambiguous in its purpose, structure and findings. Furthermore, there has also been a failure of nurse researchers to acknowledge the conflicting perspectives within phenomenology (descriptive versus interpretive). This chapter will seek to address this by providing an overview of phenomenology within nursing research and an analysis of the strengths and weaknesses associated with its use. The main types of phenomenology (descriptive and interpretive) will be examined alongside a consideration of how the philosophical underpinnings have informed the research process. Finally, some practical examples will help to elucidate how this approach has been used to explore phenomena that are central to nursing and health care.

What is phenomenology?

In its simplest form phenomenology can be described as 'the study of phenomena, the appearance of things' (Cohen 1987, p. 31). This is reflective of the fundamental principle of phenomenology articulated by Husserl – 'back to the things themselves' (Swanson-Kauffman & Schonwald 1988). This is illustrated by Van Manen (1990, p. 10) who stated 'phenomenology asks for the very nature of a phenomenon, for what makes a 'something' what it is – and without which it could not be what it is'. Husserl emphasised the importance of returning to the everyday world where people are living through various phenomena in actual situations (Giorgi 1985). Hence, phenomenology focuses on a person's lived experience as a means of uncovering meaning and generating understanding about certain 'things'. When we talk about lived experience we are referring to the events that individuals live through. By recalling the detail of these events we transform them into objects of consciousness (Kleinman 2004) that can then be re-examined. For example, in Field's (1981) phenomenological study focusing on the nurses' experience of giving an injection he identified the 'phenomenon particular' (the injection) as well as 'phenomenon perceived' (the lived experience of giving an injection).

It has been noted that nurse researchers have difficulty in understanding phenomenological language and its underpinning philosophy (Corben 1999). This has been attributed to the fact that phenomenology is described as both a philosophy and a research method (Cohen 1987). In the philosophical sense, phenomenology refers to 'a particular way of approaching the world: it implies apprehending experience as it is lived' (Parse 1995, p. 12). As a research method, phenomenology is 'governed by rigorous processes in data gathering and data analysis' (Parse 1995, p. 13). Both perspectives should not be viewed separately because the philosophical understanding of phenomenology has important implications in relation to how we use it as a research method.

Phenomenology and nursing

The use of phenomenology within nursing research has been a direct consequence of the ability of this approach to answer questions of particular relevance to nursing practice (Lawler 1998, Taylor 1993). It has been advocated that phenomenology is congruent with nursing, where humanistic knowledge is valued (Rose et al 1995). As noted by Beck (1994, p. 499), 'phenomenology affords nursing new ways to interpret the nature of consciousness in the world'. Many nurse researchers regard phenomenology as a research method that could provide understanding of the person's reality and experience, one that values individuals and the nurse–patient relationship, and one which embraces a holistic approach to the person (Benner 1994, Holmes 1990). In commenting on the use of phenomenology as a research method for nurses, Lawler (1998) suggested that:

Unless nurses know what meanings people attach to events that disrupt their lives, nurses – as practitioners and people – have a restricted capacity to help their patients or find ways to deal with their own experiences as practitioners' (p. 106)

Some examples of phenomena that have been explored using phenomenology have included:

- women's experience of acute myocardial infarction (Svedlund et al 1994);
- registered nurses' perspective of caring for adolescent females with anorexia nervosa (King & Turner 2000);
- patients' and nurses' experience of caring in nursing (McCance 2003);
- providing information to patients receiving radiation therapy (Long 2001);
- patient's experience of an intensive care unit following a liver transplant (Del Barrio et al 2004);
- nurses' experience of day hospital chemotherapy (McIlfatrick et al 2006).

In examining the implications of phenomenology for nursing knowledge development and the use of knowledge in practice, Van der Zalm and Bergum (2000) suggested that phenomenology contributes to Carper's (1978) ways of knowing, i.e. empirical, moral, aesthetic and personal knowledge development. Thus, its contribution is not in developing predictive and prescriptive theory, but in revealing the nature of human experience. In the phenomenological sense, knowledge does not inform practice, rather reflection on practice (life) results in knowledge (understanding) that in turn enlightens practice (Van Manen 1990).

Types of phenomenology

Descriptive or Husserlian phenomenology was developed by Husserl (1859–1938), and is aimed at 'uncovering and describing the essence of the phenomena of interest' (Priest 2004, p. 6). Interpretive or Heideggerian phenomenology was developed by Heidegger (1889–1976), and is aimed at 'the interpretation of phenomena to uncover hidden meanings' (Priest 2004, p. 6). These two traditions have distinct differences in relation to their philosophical underpinnings, which influence how these approaches are used as a research method. Whilst there are many phenomenological philosophers, Walters (1995) acknowledges that the phenomenological traditions drawn from the work of Heidegger and Husserl are most prominent in phenomenological nursing research. Within this section these two traditions will be described and their philosophical basis discussed, with the intention of trying to elucidate the distinct differences between these two approaches, which are summarised in Table 22.1.

Descriptive phenomenology

Husserl is considered the 'father' of the phenomenological movement. Central to his ideas was the 'fundamental recognition of experience as the ultimate ground and meaning of knowledge' (Koch 1995, p. 828). Husserl's method focused on description and explanation (Ray 1985), with the prime aim of uncovering the ultimate structures of the consciousness (essences) (Koch 1995). According to Kleinman (2004, p. 10), essence refers to 'the most essential meaning for a particular context'. It is the essence that forms the consciousness and perception of the world. Whilst Husserl did not claim himself to be a positivist, Koch (1995) argues that his emphasis on description as that which elucidates the nature of reality appeals to an empiricist's view of knowledge. Annells (1999) similarly presents a

Table 22.1 – *Summary of differences between types of phenomenology*

Descriptive phenomenology	Interpretive phenomenology
Husserlian Epistemology (questions of knowing)	Heideggerian Ontology (questions of experiencing and understanding)
Person considered as a separate mind–body person living in a world of objects	Person exists as a 'being' in and of the world
Data speaks for itself	Interpreters participate in making data
Techniques and procedures to aid rigour (adoption of analysis structures)	Own criteria for trustworthiness
Bracketing defending objectivity	Hermeneutic circle (background, pre-understanding)
Useful in uncovering the 'essence' of a phenomena	Useful in examining the contextual features of experience – values uniqueness and diversity

case for placing Husserlian phenomenology within a positivist paradigm, identifying the following assumptions:

- A phenomenon is believed to be a reality, a truth that exists as an essence (of the phenomenon), and which can be disclosed – a 'realist' belief.
- This essence of the phenomenon exists independently from the researcher – an 'objectivist' opinion.
- The phenomenologist can, and should, seek to disclose the essence of the phenomenon in its purity, untainted by the phenomenologist's preconceptions of the phenomenon – objectivity is essential (p. 14).

Phenomenological reduction is central to Husserl's approach and is associated with the idea of bracketing. Walters (1995) described phenomenological reduction as that which 'involves reducing a complex problem into its basic components by eliminating one's own prejudices about the world' (p.792). Researchers as human beings will bring their own personal experiences, preconceptions, beliefs and attitudes to the research situation, which Husserl refers to as the 'natural attitude' (Paley 1997). It is these aspects that a researcher attempts to bracket by putting aside all preconceptions. This enables the researcher to present the phenomenon exactly as the participant experiences it (Wall et al 2004). Ray (1985) describes bracketing in a nursing context, giving the example of the experience of pain. Using Husserl's approach, the clinical nurse or researcher must not impose their knowledge of pain on the client, but allow them to express their own experience of pain as lived by them.

The ability of researchers to hold in abeyance their beliefs about a phenomenon under study is a major criticism of Husserlian phenomenology (Kvale 1983, Parse 1995). Beck (1994), however, would argue that whilst 'it is impossible for a researcher to be completely free from bias in reflection of the experience being studied ... it is possible to control it' (p. 500). The processes that can be used for bracketing are not always clearly described in the literature. Wall et al (2004), in attempting to provide a guide to the novice researcher, place this process within a continuous activity of reflection, and caution that there is no standard method for undertaking bracketing. They describe the process as more of 'a psychological orientation towards oneself rather than an observable set of procedures to be adopted by a researcher' (p. 22). The critical analysis of the use of Husserlian phenomenology within nursing conducted by Paley (1997) not only questioned the idea of bracketing, but also the accurate use of this method within nursing research. He argued that nurse researchers largely misunderstand the concepts of phenomenological reduction, phenomena and essence. It is

important, however, to acknowledge the value and potential contribution that descriptive phenomenology can make to uncovering the essence of phenomena important to nursing practice.

Interpretive phenomenology

Although it is recognised that interpretive phenomenology has been informed by various philosophers, such as Gadamer (1989), Habermas (1990), Heidegger (1962) and Ricoeur (1981), this discussion will focus on the approach developed by Heidegger. Parse (1995) suggested that Heideggerian phenomenology could be viewed as an extension of Husserl's original ideas, adding meaning and interpretation to descriptions without the notion of bracketing. Heidegger did not believe that getting to know and describe the experience of individuals was enough. Instead, he stressed the importance of knowing how respondents come to experience phenomena in the way they do (Parahoo 2006). Heidegger considered that the primary focus of philosophy was on the nature of existence (ontology), while Husserl focused on the nature of knowledge (epistemology). According to Koch (1995), Heidegger focused on the 'experience of understanding', while Husserl focused on the 'experience itself'. As Moules (2002) suggested, Heidegger brought the 'something' (self/being, tradition, history, and experience) back into the 'experience of something'.

This understanding can be linked to Heidegger's emphasis on hermeneutics. Hermeneutics has been defined as the 'science of interpretation' (Allen & Jensen 1990). Hermeneutics originates from the seventeenth century and is derived from the Greek word *hermenia*, which relates to the Greek god Hermes who interpreted and conveyed messages from the gods to mortals (Mavrotataki 1997). Therefore, hermeneutic phenomenology is concerned with illuminating details of experience with the goal of creating meaning and achieving a sense of understanding (Wilson & Hutchinson 1991). An important distinction between the two types of phenomenology concerns the notion of 'letting the facts speak for themselves' or of knowledge independent of interpretation. Sandelowski (2000) argues that all enquiry entails description and all description entails interpretation.

Heidegger referred to human existence as 'Dasein', or being-there, which emphasises the 'situatedness' of human reality (Walters 1995). This indicates the need to view individuals' experience in the context in which they experience it. Munhall and Oiler (1986) noted that 'people are tied to their worlds and comprehensible only in their contexts' (p. 58). The dominant themes in interpretive phenomenology are the hermeneutic circle and the historicality of understanding (Koch 1995). Heidegger (1962) described understanding in terms of a three-fold structure consisting of:

- fore-having – something we have in advance;
- fore-sight – something we see in advance;
- fore-conception – something we grasp in advance (p. 191).

Thus, the central distinction between Husserlian and Heideggerian approaches is that presuppositions are not to be eliminated or suspended (Ray 1994). Rather, researchers acknowledge that they cannot be extracted from being-in-the-world and reject the notion of bracketing, recognising the important contribution of the researcher's experiences in the interpretive process. The researcher is, therefore, considered inseparable from assumptions and preconceptions about the phenomena under investigation, and instead of bracketing these preconceptions, they are explicated and integrated into the research findings (Lopez & Willis 2006). Linked to the fore structure of understanding is the hermeneutic circle or circle of understanding, which places us in the world in a way that presupposes understanding, enabling us to make sense of the world. The interpretive process is achieved through a hermeneutic circle, which moves from the parts of experience, to the whole of experience, and back and forth again and again to increase the depth of engagement with, and the understanding of, words or texts (Annells 1996, Koch 1996).

Criticisms of phenomenological nursing research

The use of phenomenology within nursing research has become increasingly popular (McVicar & Caan 2005). It has, however, been noted that in the nursing literature there is misuse of the term phenomenology, with no clear distinction between the use of interpretive phenomenology and descriptive phenomenology (Koch 1995, Parse 1995, Walters 1995). The main criticism centres around the detachment of key philosophical notions from the phenomenological method used in nursing research (Yegdich 2000). Misunderstandings by researchers of the philosophical issues underpinning phenomenology have led to confusion about the use and application of the method (Paley 1997). Therefore, it is important for nurse researchers to 'explore, justify and articulate the philosophical underpinnings of their selected phenomenological approach' (Priest 2004, p. 4). It is suggested that such appraisal of the philosophical underpinnings increases one's appreciation of the validity of the method and provides soundness (rigour) to the method (Corben 1999, Koch 1995). Furthermore, Lowes and Prowes (2001) state that:

> The omission of a clear statement about the philosophical underpinnings of phenomenological research results in methodological confusion that may impact on the overall quality and rigour of the research endeavour. (p. 472)

Streubert and Carpenter (1999) suggested that making explicit the school of thought that guides an inquiry will help researchers to conduct a credible study and help those who use the findings apply the results within the appropriate context.

Phenomenology and the research process

There are key methodological issues related to the research process when using phenomenology as a research method. These relate to the type of research questions posed, methods of data collection, data analysis, sampling procedures and sample size. The main steps within the research process will be discussed, with common elements and distinguishing features drawn out for both descriptive and interpretive phenomenology. Two examples of studies drawn from the nursing literature will be used to illustrate key points. Boxes 22.1 and 22.2 present an overview of the two studies – one using interpretive phenomenology (Long 2001) and the other using descriptive phenomenology (King & Turner 2000).

Articulating the research question

Starting with the phenomenon or 'thing' under study, with the clear purpose of exploring to gain a greater understanding through the experience of individuals, helps in the formulation of the research question/research aim. Nurse researchers using phenomenology often begin with a research question that focuses on the individual's experience of a particular phenomenon of relevance to nursing practice. This is reflected in the research aims presented in the exemplar studies (refer to Boxes 22.1 and 22.2), which use terms such as 'to gain insight' and 'to explore experience', consistent with the overall purpose of a phenomenological study. It is recognised that a nurse researcher's knowledge of the research literature and practice setting is what leads them to generate the research question that needs to be investigated.

Methods of data collection

The main method of data collection adopted for phenomenological studies is the research interview.

Box 22.1 – *The importance of providing information to patients receiving radiation therapy*

Phenomenological approach: interpretive phenomenology influenced by the philosophical writings of Heidegger and Gadamer.

The phenomenon: radiation therapy.
Research question or research aim: to give insight into the experience of a course of radiation therapy and to relate the findings to nurses working with patients receiving radiation therapy.
Sampling technique: purposeful sampling was used to identify participants who were receiving radiation therapy, selected based on their particular knowledge of this phenomenon.
Sample size: 20 participants (15 women and 5 men).
Data collection: open-ended interviews, which began with the question: 'Can you tell me about how you felt when the doctor told you that you needed radiation therapy?'
Data analysis: interview transcriptions of the participants' experiences were interpreted by the researcher and were reread until the researcher was able to understand what the participants were saying. Gradually, keywords fell into sub-themes, and, finally four major themes emerged. The interpretations of the transcripts became a fusion of the horizons of the participants, the interpreter, and, when relevant, the literature.
Presentation of results: the four themes identified included Being Informed, which was the umbrella theme for the three other themes: Being Supported; Everydayness and Regaining a Sense of Self. Results demonstrated deficits in the care delivered in some radiation therapy departments. Information and preparation for radiation therapy are often inadequate or do not meet the needs of the individuals. The participants considered that they needed to adopt a 'sick' or 'patient' role even though they attend treatments on an outpatient basis and this resulted in a feeling of not being in control.
Implications for practice: the clinical significance of this study indicates the need to provide ongoing information for patients undergoing radiation therapy treatment.

Reference: Long L E 2001 Being informed: undergoing radiation therapy. Cancer Nursing 24(6): 463–468.

Box 22.2 – *Caring for adolescent females with anorexia nervosa: registered nurses' perspectives*

Phenomenological approach: descriptive phenomenology.

The phenomenon: anorexia nervosa.

Research question or research aim: to explore the lived experience of registered nurses caring for female adolescent anorexics.

Sampling technique: snowball sampling was used to identify participants employed within adolescent wards of large public hospitals and who had cared for anorexic female patients in the previous 6 months.

Sample size: 5 participants (all female).

Data collection: in-depth interviews, which began with an opening request: 'Please could you describe what it is like to care for adolescent females diagnosed with anorexia nervosa?'

Data analysis: interview transcriptions were analysed using Colaizzi's (1978) procedural steps.

Presentation of results: six themes were explicated: (a) personal core values of nurses; (b) core values challenged; (c) emotional turmoil; (d) frustration; (e) turning points; and (f) resolution. These themes were taken together to describe the essence of the journey undertaken by registered nurses who cared for adolescent anorexic females and was presented as a succinct statement of the phenomenon.

Implications for practice: the study findings highlighted the need for educational programmes to support nurses to care for adolescent anorexics, the development of new regimes that focus on new ways of thinking, and greater involvement of nurses in assessing and restructuring care protocols for anorexics.

Reference: King S J, Turner D S 2000 Caring for adolescent females with anorexia nervosa: registered nurses' perspectives. Journal of Advanced Nursing 32(1): 139–147.

Access to individuals' experience of the phenomena under study tends to be through open-ended, unstructured interviews, which are audio recorded for the purposes of analysis. It is important to recognise the skills required to conduct an interview that will provide the depth of data required for a phenomenological study. Conducting phenomenological research interviews requires sensitivity and good interview skills, acknowledging the role of the researcher as the instrument through which data are collected. Beck (1994) commented that the researcher's self is the major instrument for collecting data as it is through the developing relationships that occur in the in-depth interviewing process that the meaning of a lived experience is obtained. Morse and Field (1996) maintained that 'a successful qualitative interview is more like an intimate and personal sharing of a confidence with a trusted friend' (p. 72).

A phenomenological interview usually begins with the researcher asking the participant to recount a particular experience as fully as possible. This account of their experience includes both factual information alongside feelings, attitudes and views about this experience. A useful starting point in data collection is to ask: 'Can you tell me about this experience?' (refer to Boxes 22.1 and 22.2). According to Kvale (1995), a good interview question should contribute thematically to knowledge production and dynamically to promoting a good interview interaction. Kvale (1995) also proposed six quality criteria for an interview, which can be a useful tool when examining interview transcripts (refer to Box 22.3).

There are, however, fundamental differences in conducting interviews when using descriptive phenomenology versus interpretive phenomenology. The need to bracket in descriptive phenomenology is important in the interview process. In the example presented in Box 22.2, King and Turner (2000) described how throughout the study the researcher 'deliberately pushed reflective and intruding thoughts and self-opinions out of her mind' and 'utilised reflective writing as a means of emptying her mind prior to interviewing each participant' (p. 141).

Box 22.3 – *Interview quality criteria*

- The extent of spontaneous, rich, specific and relevant answers from the interviewee
- The shorter the interviewer's questions and the longer the subjects' answers the better
- The degree to which the interviewer followed up and clarified the meaning of the relevant aspects of the answers
- The ideal interview is to a large extent interpreted throughout the interview
- The interviewer attempted to verify his or her interpretation of the subjects' answers in the course of the interview
- The interview is self-communicating – it is a story contained in itself that hardly requires much extra descriptions and explanations

In contrast, the interview process within interpretive phenomenology becomes part of the interpretive process, with the researcher bringing their preconceptions to the interview situation through the hermeneutic circle (refer to Fig. 22.1).

Methods of data analysis

Data analysis in phenomenological research is challenging and whilst there is no agreed approach there are good frameworks that present guiding principles. Colaizzi (1978) presents a seven-step procedure for analysis for use with Husserlian phenomenology used within King and Turner's study (refer to Box 22.2). Similarly, Smith (1996) presents a framework for analysis for use within interpretive phenomenology, which he terms interpretive phenomenological analysis (IPA) (see Chapter 36).

Reflecting on the process of analysis, the difference between descriptive and interpretive approaches becomes apparent. This is illustrated through King and Turner's (2000) descriptive study based on Husserl's philosophy (Box 22.2), which uses a somewhat procedural approach to data analysis with the end outcome of a description of the essence of the phenomenon (anorexia nervosa). In contrast, Long's (2001) interpretive study (Box 22.1) recognises that the researcher's preconceptions and background are integrated in the data analysis stage. Meanings that the researcher provides through interpretive data analysis are actually a blend of the meanings articulated by both the researcher and the participant (Lopez & Willis 2006). Draucker (1999), however, noted that consideration of how the experiences of the researchers and participants are converged in the research process needs to be articulated more clearly. She suggested that there is a need to consider ways in which the understanding researchers bring to the research can be vividly revealed in their hermeneutical writings. Figure 22.1 is an attempt to address this criticism, which depicts diagrammatically a process whereby the experiences and preconceptions of both the participants and the researcher are combined throughout all the stages of the research process. This extends from the time of data collection and the interview process, throughout data analysis and into the subsequent reading of this experience by others.

Sampling procedures

The basis for sampling in phenomenology is that participants have experienced the phenomenon under investigation and are willing and able to articulate their experience of this (Corben 1999, Streubert & Carpenter 1999). Kleinman (2004) identifies snowball and purposeful sampling as particularly suited to phenomenological inquiry, and it is these two techniques that have been used in the two exemplar studies presented in Boxes 22.1 and 22.2. Purposive sampling involves the researcher making a judgement about the participants for the study. According to Patton (2001), the power of purposive sampling lies in selecting information-rich cases, from which one can learn a great deal about issues of central importance of the research. Sandelowksi (1995) also commented that purposeful sampling is typically not about sampling people per se, but rather about events, incidents and experiences. Snowball sampling can be

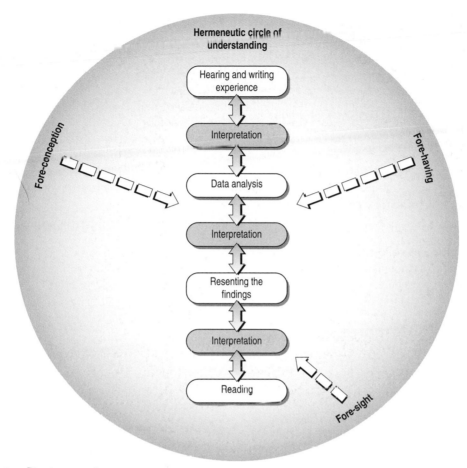

Figure 22.1 – *The interpretive process.*

described as a form of purposive sampling and is defined as 'a process of reference from one person to the next', the idea being that that the researcher is able to identify individuals who are considered credible by other participants (Streeton et al 2004, p. 37).

Conclusion

This aim of this chapter was to provide a comprehensive overview of phenomenology as a research approach, in a way that can be understood by the novice researcher, without underplaying the complexities inherent within it. The main focus was on descriptive and interpretive phenomenology, the two main traditions within phenomenological research. The philosophical underpinnings of these two approaches were described, highlighting how their distinct differences impact on its use as a research method. Conducting research using both descriptive and interpretive phenomenology was illustrated through the research process, and similarities and differences highlighted through the use of two study examples.

EXERCISES

1. Consider a phenomenon you would like to explore related to nursing practice, e.g. caring, and undertake the following activities:

   - devise your research question/research aim
   - identify the key opening interview question
   - undertake a mock interview with a colleague
   - reflect on the process and the skills required to be an effective interviewer.

2. Using a process of reflection, consider your own values and beliefs regarding your chosen phenomenon in Exercise 1, and consider the challenges in bracketing these 'preconceptions' if you were to undertake a descriptive phenomenological study.

3. Search the literature and identify a phenomenological study and critique it, considering the following:

   - type of phenomenology
   - research question/aim
   - sampling procedures
   - methods of data collection
   - data analysis.

References

Allen M N, Jensen L 1990 Hermeneutical inquiry; meaning and scope. Western Journal of Nursing Research 12: 241–253

Annells M 1996 Hermeneutic phenomenology: philosophical perspectives and current use in nursing research. Journal of Advanced Nursing 23: 705–713

Annells M 1999 Evaluating phenomenology: usefulness, quality and philosophical foundations. Nurse Researcher 6(3): 5–19

Barkway P 2001 Michael Crotty and nursing phenomenology: criticism or critique? Nursing Inquiry 8: 191–195

Beck C T 1994 Phenomenology: its use in nursing research. International Journal of Nursing Studies 31: 499–510

Benner P 1994 Interpretive Phenomenology. Sage, London

Carper B A 1978 Fundamental patterns of knowing in nursing. Advances in Nursing Science 1: 13–23

Cohen J 1987 A Historical overview of the phenomenologic movement. IMAGE: Journal of Nursing Scholarship 19: 31–34

Colaizzi P F 1978 Psychological research as the phenomenologist views it. In: Valle R, King M (eds) Existential Phenomenological Alternatives for Psychology. Oxford University Press, Oxford

Corben V 1999 Misusing phenomenology in nursing research: identifying the issues. Nurse Researcher 6(3): 52–66

Crotty M 1996 Phenomenology and Nursing Research. Churchill Livingstone, Melbourne

Del Barrio M, Lacunza M, Armendariz A C, et al 2004 Liver transplant patients: their experience in the intensive care unit: a phenomenological study. Journal of Clinical Nursing 13: 967–976

Draucker C B 1999 The critique of Heideggerian hermeneutical nursing research. Journal of Advanced Nursing 30: 360–373

Field P A 1981 A phenomenological look at giving an injection. Journal of Advanced Nursing 6: 291–296

Gadamer H G 1989 Truth and Method. Continuum, New York

Giorgi A 1985 Phenomenology and Psychological Research. Duquesne University Press, Pittsburgh

Habermas J 1990 The Philosophical Discourse of Modernity. MIT Press, Cambridge MA

Heidegger M 1962 Being and Time (Reprinted version 1980). Basil Blackwell, Oxford

Holmes C A 1990 Alternatives to natural science foundations for nursing. International Journal of Nursing Studies 27: 187–198

King S J, Turner D 2000 Caring for adolescent females with anorexia nervosa: registered nurses perspectives. Journal of Advanced Nursing 32: 139–147

Kleinman S 2004 Phenomenology: to wonder and search for meanings. Nurse Researcher 11(4): 7–19

Koch T 1995 Interpretative approaches in nursing research: the influence of Husserl and Heidegger. Journal of Advanced Nursing 21: 827–836

Koch T 1996 Implementation of hermeneutic inquiry in nursing: philosophy, rigour and representation. Journal of Advanced Nursing 24: 174–184

Lawler J 1998 Phenomenologies as research methodologies for nursing: from philosophy to researching practice. Nursing Inquiry 5: 104–111

Kvale S 1983 The qualitative research interview: a phenomenological and hermeneutic mode of understanding. Journal of Phenomenological Psychology 14: 171–196

Kvale S 1995 Interviews: An Introduction to Qualitative Research Interviewing. Sage, Thousand Oaks, CA

Long L E 2001 Being informed: undergoing radiation therapy. Cancer Nursing 24; 463–468

Lopez K A, Willis D G 2006 Descriptive versus interpretive phenomenology: their contributions to nursing knowledge. Qualitative Health Research 14: 726–735

Lowes M L, Prowse M A 2001 Standing outside of the interview process? The illusion of objectivity in phenomenological data generation. International Journal of Nursing Studies 38: 471–480

McCance T V 2003 Caring in nursing practice: the development of a conceptual framework. Research and Theory for Nursing Practice: An International Journal 17: 101–116

McIlfatrick S J, Sullivan K, McKenna H P 2006 Nursing the clinic vs nursing the patient: nurses' experience of a day hospital chemotherapy service. Journal of Clinical Nursing 15(9): 1170–1178

McVicar A, Caan W 2005 Research capability in doctoral training: Evidence for increased diversity of skills in nursing research. Journal of Research in Nursing 10: 627–646

Mavrotataki M 1997 Greek Mythology and Religion. Hattalis, Athens

Morse J M, Field P A 1996 Nursing research: the application of qualitative approaches, 2nd edn. Chapman & Hall, London

Moules N J 2002 Hermeneutic inquiry: paying heed to history and Hermes – an ancestral, substantive and methodological tale. International Journal of Qualitative Methods 1(3): Article 1. Online. Available: http://www.alberta.ca/~ijqm/ 6 sept 2002

Munhall P, Oiler C 1986 Nursing Research: A Qualitative Perspective. Appleton, New York

Paley J 1997 Husserl, phenomenology and nursing. Journal of Advanced Nursing 26: 187–193

Paley J 1998 Misinterpretive phenomenology: Heidegger, ontology and nursing research. Journal of Advanced Nursing 27: 817–824

Parahoo K 2006 Nursing Research: Principles, Process and Issues, 2nd edn. Macmillan, London

Parse R R 1995 Building knowledge through qualitative research: the road less travelled. Nursing Science Quarterly 9: 10–16

Patton M Q 2001 Qualitative Evaluation and Research Methods. Sage, Newbury Park

Priest H 2004 Phenomenology. Nurse Researcher 11(4): 4–6

Ray M A 1985 A philosophical method to study nursing phenomena. In: Leininger M M (ed) Qualitative Research Methods in Nursing. Grune & Stratton, Orlando: 81–92

Ray M 1994 The richness of phenomenology: philosophic, theoretic and methodological concerns. In: Morse J M (ed) Critical Issues in Qualitative Research Methods. Sage, Thousand Oaks, CA: 117–133

Ricoeur P 1981 Hermeneutics and Human Sciences: Essays on Language, Action and Interpretation. Cambridge University Press, New York

Rose P, Beeby J, Parker D 1995 Academic rigour in the lived experience of researchers using phenomenological methods in nursing. Journal of Advanced Nursing 21: 1123–1129

Sandelowski M 1995 Focus on qualitative methods: sample size in qualitative research. Research in Nursing and Health 18: 179–183

Sandelowski M 2000 Whatever happened to qualitative description? Research in Nursing and Health 23: 334–340

Smith J A 1996 Beyond the divide between cognition and discourse: using interpretative phenomenological analysis in health psychology. Psychology and Health 11: 261–271

Streeton R, Cooke M, Campbell J 2004 Researching the researchers: Using a snowballing technique. Nurse Researcher 12(1): 35–45

Streubert H J, Carpenter D R 1999 Qualitative Research in Nursing: Advancing the Humanistic Perspective. Lippincott, Philadelphia

Svedlund M, Danielson E, Norberg A 1994 Women's narratives during the acute phase of their myocardial infarction. Journal of Advanced Nursing 35: 197–205

Swanson-Kauffman K, Schonwald E 1988 Phenomenology. In: Sarter B (ed) Paths to Knowledge: Innovative Research Methods for Nursing. National League for Nursing, New York: 97–105

Taylor B 1993 Phenomenology: one way to understand nursing practice. International Journal of Nursing Studies 30: 171–179

Van der Zalm J E, Bergum V 2000 Hermeneutic phenomenology: providing living knowledge for nursing practice. Journal of Advanced Nursing 31: 211–218

Van Manen M 1990 Researching Lived Experience: Human Science for An Action Sensitive Pedagogy. State University of New York Press, New York

Wall C, Glenn S, Mitchinson S, Poole H 2004 Using a reflective diary to develop bracketing skills during a phenomenological investigation. Nurse Researcher 11(4): 20–29

Walters A J 1995 The phenomenological movement: implications for nursing research. Journal of Advanced Nursing 22: 791–799

Wilson H, Hutchinson S 1991 Triangulation of qualitative methods: Heideggerian hermeneutics and grounded theory. Qualitative Health Research 1: 263–276

Yegdich T 2000 In the name of Husserl: nursing in pursuit of the things-in-themselves. Nursing Inquiry 7: 29–40

Chapter 23

Ethnography

Anne Williams

Introduction

Ethnography has the potential to make a strong contribution to researching nursing practice insofar as observation which lies at its heart provides access to aspects of practice that are not immediately visible when other research methods are used. Deirdre Wicks, a nurse and sociologist writing in 1998 about her ethnographic research to explore nurses and doctors at work in acute hospital settings, recalls an instance when she observed how nursing skills and knowledge involved in assessing the critical time to call a doctor to see a severely ill patient disappeared in the institutional process of reportage and documentation. The doctor's words written in his notes were recorded as follows: 'called to the ward to see ...'. Wicks tells us that 'the anonymous nurse's role in this disappeared in the medical actions that would now unfold' (p. 140).

Wicks' ethnography reports on aspects of practice which otherwise might have been taken for granted, and conveys the detail and complexity of relationships and processes involved in shaping nursing practice. It demonstrates how important it is to note what is seen *in situ* by researchers, if we are to understand a situation or event fully. Equally important as what is seen is what is heard, for what people say they do and what they believe and think about a given situation offers insights into the expectations, values and ideas that patients, professionals and others occupying the settings draw on in order to make sense of nursing practice.

This chapter focuses on the question, what is the nature of ethnography's contribution to researching nursing practice? In order to answer the question it is useful first of all to give a brief if inevitably partial account of the background from which ethnography has emerged. Following this, the contributions of a number of ethnographies which were undertaken to explore the organisation of nursing practice are discussed. I then draw from the discussion some key issues for us to consider if ethnography is to sustain its contribution to researching and understanding practice within the context of nursing.

Background: what is ethnography?

There are a number of ways of explaining ethnography. Brewer (1994, 2000), for example, has made a distinction between ethnography as methodology and ethnography as method. The former refers to a philosophical imperative to 'understand' how people experience their world and the latter to what ethnographers actually do, namely: to observe and listen through participant observation which, as others have observed, may involve observation alone or a more participative approach whereby researchers talk, work or even live in the company of those they encounter in the field of study (Burgess 1984, Hammersley & Atkinson 1995). In trying to define ethnography, this section of the chapter refers to both the idea of ethnography as methodology and to the methods that ethnographers actually use. The account given is influenced by my own experiences of studying anthropology, engaging with feminist ideas and above all my work as a nurse.

Roughly translated the word 'ethnography' means 'writing culture'. Ethnography refers to a long-established research tradition within the discipline of social anthropology, whereby early anthropologists sought to understand cultures other than their own through participant observation over a period of months and sometimes years. Typically research was conducted amongst relatively small groups of people or fairly self-contained societies, often previously unknown to the so-called developed world. The anthropologists wrote about what they observed and heard in these groups and societies, at the same time reflecting on this. The latter practice of reflecting was important as it allowed anthropologists not only to describe what they heard and saw in the field but also to analyse expectations, ideas, values and beliefs, in short the 'culture' characterising the groups of people they studied. Their analyses also allowed them to compare and contrast between and across a range of cultures. Furthermore, it allowed them to explore the differences and similarities between their own and other cultures. Classic accounts of the practice of ethnography include Malinowski's *Argonauts of the Western Pacific* (1922) in which, to summarise crudely, he describes a system of ceremonial exchange amongst the Trobriand Islanders. His work laid the foundation for further work on the importance of exchange, and the principle of reciprocity, as a means of maintaining social relationships and social control. Above all, despite the paternalism, colonialism and sexism inherent in much of the work undertaken in the early twentieth century (a criticism that could be levelled at far more recent ethnographic work), his wish was, as Kuper (1983) notes, to discover the Islanders' 'passions' and 'deepest ways of thinking'.

Since the early years of the discipline, anthropologists have extended their studies of culture and social organisation to include exploration within their own societies. This process was partly driven by critiques made by groups of people whom earlier anthropologists had studied. While they may have appreciated anthropologists' quests to explore other ways of life (a point noted by Mead in her autobiographical book *Blackberry Winter* (1972)), the legitimacy of statements made about the ideas and values of a group of people hitherto completely unknown to the anthropologist was questioned. Indeed the very process of going out to study another culture came to be viewed by some anthropologists themselves as a way of expropriating knowledge for gain which did not necessarily benefit the society studied, and which was then reconstructed to produce a 'Western' version of the society. Some thirty years ago Said in his magnificent book *Orientalism* (1978) referred to how this approach had constructed a particular discourse; Western anthropologists were producing Western versions or constructions of those they encountered. The critique led anthropologists to strive to 'see themselves' in their work (Wheeler 1973) and to consider how they, themselves, actually constructed 'otherness and 'other cultures', both 'at home' and 'abroad', drawing on their own ideas and values.

The movement to question the conduct and purpose of ethnography was given impetus by so-called radical anthropologists writing in the USA and the UK in the 1980s and 1990s, for example Clifford and Marcus (1986) in the USA, Atkinson (1990) in the UK. These and other authors drew attention to the devices used by anthropologists and others to persuade readers about the authenticity and truth of their observations as well as noting how what was written about other cultures could also be read as a statement about the anthropologist and the research community producing the knowledge. This written reflexivity was strengthened by the writings of feminists both in anthropology and sociology who drew attention to the diversity of possible ethnographies, even within one's own culture and society. For example, Stanley and Wise (1983) have drawn attention to how in some writings ostensibly conveying 'women's experiences' the category of 'women' is presented as homogeneous. Consequently some women may not recognise their experiences in the often very particular accounts written by social scientists with a specific purpose in mind and who are writing within a particular theoretical framework. Critiques such as these drew attention to how the ways in which ideas are interpreted and shaped and how they inform everyday life depends on a number of factors, not least the gender, race/ ethnicity, age and socio-economic status of the anthropologist.

Ethnographic research in nursing

Ethnographic research has been conducted within the various fields of nursing by nurses including those with anthropological or sociological training, and by other researchers. A classic early example from the USA is Oleson and Whittaker's *The Silent Dialogue* (1968) and, from the UK, Dingwall's *Social Organisation of Health Visitor Training* (1977). In the 1980s, accounts of nursing based on ethnographic research within the UK included David Hughes (1988) study of aspects of interaction between nurses and doctors and James' (1984) account of nurses working in palliative care. Work inspired by ethnography includes Melia's (1981) research on student nurses' understandings of their work, and work reflecting on how an ethnographic account is constructed includes the monograph *Reflections on the making of an ethnographic text* (Williams 1990), which draws on an ethnography of nursing in a London teaching hospital. In the 1990s there was a proliferation of ethnographic research including Smith's (1992) account of how nurses care and the emotional labour involved. Porter's work and his exposition of critical realist ethnography based on his ethnography of nursing's relationship with medicine (1993, 1994, 1995) is another example.

The scope and depth of ethnographic research is such that much of the work mentioned was produced first as PhD theses. Typically, periods of observation in ethnographic research may extend from six months or so to 18 months or more. The trend for conducting ethnographic research for the PhD degree has gained momentum, producing work spanning a variety of settings from acute care to primary care. Examples of the former include ethnographies carried out in intensive care settings, exploring the contemporary nursing role in relation to medicine (Coombs 2000) and ritual and symbolism in this setting (Philpin 2004). Also included in this category is Wiseman's study of the use of empathy in oncology wards (Wiseman 2003).

Examples of ethnographies conducted in primary care settings include Hughes' (2005) ethnography of nurses' experiences of strategic decision-making in local Health Boards in Wales, and Clark's (2001) ethnography of nursing care in Ethiopia. Ethnographic work has also been conducted in midwifery and related areas, for example Hunter's study of the emotional labour experienced by midwives (2002), Mills' research on aspects of contraception practices and meaning in Australia (2003) and Speier's highly reflexive, ethnographic account of the childbirth educator as ethnographer (2002).

These are only a few examples of the use of ethnography in answering questions about role and practice mainly but not exclusively within nursing and on its boundaries with other professions. A feature of much of this work is the attention paid to the role of the researcher who may enter the field as both researcher and practitioner. The challenges and opportunities this presents are for the most part described in detail in the theses themselves. While I do not intend to discuss these in this chapter, it is worth mentioning that taken as a whole they contribute to a critique of assumptions made about the nature of researcher–researched relationships, researcher identity and the construction of knowledge. They are sources worth reading for those contemplating ethnographic research insofar as they document in detail how the position of the researchers in relation to the fields of study affects the products of research. In short they deal with the issue of reflexivity.

Reflexivity in the context of ethnography

Seeing and hearing within the context of an ethnography are not simple matters. They are possible, as Whittaker (1986, p. xvi) suggests, 'through decisions and strategies, which in their turn demand a highly developed sense of what are data and what are irrelevancies'. An ethnographer goes into the field of study with a working frame of reference, however underdeveloped it may be. To take Wicks as an example, her frame of reference rested in part on an interest in competing discourses: the dominant discourses of scientific medicine, on the one hand, and holistic, bedside healing, on the other. Her interest in these inevitably helped to filter out aspects of what was going on in the wards she visited as well as making other aspects highly significant. In short, the account she gives is very particular.

As in other methods discussed in this collection, reflexivity in assessing an ethnographer's theoretical position is by now taken as axiomatic to rigorously conducted ethnographic research. This is so even though some might suppose that the outputs of observation or what is seen promise greater objectivity than the products of interviews or what is heard from people accounting for their actions. For example, actions captured on videotape may appear to be more objective than 'subjective' accounts given by those involved in those actions. Degrees of objectivity within ethnographic fieldwork are debatable; however, an ethnographer's frame of reference (like a photographer's frame) inevitably affects perspective and even when the evidence seems incontrovertible the representation of that evidence and its interpretation may differ between ethnographers. Cross referencing between researchers (inter-rater reliability) may help ameliorate uncertainties about truth. However, researcher reflexivity indicates recognition of the possibility that the product or ethnographic account produced is affected by the position of the researcher in relation to the field of study, and shows how this is so. This is not simply in relation to preferences and personality but rather in relation to the theories and ideas held by the researcher which form the backdrop against which she or he understands the data and findings are discussed.

Thus reflexivity is part of the process of addressing the strength or weight of evidence insofar as situating ethnographic findings within the context of the ethnographer's interests and perspective gives the reader a sense of how the findings have been shaped. It is a necessary part of the process of showing through discussion and debate how project findings either confirm or challenge existing knowledge already published about the topic in question.

A case illustration: exploring what nurses do when they go to work

Amongst recent reviews of ethnographic work, Allen's (2004) *Re-reading nursing and rewriting practice: towards an empirically based reformulation of the nursing mandate* is concerned with ethnographic evidence that answers the question, what do nurses do when they go to work? The review is highlighted in this chapter because it provides a rigorous, evidence-based illustration of how a number of ethnographies not only reveal taken-for-granted aspects of practice but, taken together, provide the basis for a critique of long-established theories upon which we base and understand our practice as nurses.

As Allen notes, her review of ethnographic work questions the idea that nursing practice is based on an individualised, unmediated, caring relationship which has for many generations acted as the theoretical, if not always evidence-based, foundation for how we educate nurses. Indeed, her review of a decade of ethnographic studies of nursing leads her to conclude that contemporary nursing may be better described as being shaped by interrelated bundles of activity', namely: managing multiple agenda, circulating patients, bringing the individual into the organisation, managing the work of others, mediating occupational boundaries, communicating information, maintaining a record, and prioritising care and rationing resources. Within and across these bundles of activity nurses are constituted as heath care intermediaries who negotiate care with patients and other health care professionals. From this perspective nurses reconcile requirements of the organisation with patients' wishes; they broker, interpret and translate clinical,

social and organisational information. Further, nurses are blurring the jurisdictional boundaries of their practice with other groups' boundaries – patients and professionals – in order to ensure continuity of care (Allen 2004, pp. 273–280).

This picture of nursing work may appear to be less inspirational than the idea of a special and intimate relationship between nurse and patient; however, it does help to explain why it is sometimes so difficult for nurses to clearly articulate what it is they do. An important point for the present discussion is that the evidence for Allen's assertions is based on systematic and sustained observations across a range of settings and from a variety of perspectives, both of which, in conjunction with a reflexive approach, are recognised across qualitative methodologies and methods at least as ways of establishing research rigour and credibility. The range and diversity of approaches in the research referred to in this particular review are outlined below.

One methodology, different approaches

Allen takes as her evidence ethnographic field studies where observation was the central component of investigation. As Allen notes (2004, p. 272), the ethnographies analysing the social organisation of nursing practice covered many settings including hospitals, community and nursing homes in a number of countries including the UK, USA, Canada, Sweden and Belgium. The majority of the research was conducted in hospital settings (Allen 2004, p. 272). There is variation, as she also points out, in the approaches taken by the researchers in conducting their research. Some undertook the research as a detached non-participant observer (Tjora 2000); some as a paid member of nursing staff and therefore as participant (Henderson 1995, Porter 1995), with most researchers falling between these two extremes.

With regard to the ways in which the ethnographies were framed theoretically, some studies had a single theoretical framework (Sbaih 2002, Vukic

& Keddy 2002). Others employed more than one to develop theory (Savage 1995, Wicks 1998) and a number provided descriptive accounts (Jervis 2002, Kneafsey & Long 2002, Waters & Easton 1999). There was also variation in the ways in which the research was represented. Some authors made a very clear separation between the field data and analysis, pressing home the importance of objectivity and accuracy, for example Allen (2001), Purkis (1996), Purkis (2001a, 2001b). Others adopted a narrative style which, as Allen suggests, reflects a concern to convey a particular way of viewing nursing work rather than painstaking accuracy. These authors include Annandale et al (1999), Foner (1994), Henderson (1995) and Latimer (2000).

Diversity of approach is a distinguishing feature of ethnographic research and those who write about the conduct of ethnography within health care settings, and more broadly, have grappled with the issue of how best to categorise and understand the various approaches taken. Useful reading includes many articles and texts, written from varying discipline perspectives, notably anthropology and sociology; some politically motivated and some pursuing the subject from the standpoint of the health care professional. Readings include those which by now have acquired the status of a 'classic text', for example *The Ethnographic Imagination* (Atkinson 1990), *Ethnography, Principles in Practice* (Hammersley & Atkinson 1995) and *What's Wrong with Ethnography* (Hammersley 1992).

Building on ethnographic insights

Despite the different settings, perspectives and research questions posed within the studies she reviewed, Allen (2004, p. 272) notes that the observational studies showed remarkable similarities. However, she writes: 'an interesting feature of the literature reviewed was the relatively low level of cross referencing between publications'. She continues in a footnote to the study:

This might reflect the fact that a number of studies were carried out simultaneously and therefore the authors may have been unaware of each other's work. It might also reflect dominant intellectual trends in the ethnographic tradition, which tend to emphasise the cultural uniqueness of social settings rather then their points of connection with similar contexts.

She makes the useful point that the interlinkages she recognised by looking across a body of work adds weight to the argument that future studies would do well to take greater account of existing knowledge, adding that there is also a need to build on and develop prior ethnographic work. This latter comment may at first glance appear to run counter to the current steer towards multiple methods as a feature of programme building. Read another way it emphasises the importance of developing strength within methodologies in order to contribute more effectively to multi-method research programmes. Allen's review, itself, shows how observation can identify aspects not readily apparent using other methods. It also is an important example of how analyses of a critical mass – in this case a number of ethnographies – provides a platform for questioning taken-for-granted assumptions about the theories upon which we base our practice as nurses. Specifically it provides a critique of the theory that practice is based on the 'unmediated care of *individuals*' to consider practitioners' relationship to health care *systems* and their role in constituting *contexts of care* '(Allen 2004, p. 279, her emphasis). As such it potentially provides a platform from which to reassess how we prepare nurses for what they will actually encounter on the wards.

Insofar as Allen bases her argument on evidence provided by studies in which observation was identified as the central component of exploration, there is a sense in which 'looking' and 'seeing' are privileged, theoretically at least, over 'listening' and 'hearing', although we cannot assume the latter actions and senses involved were totally absent in the conduct of individual ethnographies. There is, however, a case to be made for the importance of understanding what drives and motivates nurses in what they actually do, how they understand their work and how they justify what they do as 'nursing practice', Furthermore, it may be the case that what nurses (and others) say they do or say they ought to do illuminates what we see and how we understand nursing practice.

What is ethnography's contribution to researching nursing practice?

Ethnography offers methods which allow researchers insights into the taken-for-granted details of the everyday and often mundane practices of nursing. It offers an approach which gives a better reflection of the complexity of practice than methods which rely solely on numerical analyses. Nursing colleagues in clinical practice quite often pose questions involving a degree of complexity that is difficult to respond to using methods such as the randomised controlled trial or surveys. Ethnography is a resource that can be used to build an evidence base that allows the extraordinariness of ordinary, everyday nursing practice to be given due consideration. As the case illustration discussed in this chapter demonstrates, one of the outcomes may be that we are challenged to reassess our assumptions about nursing practice.

Moreover, if data within such studies are scrutinised and treated rigorously, taking account of their complexity; if due care is given to establishing the grounds on which knowledge claims are being met and rigour and reflexivity are applied at all stages of the research, then we can begin to build

high quality evidence and critical mass in areas of nursing practice that other methods find hard to reach. This in turn provides a potentially strong basis for synthesis, theorising and debate on issues of substance which affect the ways in which we prepare and educate nurses of the future.

Conclusion

In attempting to answer a question about the nature of ethnography's contribution to researching nursing practice the chapter has limited itself to exploring the emergence of ethnography essentially within the boundaries of the discipline of anthropology. Those who wish to pursue the aetiology of ethnography may wish to look outside the boundaries set. Similarly the discussion of ethnography within the context of nursing and health care organisation and practice is partial; however, it is hoped that the case illustration is illuminating and will prompt further exploration. Indeed, the selected issues highlighted in the chapter take us beyond the inevitable limits of the chapter's scope to consider the potential of ethnography for sustaining its contribution to researching and understanding practice within the context of nursing.

Acknowledgements

I would like to thank Davina Allen for generously allowing me to use her review of ethnographic work. I would also like to thank both Davina Allen and John Keady for their helpful comments on an earlier draft of the chapter.

References

Allen D 2001 The Changing Shape of Nursing Practice: the Role of Nurses in the Hospital Division of Labour. Routledge, London

Allen D 2004 Re-reading nursing and rewriting practice: towards an empirically based reformulation of the nursing mandate. Nursing Inquiry 11: 271–283

Annandale E, Clark J, Allen E 1999 Interprofessional working: an ethnographic case study of emergency health care. Journal of Interprofessional Care 13: 139–150

Atkinson P 1990 The Ethnographic Imagination: Textual Constructions of Reality. Routledge, London

Brewer T 1994 The ethnographic critique of ethnography: sectarianism in the RUC. Sociology 28(1): 231–244

Brewer T 2000 Ethnography. Open University Press, Buckingham

Burgess R G 1984 In the Field: An Introduction to Field Research. George Allen and Unwin, London

Clifford J, Marcus G E 1986 Writing Culture: The Poetics and Politics of Ethnography. University of California Press, Berkeley

Clark J 2001 Oppression and caring: a feminist ethnography of working to improve patient care in Ethiopia. Unpublished PhD thesis, Trinity College, Dublin

Coombs M 2000 Medicine, nursing and policy development in intensive care: an ethnography to explore the contemporary nursing role. Unpublished PhD thesis, Oxford Brookes University.

Dingwall R 1977 The Social Organisation of Health Visitor Training. Croom Helm, London

Foner N 1994 The Care Giving Dilemma, Work in an American Nursing Home. University of California Press, Los Angeles

Hammersley M 1992 What's Wrong with Ethnography. Routledge, London

Hammersley M, Atkinson P 1995 Ethnography: Principles in Practice, 2nd edn. Routledge, London

Henderson J N 1995 The culture of care in a nursing home: effects of a medicalized model of long term care. In: Henderson J (ed) Nursing Home Ethnography. Bergin and Garvey, Westport, CT: 37–54

Hughes A 2005 The experiences of nurses on Local Health Group Boards in Wales: a gendered analysis. Unpublished PhD thesis, University of Wales, Swansea

Hughes D 1988 When nurse knows best: some aspects of nurse/doctor interaction in a casualty department. Sociology of Health and Illness 10: 1–22

Hunter B 2002 Emotion work in midwifery: an ethnographic study of the emotional work undertaken by a sample of student and qualified midwives in Wales. PhD, University of Wales, Swansea

James N 1984 'Postscript to nursing'. In: Bell C, Roberts H (eds) Social Researching. Routledge and Kegan Paul, London

Jervis L L 2002 Working in and around the chain of command: power relations among nursing staff in an urban nursing home. Nursing Inquiry 9: 13–24

Kneafsey R, Long A F 2002 Multidisciplinary rehabilitation teams: the Nurse's role. British Journal of Therapy and Rehabilitation 9: 24–29

Kuper A 1983 Anthropology and Anthropologists: The British Modern School. Routledge and Kegan Paul, London

Latimer J 2000 The Conduct of Care: Understanding Nursing Practice. Blackwell, Oxford

Malinowski B 1922 Argonauts of the Western Pacific. E P Dutton, New York

Mead M 1972 Blackberry Winter: My Earlier Years. William Morrow, New York

Melia K 1981 Student nurses' accounts of their work and training: a qualitative analysis. Unpublished PhD Thesis, University of Edinburgh

Mills A 2003 Knowing contraception: exploring meanings and practices. Unpublished PhD thesis, University of Technology, Sidney, Australia

Oleson V, Whittaker E 1968 The Silent Dialogue: a Study in the Social Psychology of Professional Socialization. Jossey-Bass, San Francisco

Philpin S 2004 An interpretation of ritual and symbolism in an intensive therapy unit. Unpublished thesis, University of Wales, Swansea

Porter S 1993 Critical realist ethnography: the case of racism and professionalism in a medical setting. Sociology 27: 591–609

Porter S 1994 The occupation of nursing and its relationship to medicine (Dept Sociology). Unpublished PhD thesis, The Queen's University, Belfast

Porter S 1995 Nursing's Relationship with Medicine. Avebury, Aldershot

Purkis M E 1996 Nursing in quality space: technologies governing experiences of care. Nursing Inquiry 3: 101–111

Purkis M E 2001a Governing the health of populations: the child, the clinic and the 'conversation'. In: Young L E, Hayes E (eds) Transforming Health Promotion Practice: Concepts, Issues and Applications. FA Davies, Los Angeles CA: 190–206

Purkis M E 2001b Managing home nursing care: visibility accountability and exclusion. Nursing Inquiry 8: 141–150

Said E 1978 Orientalism. Random House, New York

Savage J 1995 Nursing Intimacy: An Ethnographic Approach to Nurse Patient Interaction. Scutari Press, London

Sbaih L C 2002 Meanings of the immediate: the practical use of the patients charter in the accident and emergency department. Social Science and Medicine 54: 1345–1555

Smith P 1992 The Emotional Labour of Nursing: How Nurses Care. Macmillan, London

Speier D 2002 The childbirth educator as ethnographer: a feminist retrospective ethnography of a professional practice. Unpublished PhD thesis, University of Manchester

Stanley L, Wise S 1983 Breaking Out: Feminist Consciousness and Feminist research. Routledge and Kegan Paul, London

Tjora A H 2000 The technological mediation of the nursing–medical boundary. Sociology of Health and Illness 22: 721–741

Vukic A, Keddy B 2002 Northern nursing practice in a primary health care setting. Journal of Advanced Nursing; 40: 542–548

Waters K, Easton N 1999 Individualised care: is it possible to plan and carry out? Journal of Advanced Nursing; 29: 79–87

Wheeler T 1973 To See Ourselves; Anthropology and Modern Social Issues. Scott, Foresman and Company, Glenview, IL

Whittaker E 1986 The Mainland Haole; The White Experience in Hawaii. Columbia University Press, New York

Wicks D 1998 Nurses and Doctors at Work: Rethinking Professional Boundaries. Open University Press, Buckingham

Williams A 1990 Reflections on the Making of an Ethnographic Text. Studies in Sexual Politics Monograph No 1, University of Manchester.

Wiseman T 2003 An ethnographic study of the use of empathy on an oncology ward. Unpublished PhD, RCN Institute/University of Manchester.

Chapter 24

Delphi Studies

Hugh McKenna and Sinead Keeney

Introduction: what is the Delphi technique?

I have brought golden opinions from all sorts of people. (Macbeth vii: *31*)

The Delphi technique is a structured process, which uses a series of questionnaires (or rounds) to gather information. The process continues until 'group' consensus is reached (Beretta 1996, Green et al 1999). It has grown in popularity recently within nursing research (McKenna 1994a). Like questionnaires, it allows the inclusion of a large number of individuals across diverse geographic locations and expertise; unlike questionnaires, the Delphi aims to gather consensus of opinion, judgement or choice. In face-to-face meetings a specific member or members might dominate the discussions. One of the advantages of the Delphi is that the members (experts) do not meet and their comments and preferences are gained through anonymised surveys leading towards consensus (Jaiarth & Weinstein 1994).

Background

The Delphi technique was originally developed by the RAND Corporation where its initial purpose was technological forecasting for the military. Since its inception the Delphi technique has evolved into a number of modifications. Each type of Delphi has the same aim – to gain consensus on the issue at hand – but differs in the process used to reach this consensus. The different types of Delphi include the classic Delphi (McIlfatrick & Keeney 2003), the modified Delphi (McKenna 1994a), the policy Delphi (Crisp at al 1997), the real-time Delphi or conference Delphi (Beretta 1996) and, more recently, the e-Delphi (Avery et al 2005). There are many studies reporting on these different manifestations, demonstrating the flexibility of the method.

The Delphi process

The classic Delphi involves the presentation of a questionnaire to a panel of 'informed individuals' in a specific field of application, to seek their opinion on a particular issue. Data are summarised and a new questionnaire is designed based solely on the results obtained from the first application. This second instrument is returned to each subject and they are asked (in the light of the first round results), to reconsider their initial opinions. Repeat rounds may be carried out until consensus of opinion, or a point of diminishing returns, has been reached.

In essence, the Delphi technique is a multistage approach with each stage building on the results of the previous one. Hitch and Murgatroyd (1983) see it as resembling a highly controlled meeting of experts, controlled by a chairperson who is adept at summing up the feelings of the meeting by reflecting the participants' own views back to them in such a way that they can proceed further – the only difference is that the individual responses of the members are unknown to one another. In the first round of any Delphi investigation, a wide divergence of individual opinion is typical. Nevertheless, after several iterations there is a tendency for subjects to converge towards consensus.

The modified Delphi is similar to the classic Delphi but uses interviews or focus groups to gather the first round opinions (McKenna 1994a). The policy Delphi is used mostly within organisations to examine and explore policy issues (Turoff & Linstone 2002) with 10 to 50 people as a precursor to a committee meeting and used to explore the advantages and disadvantages of a certain issue. A face-to-face committee would then use the Delphi results to formulate the required policy.

The real-time or conference Delphi uses the Delphi process in a 'real-time' setting, eliminating the delay caused by the pen-and-paper type Delphi. It takes the form of panel members undertaking rounds face-to-face and analysis being undertaken in situ between each round (Linstone & Turoff 2002). The e-Delphi is a newer approach and has developed as a result of advancing technology. This is the administration of either the classic or modified Delphi electronically by email or completion of an online form (Avery et al 2005).

Defining the Delphi

According to Dalkey and Helmer (1963), the Delphi technique is 'a method used to obtain the most reliable consensus of opinion of a group of experts by a series of intensive questionnaires interspersed with controlled feedback' (p. 458). With increasing usage, broader definitions have been put forward. For instance, Reid (1998) believes the 'Delphi' is a method for the systematic collection and aggregation of informed judgement from a group of experts on specific issues.

Lynn et al (1998) defined the Delphi technique as an iterative process designed to combine expert opinion into group consensus. Most definitions attempt to encompass or highlight the ever-adapting Delphi process in one sentence, resulting in broad and varying interpretations. Regardless of definition, the purpose of the technique is to achieve consensus among a group of experts on a certain issue where no agreement previously existed.

The lack of uniformity in the use of the technique has spawned criticism from some researchers stating that the emergence of modifications of the technique poses a threat to its credibility and to the validity and reliability of the research findings (Sackman 1975). Box 24.1 outlines the characteristics of the original classic Delphi (McKenna 1994a), from which modifications have developed.

Sampling and the use of experts

The Delphi does not use a random sample which is representative of the target population, but rather employs 'experts' as panel members. This means that each panel member is an expert in the area of

Box 24.1 – *Characteristics of a classic Delphi (McKenna 1994a)*

1. The use of a panel of 'experts' for obtaining data
2. Participants do not meet in face-to-face discussions
3. The use of sequential questionnaires and/or interviews
4. The systematic emergence of a concurrence of judgement or opinion
5. The guarantee of anonymity for participants' responses
6. The use of frequency distributions to identify patterns of agreement
7. The use of two or more rounds, between which a summary of the results of the previous round is communicated to and evaluated by panel members

interest. Experts have been defined as: a group of 'informed individuals' (McKenna 1994a); 'specialists' in their field (Goodman 1987); and someone who has knowledge about a specific subject (Green et al 1999). For example, a study that investigates the changing role of the midwife may include midwives who are knowledgeable about the subject under consideration (Lemmer 1998).

Sackman (1975) and Linstone and Turoff (1975) criticised the use of experts, as did Strauss and Zeigler (1975) who claimed that valid expert opinion is scientifically untenable and overstated. Similarly, in her critical examination of the Delphi, Goodman (1987) noted that:

It would seem more appropriate to recruit individuals who have knowledge of a particular topic and who are consequently willing to engage in discussion upon it without the potentially misleading title of 'expert' (p. 732).

One other criticism of the selection of experts is the potential for selection bias affecting the results. For example, if you were seeking consensus on whether the Labour Party should lead the UK government in the next 10 years, there is obvious bias in having the panel composed entirely of Labour Party members!

Panel selection

Deciding on the experts to include in the Delphi panel is regarded as the 'linchpin of the method' (Green et al 1999). There is little agreement in the literature regarding the relationship of the panel to the larger population of experts and the sampling method used to select such experts (Green et al 1999, Williams & Webb 1994). Guidance from the literature suggests that, when using the Delphi, it is not necessary to calculate sample size using power calculations. Beretta (1996) stated 'representative sample techniques may be inappropriate when expert opinions are required' (p. 83). Previously, Goodman (1987) pointed out that, originally, the Delphi 'tends not to advocate a random sample of panellists' (p. 730). Moreover, Helmer (1977) argued that:

... a Delphi inquiry is not an opinion poll, relying on a random sample ... rather once a set of experts has been selected (regardless of how) it provides a communication device for them, that uses the conductor of the exercise as a filter in order to preserve anonymity of responses. (p. 17).

In contrast, Reid (1998) maintained that the generalisability of results cannot be claimed unless it can be stated that these panels constitute a genuine population.

The importance of using 'criteria' to select a Delphi sample is an area that has grown in popularity (Keeney et al 2006). For example, these may include having published at least one paper in the area of investigation if it is an academic issue, or having 10 years' clinical experience in a certain role if the area of investigation requires specific clinical knowledge. Criteria can be simple or multilayered depending on necessity. Simple criteria can denote gender, age or educational attainment.

Panel size

There is no universal agreement on what size the sample should be when using the Delphi technique.

Box 24.2 – *Factors to consider regarding sample size*

- Consider the number of experts in the field and purposively select a sample, taking into account location, grade etc. (see below under sample selection).
- Select a manageable sample – there is considerable administration with a Delphi and the larger the sample the more work will be needed.
- Consider time constraints as this will have an impact on the sample size – the larger the sample, the more time will be spent following up people to return the questionnaire as you will want to maximise the response rate as much as possible.
- Generally the larger the sample, the poorer the response rate. If the sample can be kept small and incorporate interested experts, a good response rate is more likely, which in turn will increase the chances of a good level of consensus.

Linstone (1978) reported on studies using several hundred panellists and a Japanese Delphi that had several thousand panellists. Dalkey and Helmer (1963) stated that a suitable number is seven and that accuracy deteriorates with less and improves with more. Alexander and Kroposki (1999) asserted that the sample size should be over 60, while Burns (1998) argued for 15. Beech (1999) suggested that this disagreement over sample size is one of the disadvantages of conducting a Delphi study, whereas Box 24.2 outlines the important factors to consider when deciding on the size of the sample for the Delphi technique.

Anonymity and confidentiality

It should be noted that complete anonymity is not possible when using the Delphi technique. However, lack of complete anonymity is a fact that many researchers who use the Delphi do not address. The researcher needs to be able to link panel members with their responses, which threatens true anonymity. The reason for this is that the researcher may provide feedback in the form of individual response to the previous round as well as the overall group response.

This lack of complete anonymity may raise ethical issues in relation to confidentiality. It is vital that the researcher makes it clear that responses will be visible to the researcher but not to the other panel members. This will ensure that the participant is fully informed before deciding whether to participate.

Panel members often know other panel members, but cannot attribute responses. It is like being in an elite 'expert' club where the membership is known but they do not meet face-to-face. McKenna (1994a) uses the term 'quasi-anonymity' to describe this situation. Sackman (1975) argued that this can lead to a lack of accountability for the views expressed, while Goodman (1987) maintained that it encourages hasty ill-considered judgements. However, Rauch (1979) postulates that knowing who the other subjects are should have the effect of motivating the panellists to participate.

This promise of quasi-anonymity also facilitates panel members to be open and truthful about their views; this, in turn, provides insightful data for the researcher. The only difficulty may be if a panel member and the researcher know each other and the former's responses are influenced because of this. Such panel members may be excluded from the study.

The basis of the Delphi is that panel members alter their views towards consensus as the study progresses. However, it is unclear whether they do this on the basis of new information or, despite the protection of quasi-anonymity, feel pressurised to conform to the 'group think'.

Delphi rounds

Within the Delphi technique the number of rounds depends upon the time available and what type of Delphi the researcher has employed, raising the question of how many rounds it takes to reach consensus. The original classic Delphi used four rounds (Young & Hogben 1978). However, this has been modified by many to suit individual research aims and in some cases it has been shortened to two or three rounds (Beech 1997, Green et al 1999) by using focus groups or interviews as a substitute for the first qualitative round (Keeney et al 2006). The difficulty with a three or four rounds Delphi is keeping the panel members interested and committed to returning each round. The topic needs to be of great interest to the panel members or they have to be rewarded in other ways, otherwise the response rate can suffer.

Round one

The purpose of round one, regardless of the type of Delphi, is to generate ideas. The panel members are asked for their responses to, or comments about, an issue. In the classic Delphi the questions are open-ended, allowing panel members freedom in their responses. The number of responses generated from this can be large, especially if the researcher opts to include all responses in round two and maintain the original language. While this is adhering strictly to the original Delphi format, difficulties may include alienation of the sample due to the length of subsequent questionnaires and the time required to complete it (Green et al 1999, Keeney et al 2006). Furthermore, if questions are poorly phrased or rephrased inappropriately by the researcher, the reliability and validity of data may be compromised.

The modified Delphi often uses focus groups, interviews, statements derived from the literature or case study scenarios to replace this first qualitative round (Endacott 1998, Keeney et al 2006, McKenna 1994b). Here data can be content analysed into specific statements and the numbers of statements can be controlled. However, researcher bias in interpretation could be a difficulty.

There is now some support for revising these approaches and providing pre-existing information to help in the ranking of responses, for example,

from the existing literature or recent relevant empirical research. This approach could introduce bias, limit the available options, or omit recent opinion that may not be publicly available. Nonetheless, a clear advantage in this approach is that it could introduce efficiency in a technique that has the potential to be extremely time-consuming (Jenkins & Smith 1994).

Subsequent rounds

Subsequent rounds generally use the format of structured questionnaires and include individual and group feedback. Panel members can change their responses in the light of the group's views. Responses are analysed and used to form a new questionnaire. It has been illustrated that this iterative process encourages involvement, motivation, ownership and acceptance of the findings (McKenna & Keeney 2004, Walker & Selfe 1996).

Response rate

A poor response rate in the final rounds of the Delphi technique is a difficulty that most researchers using the method will encounter. For example, in Farrell and Scherer's research (1983) into identifying consensus on suitable nursing standards, returns were disappointing. Of a sample of 1441 nurses, 662 agreed to participate; only 472 returned the questionnaires in round one and 141 responded to the second. This is a common occurrence, but seldom discussed in any report of results.

It is important to achieve a high response rate in the first round as it is inevitable that panel members will drop out. Furthermore, the more rounds undertaken, the greater the potential for dropout. To achieve consensus, it is important that those panel members who have agreed to participate stay involved until the process is completed (Buck et al 1993). On the other hand, McKenna (1994b) found that using face-to-face interviews in the first round increased the return rates of postal questionnaires in the second. This minimised the number of postal rounds and increased the commitment of the panel members who felt more involved in the process. McKenna's (1994b) study achieved a 100% response rate, which is very rare in Delphi studies.

Consensus

Achieving consensus on a certain issue does not mean that the correct answer has been found. It means that consensus has been reached among a panel of participants. In addition, the Delphi has been criticised as a method which forces consensus and is weakened by not allowing participants to discuss issues; no opportunity arises for respondents to elaborate on their views (Goodman 1987, Walker & Selfe 1996). However, bearing this in mind, consensus can be gained and the Delphi can be used as a useful, integral consensus technique.

Lindeman (1975) maintained that the Delphi is especially effective in difficult areas which can benefit from subjective judgements on a collective basis, but for which there may be no definitive answer. Therefore, it would be difficult, if not impossible, to achieve 100% consensus between any group of people on such issues and experts are no exception. A key concept within the Delphi and one which has stimulated much debate is what percentage constitutes consensus. Loughlin and Moore (1979) believed that 51% was an acceptable consensus level. Other researchers have set much higher levels including Green et al (1999), who set their consensus level at 80%, and McKenna and Hasson (2001), who used a level of 75%. While there is no universal agreement or guidelines on the level of consensus, Keeney et al (2006) suggested that researchers should decide on the consensus level before commencing the study and consider using a high level of consensus such as 75%.

Application of the Delphi in nursing research

In recent years the Delphi technique has become increasingly prevalent in nursing research. The classic or modified Delphi are the types most preferred by nurse researchers, although the e-Delphi appears to be increasing in usage. For example, Gibson (1998) used a three-round classic Delphi to identify the content and context of nurses' continuing professional development needs. Irvine (2005) also used a three-round classic Delphi to gain consensus on the competencies necessary for district nurses in health promotion. McKenna (1994b) used a modified Delphi to gain consensus on the essential elements of a practitioner's nursing model.

The Delphi is often used to identify guidelines or set priorities. Bond and Bond (1982) used the technique to establish clinical nursing research priorities, as did others (Annells et al 2005, Cohen et al 2004, Daniels & Ascough 1999, Forte et al 1997, Lindeman 1975, Lynn et al 1998, Soanes et al 2000). Boxes 24.3 and 24.4 outline a Delphi study undertaken by McIlfatrick and Keeney in 2003.

Reliability and validity

As with any study, issues of rigour and trust are important. At present there is no evidence of the reliability of the Delphi as a method. No study has yet been undertaken to determine whether the results would be the same if the same information was given to more than one panel made up of experts from the same field. Keeney et al (2006) suggested that for this reason, Lincoln and Guba's (1985) criteria for rigour in qualitative studies could be applied. These are: credibility (truthfulness), fittingness (applicability), auditability (consistency) and confirmability.

Validity is also an area of difficulty for the Delphi. Hill and Fowles (1975) suggested that threats to validity emerge from the pressures put on panel members to change their opinion in line with the group response. However, Goodman (1987) believed that because panel members have in-depth knowledge of the issue under investigation, content validity is assured. Furthermore, she states that the use of successive rounds increases concurrent validity.

Box 24.3 – *Identifying cancer nursing research priorities using the Delphi technique (McIlfatrick & Keeney 2003)*

Aim: the aim of the study was to facilitate a strategic approach to cancer nursing research by identifying the research priorities of cancer nurses.

Sample: the sample was constituted of 60 panel members recruited at a cancer nursing conference.

Method: a three-round Delphi was used. While it was a 'pen-and-paper' Delphi, the first round was circulated to the panel members at a cancer nursing conference. Rounds two and three were administered as postal rounds. The first round was the classic Delphi but administered at a conference. Box 24.4 outlines the question posed to panel members in round one. The results were summarised and formed the basis for round two where panel members were asked to rate each research priority for importance on a Likert scale of 1–7, with 1 being high importance and 7 being low importance. The researchers set the consensus level at 65%. The third round questionnaire was formulated from the round two responses.

Results: the response rates for rounds two and three were 78% and 91% respectively. Feedback was provided within round three incorporating individual and group feedback. For all items in round three a higher level of consensus was gained than in round two. All items except one achieved consensus. The top priority areas for research were psychosocial issues, for example communication and information needs; professional issues relating to nurse burnout, stress and nurse-led care; and context of care issues including continuity of care.

Outcome: the identified priorities helped to provide direction and focus for the development of a cancer nursing strategy for Northern Ireland.

Box 24.4 – *Round one questionnaire (McIlfatrick & Keeney 2003)*

Survey of cancer nursing research priorities: Round one

Please list below five important questions or problems relating to oncology/palliative nursing practice which you consider need to be researched. The questions might relate to a current area of patient care or a new idea or innovative technique.

You may have difficulty identifying as many as five problems. However, we encourage you to return the questionnaire, irrespective of how many problems you can identify, so that you may be involved in reviewing the ideas expressed by others.

When writing the problems, please be as specific as you can. For example instead of 'Investigate the treatment of stomatitis', the question 'Is Corsodyl mouthwash effective in the prevention and treatment of stomatitis?' is more specific and useful. Other examples might be 'Compare a selection of dressings for ability to control odour from malignant wounds' or 'What are the informational needs of a patient at the start and during chemotherapy?'

Conclusion

This chapter has presented a critical exploration of the Delphi technique. The process and the problems of definition have been explored. Sampling issues have been discussed including the use of expert panels, defining expertise and advising on the best use of the expert panel. Anonymity has been scrutinised and the concept of quasi-anonymity introduced. Consensus levels have been debated, as has the importance of the researcher understanding that achieving consensus may not be the same as finding the correct answer. Finally, response rates have been considered, as has the concept of rigour.

EXERCISES

1. Access examples of each type of Delphi from the literature and explore the common themes across each type and the differences between them. Assess which type of Delphi would be most suitable for different research questions in nursing and list the reasons why this is the case.
2. Decide which type of Delphi you are going to use for your study. Write inclusion criteria for your expert panel. Identify whom you would invite to participate in your panel and how they meet the criteria that you have set. It may be necessary to adjust your criteria depending on the numbers of experts required.
3. Design the first round of your Delphi. This could be an open-ended postal questionnaire, a list of statements derived from the literature in the form of a Likert scale, an interview schedule for face-to-face interviews, a focus group schedule or a case study scenario.

References

Alexander J, Kroposki M 1999 Outcomes for community health practice. Journal of Nursing Administration 29: 49–56

Annells M, Deroche M, Koch T, et al 2005 A Delphi study of district nursing research priorities in Australia. Applied Nursing Research 18: 36–43

Avery A J, Boki S P, Sheikh A, et al 2005 Identifying and establishing consensus on the most important safety features of GP computer systems: e-Delphi study. Informatics in Primary Care 13: 3–12

Beech B F 1997 Studying the future: A Delphi survey of how multi-disciplinary clinical staff view the likely development of two community mental health centres over the course of the next two years. Journal of Advanced Nursing 25: 331–338

Beretta R 1996 A critical review of the Delphi technique. Nurse Researcher 3(4): 79–89

Bond S, Bond J 1982 A Delphi survey of clinical nursing research priorities. Journal of Advanced Nursing 7: 565–567

Buck A J, Gross M, Hakim S, et al 1993 Using the Delphi process to analyse social policy implementation – a post hoc case study from vocational rehabilitation. Policy Sciences 26(4): 271–288

Burns F M 1998 Essential components of schizophrenia care: a Delphi approach. Acta Psychiatrica Scandinavica 98: 400–405

Cohen M Z, Harle M, Woll A M, et al 2004 Delphi survey of nursing research priorities Oncology Nursing Forum 31: 1011–1018

Crisp J, Pelletier D, Duffield C, et al 1997 The Delphi method? Nursing Research 46: 116–118

Dalkey N, Helmer O 1963 Delphi Technique: characteristics and sequence model to the use of experts. Management Science 9: 458–467

Daniels L, Ascough A 1999 Developing a strategy for cancer nursing research: identifying priorities. European Journal of Oncology Nursing 3: 161–169

Endacott R 1998 Needs of the critically ill child: a review of the literature and report of a modified Delphi study. Intensive Critical Care Nursing 14: 66–73

Farrell P, Scherer K 1983 The Delphi Technique as a method for selecting criteria to evaluate nursing care. Nursing Papers 15: 51–60

Forte P S, Ritz L J, Balestracci Jr M S 1997 Identifying nursing research priorities in a newly merged healthcare system. Journal of Nursing Administration 27(6): 51–55

Gibson J M E 1998 Using the Delphi to identify the content and context of nurses continuing professional development needs. Journal of Clinical Nursing 7: 451–459

Goodman C M 1987 The Delphi technique: a critique. Journal of Advanced Nursing 12: 729–734

Green B, Jones M, Hughes D, et al 1999 Applying the Delphi Technique in a study of GPs' information requirement. Health and Social Care in the Community 7: 198–205

Hill K Q, Fowles J 1975 The methodological worth of the Delphi forecasting technique. Technological Forecasting and Social Change 7: 193–194

Hitch P J, Murgatroyd J D 1983 Professional communications in cancer care: a Delphi survey of hospital nurses. Journal of Advanced Nursing 8: 413–422

Helmer O 1977 Problems in Futures research: Delphi and casual cross-impact analysis. Futures 9: 17–31

Irvine F 2005 Exploring district nursing competencies in health promotion: the use of the Delphi technique. Journal of Clinical Nursing 14: 965–975

Jairath N, Weinstein J 1994 The Delphi methodology (Part One): A useful administrative approach. Canadian Journal of Nursing Administration 7: 29–40

Jerkins D, Smith T 1994 Applying Delphi methodology in family therapy research. Contemporary Family Therapy 16: 411–430

Keeney S, Hasson F, McKenna H P 2000 Consulting the oracle: ten lessons from using the Delphi technique in nursing research. Journal of Advanced Nursing 53: 1–8

Lemmer B 1998 Successive surveys of an expert panel: research in decision making with health visitors. Journal of Advanced Nursing 27: 538–545

Lindeman C A 1975 Delphi survey of priorities in clinical nursing research. Nursing Research 24: 434–441

Lincoln Y S, Guba E G 1985 Naturalistic Inquiry. Sage, London

Linstone H A 1978 The Delphi technique. In: Fowles R B (ed) Handbook of Futures Research. Greenwood, Westport, CT

Linstone H A, Turoff M 1975/2002 The Delphi Method: Techniques and Applications. Addison-Wesley, Reading, MA (republished 2002)

Loughlin K G, Moore L F 1979 Using Delphi to achieve congruent objectives and activities in a paediatrics department. Journal of Medical Education 54: 101–106

Lynn M R, Layman E L, Englebardt S P 1998 Nursing administration research priorities: a national Delphi study. Journal of Nursing Administration 28(5): 7–11

McIlfatrick S J, Keeney S 2003 Identifying cancer nursing research priorities using the Delphi technique. Journal of Advanced Nursing 42: 629–636

McKenna H P 1994a The Delphi technique: a worthwhile approach for nursing? Journal of Advanced Nursing 19: 1221–1225

McKenna H P 1994b The essential elements of a practitioners' nursing model: a survey of clinical psychiatric nurse managers. Journal of Advanced Nursing 19: 870–877

McKenna H P, Hasson F 2001 A study of skills mix issues in midwifery: a multi method approach. Journal of Advanced Nursing 37: 95–113

McKenna H P, Keeney S 2004 Leadership within community nursing in Ireland north and south: the perceptions of community nurses, GPs, policy makers and members of the public. Journal of Nursing Management 12: 69–76

Rauch W 1979 The decision Delphi. Technological Forecasting and Social Change 15: 159–169

Reid N 1998 The Delphi Technique: its contribution to the evaluation of professional practice. In: Ellis R (ed) Professional Competence and Quality Assurance in the Caring Profession. Chapman and Hall, London

Sackman H 1975 Delphi Critique. Lexington Books, Lexington, MA

Soanes L, Gibson F, Bayliss J, et al 2000 Established nursing research priorities on a paediatric haematology, oncology, immunology and infectious diseases unit: a Delphi survey. European Journal of Oncology Nursing 4: 108–117

Strauss H J, Ziegler L H 1975 The Delphi technique: An adaptive research tool. British Journal of Occupational Therapy 61: 153–156

Turoff M, Linstone H A 2002 The Delphi Technique: Techniques and Applications. Digital Version. Online. Available: http://www.is.njit.edu/pubs/delphibook/ 5 Sept 2006 (originally published in 1970)

Walker A M, Selfe J 1996 The Delphi method: a useful tool for the allied health researcher. British Journal of Therapy and Rehabilitation 3: 677–681

Williams P L, Webb C 1994 The Delphi technique: An adaptive research tool. British Journal of Occupational Therapy 61: 153–156

Young W H, Hogben D 1978 An experimental study of the Delphi technique. Education Research Perspective 5: 57–62

Chapter 25

Longitudinal Studies

Roger Watson

Introduction

Chapter 17 was concerned with the ways data can be obtained using a range of non-experimental methods using cross-sectional studies. An extension of the use of survey methods, longitudinal studies, are considered in this chapter. If you wish to know how something changes over time either as a result of an intervention or for no other reason than the passage of time – a prime example being ageing (see, for example, Wenger et al 1999) – then longitudinal studies are required.

Longitudinal studies are characterised, as distinct from cross-sectional studies, by the collection of data at two or more time points (Watson 1998). Two or three time points – although there are exceptions – are common because there are many difficulties associated with gathering data across more time points (McKenna et al 2006). This chapter will consider some of the analytical methods associated with longitudinal studies but will mainly be concerned with addressing the practical aspects of longitudinal studies.

Why do we need longitudinal studies?

It is possible to study ageing, for example, using cross-sectional or longitudinal studies. If we wish to study whether or not age and cardiovascular disease are linked we could take a large sample of people with a wide range of ages at one time. We are very likely to find that there is a link between ageing and cardiovascular disease but we may be limited in the use to which that information could be put. If we wish to make short-term projections about use of health service resources then the data may be useful. However, if we wish to make long-term projections about the link between age and cardiovascular disease the data are less useful. In any such study, the older people who were included have lived through very different times and experiences from the younger people in the study who would, in turn, become the older people of the future. During the lifetime of the older people in the study, many changes influencing cardiovascular disease will have taken place such as nutrition, improvements in health services, awareness of smoking and sedentary lifestyles and these will, possibly, have had more influence on the younger than the older people in the sample. Therefore, it may not be valid to compare young and old people sampled at the same time and this is referred to as a 'cohort effect' (Polit & Hungler 1995). The influence of such a cohort effect on any future predictions of the link between age and cardiovascular disease is very hard to predict. For example, it may lead to fewer older people having cardiovascular disease due to better health education and health care. Conversely, it may also lead to more older people with cardiovascular disease in future as improvements in health care increase the survival time of those with cardiovascular disease.

The way to overcome the cohort effect is to carry out a longitudinal study whereby the same group of people is followed over a long time with several data collection points. Cross-sectional studies are still used, however, especially in studies of ageing. They are quick and relatively cheap. If we wanted to study the effect of ageing over a 50-year period, the person initiating the study is unlikely to be alive at its conclusion and few researchers would be willing to commit to this. However, a notable exception is the Baltimore Longitudinal Study on Ageing established in 1958 by Nathan Shock (http://www.grc.nia.nih.gov/branches/blsa/blsa.htm – accessed 30 April 2007). On the other hand, in educational studies, where the progress of students

is being followed over a programme there is little excuse for not conducting a longitudinal study, especially when personnel changes, curriculum changes and so forth may induce a profound cohort effect.

Who should be included in longitudinal studies?

Longitudinal studies can include repeated cross-sectional studies where the same data are gathered at subsequent times regardless of who is included at each time. Such studies are favoured by the organisations that test political affiliations. However, such a design is relatively weak because the same people are not necessarily sampled at each time (Watson 1998). Such studies are called trend studies (Polit & Hungler 1995). The purpose of longitudinal studies is to measure change and the weaknesses in repeated cross-sectional studies are obvious and mainly relate to the fact that any change that is observed may simply be due to the fact that different people have been included in the cross-sectional samples. While efforts should be made to ensure that such samples are representative of the population and that bias is minimised, it is impossible to be certain that what is observed is not an artefact of who has been included at each time.

The strongest design in longitudinal studies is one where the same people are included at each time (Watson 1998). These studies are called cohort studies (Parahoo 2006, Polit & Hungler 1995). This is especially true where the effect of an intervention is being studied. In such a study, only those who have had the intervention, and possibly a control group, could possibly be of interest and, to be certain that it was the intervention that was being studied, only people studied before the intervention or at the first point in the study should be included (Elliott & Hayes 2003). A baseline for each subject has to be established to provide a mean baseline for the group receiving the intervention and for the control group. The introduction of other subjects later in the study would threaten the validity of the results.

Longitudinal studies are not easy

However, despite the superiority of longitudinal over cross-sectional or even repeated cross-sectional designs, they are inherently difficult to conduct. They are expensive due to their length and it can be difficult to obtain funding; they do not offer a very 'quick return' for research funding investment, making them unattractive to some researchers and research funding bodies. However, the primary problem with longitudinal studies is that of attrition (Polit & Hungler 1995): the loss of subjects throughout the study and the concomitant difficulty of finding people who are, initially, willing to enter into a long-term relationship with a research team and, thereafter, willing to remain in the study. Even if people enter a longitudinal study, with the best will in the world, it may be difficult or impossible to find them in subsequent waves of a study – especially if the time between waves is significant (years) and the study is very long. The reasons are obvious: apart from dying or not wishing to remain in the study, people move home during the course of a study. In addition, the research team may change or funding may not be secure for the proposed duration of the study.

Attrition

The problem of attrition is the main consideration in any longitudinal study. Given that it is quite possible to have 50% attrition in a study with relatively short periods between waves and with a population that is not mobile (Watson et al 1999a and 1999b), then you can imagine the problem in studies with extended periods between waves and including mobile populations. There is no easy solution to this problem. The solution most often applied is to ensure that the initial wave of the study begins with a sample size that is sufficient to withstand attrition over several waves, leaving a sufficient sample size for analysis across all the time waves. Clearly, with no effort to stem attrition between waves, this is very expensive and wasteful. For example, if the aim is to have a sample size of 200 people in the final wave of a study to permit robust statistical analysis and there are four waves in the study, then the initial sample size, if attrition is estimated at 50% between each wave of the study, would have to be 1600 people. If we also take into account that there may only be a 50% return rate of data at any of the waves of the study, then the problem is further compounded and the initial sample size needs to be 3200. This is a very large sample size for any research study and the initial expense will be very high. The likelihood of conducting a study which requires the above numbers will also be dependent on the group that is being studied. For example, if you wish to study the general population, then this could relatively easily be carried out in one city. However, if you wanted to study student nurses, then you would have to include nearly all of the departments of nursing in the UK.

Addressing attrition

It is clear that one of the major problems to be addressed in longitudinal studies is attrition. The most cost-effective way of conducting a longitudinal study is to keep the initial sample size as small as possible and then to maintain a high proportion of that sample for the duration of the study. In addition, the duration of the study should be as long as necessary to gather the data of interest and no longer. For example, if two waves of a longitudinal study will provide you with all the information you need about some phenomenon then a third wave is unnecessary. Several strategies can be applied to maintain a sample in a longitudinal study. However, the key strategy is to ensure the commitment of the people who are entering at the start of the study. In effect, this is no different from ensuring that people participate in any study, whether cross-sectional or longitudinal. However, any negative experiences of participating in the first wave of a longitudinal study will compound any deficiencies in your strategy to get people to participate in the first place. Most of what follows is based on experience of conducting longitudinal studies with nursing students (Watson et al 1999a and 1999b); the BMJ (http://bmj.bmjjournals.com/epidem/epid.7.html – accessed 30 April 2007) and the Centre for Longitudinal Studies also offer excellent advice (http://www.cls.ioe.ac.uk – accessed 30 April 2007).

Therefore, when inviting people to participate in a longitudinal study it must be made clear to them at the outset that their participation will be required for a period of time – maybe years. Comprehensive and clear information must be provided to potential participants and this should be written such that it is readable by all of the participants – the same level of education and ability with language as the researchers must not be assumed and readability indices (e.g. Flesch index (http://csep.psyc.memphis.edu/cohmetrix/readabilityresearch.htm – accessed 30 April 2007)) can be used for this purpose to make sure that sentences are not too long and paragraphs are not too complex. Jargon should be avoided and any necessary technical terms should be explained. If the above information appears in a separate information sheet, then this should be accompanied by a friendly, short and informative covering letter; again this should be readable. The letter should be headed by an appropriate logo and the name and address and contact details of the person writing the letter – to whom any enquiries should be invited – should be clear. The letter should be signed – personally if possible. Participants will have to provide their consent to take part in the study and the key features of the study, any inconvenience that may arise and any reward or incentive that may be provided should have been clearly explained in the information about the study, so that potential participants can provide informed consent. All the usual assurances about confidentiality and security of research data and their ability to withdraw from the study at any point must be provided. Finally, in the process of obtaining informed consent, opportunity to ask questions and to have them answered should be provided. The value of the person to the study and the necessity for its longitudinal nature should also be emphasised.

Keeping people in the study

Once the study is under way, i.e. once the first wave of data has been collected, it is essential to maintain contact with the participants – using almost any excuse to do so. It is an excellent idea to write to all those who took part in the first wave thanking them for taking part and reminding them of their importance to the study and when they can expect to hear from you again. If you promised to provide them with feedback from the first wave – if this is possible and does not compromise the study – then it is essential that you follow through with this. If feedback on actual data and analysis is not possible, then you could let them know how many people actually took part in the first wave and how well the data were collected. If the sample is likely to be mobile – and the longer the time between waves of a study is then the more essential this becomes – you should ask participants to let you know if they change address or employment; anything that may make it more difficult for you to trace them in subsequent waves. This should be made as easy as possible for participants by, for example, providing them with a prepaid return envelope and a card to complete. However, you should also give them the chance to phone you or email you if they prefer. You cannot expect participation in the study to be the priority of people who may be busy, moving house or changing jobs; therefore, you may consider contacting them on a regular basis to find out if their contact details remain the same. If you have established a website for the study then they should be given the web address.

Methodological considerations

The above are very practical, almost common sense, aspects of a longitudinal study but there are also methodological considerations to make the outcome of your study as successful as possible. Meticulous planning is required and, if possible, at the beginning of the study, the precise details of data collection at each time wave should have been planned. Put simply, you want to make the data collection process as easy as possible for yourself and your participants. To do this you need to consider what data you need to collect and why. The most basic consequence of this is that you should gather every piece of data that you need and no data that you do not need. You must resist the temptation to gather additional, unplanned data, as the study progresses. Moreover, this may have ethical implications as you will have been granted permission to gather certain data and if you have to gather more, then a renewed ethical application may be required.

Without good reason only one questionnaire on one aspect of a study should be included. For example, it could be unnecessary to administer two questionnaires measuring psychological morbidity or quality of life, respectively. You should decide which of several options is best for your study and only administer that one. Again, unless absolutely necessary, the same questionnaire should not be administered more than once in a study. Clearly, the phenomenon of interest will have to be measured at each point but the basic demographics should only be gathered at the start and any questionnaire gathering data such as personality or mental ability should only be administered at the start as these are unlikely to change. This is demonstrated in the study by Deary et al (2003). Similarly, if you are only interested in a phenomenon such as burnout at the end of the study and not on how it changes during the study, then this should only be gathered at the end of the study. Clearly, the best point at which to administer most questionnaires is at the start of the study when you have most participants and they are most motivated to participate. The strategy used in a longitudinal study of nursing students in Scotland illustrates this (Watson et al 199a, 1999b). Repeated and redundant questionnaires indicate a poor design and will also lessen people's desire to remain in the study – make it as easy as possible to be a participant.

Questionnaires

One way to avoid unnecessary questionnaires is to revisit the aims and objectives of the study

repeatedly at the design stage. You must avoid, at all costs, the problem of simply adding another questionnaire because someone in the research group or even outside it thinks it is a good idea. Do not allow the study to be used to gather data not central to what you are trying to achieve. The development of questionnaires is considered in Chapter 29.

If possible you must avoid altering questionnaires – other than for obvious errors, during the course of a study. Some longitudinal studies – over many years – suffer from this and by the end of the study the data that are being gathered bear little relationship to the data gathered at the start of the study; again, this indicates poor design and a drift away from the initial research questions. A good strategy is to decide upon a minimum data set and adhere to it throughout. If alterations to questionnaires do become necessary – perhaps as a result of a change in policy in the area you are investigating or a change in job titles or clinical practice, then ensure that the minimum data set is not compromised.

Good record keeping is essential and good filing of hard copy returned questionnaires is also essential. The best time to enter data onto a database is immediately upon completion of a wave of the study and the labelling of items in the database should be consistent, clear and logical. For example, if you have used the GHQ-12 at each time point, the data should be entered in the same way each time, in the same order and using the same labels, except to indicate the time wave. Thus, for the first item of the GHQ, you could label it GHQ1 and for the first time wave it could be GHQ1T1 and for the same item at time 2 it could be GHQ1T2 and so on. Scales should be totalled and psychometrics, such as internal consistency and factor structure, done at each time wave to ensure that the questionnaires have been administered and completed, and data entered properly.

Analysis

Analysing longitudinal studies is more complex than analysing cross-sectional studies because, in addition to any relationships between variables at the same time, the relationship of variables across time has to be analysed. In fact, it is precisely this relationship that is made possible by longitudinal studies (Watson 1998).

One of the most basic pieces of information that has to be reported, as with any study, is the number of people in the study and the demographic data: in a longitudinal study you need to report these at each wave of the study. These data will help you to see how many people have dropped out of the study across time (this will be inevitable regardless of your best efforts to retain participants) and also if any particular group has been more subject to attrition than another, for example men or women, young or old.

Simple experiments are really basic forms of longitudinal study either where there is a simple before and after design (pre-test/post-test) or where a treatment group and a control group are being compared, as in a randomised controlled trial (RCT). In both cases data will be gathered at two points in time: either before and after for the whole group or before and after for both groups – to compare change in a treatment group with the control group. As explained in Chapter 35, either a dependent t-test or an independent t-test would be appropriate, respectively, to test if the difference in the mean value of the dependent variable has either changed significantly between pre- and post-test, or between the treatment and the control group. The pre-test/post-test design and the RCT can both be extended over time to more than two time waves and, in such a truly longitudinal study, it is possible – but not advisable – to carry out t-tests between each wave of the study and/or between the treatment and control group at each time wave. However, this strategy is likely to be very confusing and hard to interpret due to the multiple t-tests that would have to be performed. You could measure the difference between the first and final waves of the study but then you would lose a great deal of information contained in the intermediate waves – and this would negate the point of conducting the longitudinal study in the first pace.

Where change in an independent variable is being studied across several waves, an appropriate test is a repeated measures ANOVA; this is analogous to the ANOVA described in Chapter 35. Either a single factor repeated measures ANOVA or a two factor repeated measures ANOVA is used depending on whether a single group is being followed across time or two groups are being compared as in a study of the effect of counselling on psychological morbidity in inflammatory bowel disease (Smith et al 2002). The repeated measures ANOVA takes time into account and provides a solution which tells you if the change in the independent variable is significant across the whole study. This is useful as the difference between the two groups at each time may not be the same. For instance, the difference between the two groups may become greater over time or it may become less and, in the case of therapies such as counselling, the difference may become apparent after one wave of the study but as the effect of intervention wears off, the difference may become smaller. It would be very easy for someone trying to convince you that the therapy worked to select the waves where the difference was greatest and ignore the waves where the effect was reduced.

Single-case studies

Sometime referred to as time-series analysis, single-case studies, or single-case experiments provide another way of analysing longitudinal data. These studies are considered in more detail in Chapter 19 and are principally concerned with interventions. The name single case can be misleading as a single case can be an individual or a unit. In one sense, the single-case study is a series of before and after studies with a case being defined and studied prior to an intervention – the baseline period – an intervention being introduced and the case being studied after the intervention for any change in a variable of interest. There are many variations on the single-case study and the above would be described as an AB study. The simplest variation is the ABA study where the intervention is withdrawn and the variable of interest studied again. More complex variations are possible with the use of multiple baselines for different variables and the introduction of more than one intervention.

Multivariate analysis

There are several advanced statistical methods of analysing longitudinal studies which take into account several variables simultaneously. These methods have largely been subsumed within and superseded by multilevel modelling, which is likely to become routine in the analysis of longitudinal studies. Multilevel modelling, as the name suggests, is a technique for modelling data at several levels. Therefore, if a study measures outcomes such as general health and includes demographic variables such as age, gender and occupation and is also longitudinal, then multilevel modelling is applicable (Campbell 2001). An additional advantage of multilevel modelling is its ability to handle missing data.

Conclusion

Longitudinal studies are essential if phenomena are to be studied over time. However, special attention needs to be paid to a range of factors when establishing a longitudinal study. The most important consideration in a longitudinal study is the retention of subjects and the prevention of attrition and, while this is an inevitable aspect of any longitudinal study, there are many ways of addressing it. Principally, a well-designed study which inconveniences participants the least will have the greatest chance of success.

A range of analytical strategies is available for longitudinal studies but the essential feature of any analysis is to obtain good data. Again, this will be largely dependent upon your design and on the instruments you use to obtain the data. Missing data detract from longitudinal studies and, again, design is important. Well-designed instruments that are easy to complete will ensure good data; it is pointless retaining people in a study if the data they provide are poor.

EXERCISES

1. Make two columns on a sheet of paper headed 'cross-sectional' and 'longitudinal', respectively. List the advantages of each and then draw a line across the paper below which you should list the disadvantages of each.
2. Design a longitudinal study to investigate a topic of your choice and try to build in features which will overcome some of the disadvantages of longitudinal studies.
3. Multilevel modelling is now the statistical method of choice for analysing longitudinal data; find out as much about this method on the internet as you can, bearing in mind that it is also referred to as random effects and mixed effects modelling. Try to understand what advantages it offers over more traditional analyses.

References

Campbell M J 2001 Statistics at Square Two: Understanding Modern Statistical Applications in Medicine. BMJ Books, London
Deary I J, Watson R, Hogston R 2003 A longitudinal study of burn out and attrition in nursing students. Journal of Advanced Nursing 43: 71–81
Elliott D, Hayes L 2003 Observational designs and methods. In: Schneider Z, Elliott D, LoBiondo-Wood G, Haber J Nursing Research: Methods, Critical Appraisal and Utilisation, 2nd edn. Mosby, Sydney: 295–315

McKenna H, Hasson F, Keeney S 2006 Surveys. In Gerrish K, Lacey A (eds) The Research Process in Nursing, 5th edn. Blackwell, Oxford: 260–273

Parahoo K 2006 Nursing Research: Principles, Process and Issues, 2nd edn. Palgrave, London

Polit D F, Hungler B P 1995 Nursing Research: Principles and Methods, 5th edn. Lippincott, Philadelphia

Smith G D, Watson R, Roger D, et al 2002 Inflammatory bowel disease patients: impact of a nurse led counselling service upon quality of life. Journal of Advanced Nursing 38: 152–160

Watson R 1998 Longitudinal quantitative research designs. Nurse Researcher 5(4): 41–54

Watson R, Deary I J, Lea A 1999a A longitudinal study into the perceptions of caring and nursing among student nurses. Journal of Advanced Nursing 29: 1228–1237

Watson R, Deary I J, Lea A 1999b A longitudinal study into the perceptions of caring among student nurses using multivariate analysis of the Caring Dimensions Inventory. Journal of Advanced Nursing 30: 1080–1089

Wenger G C, Burholt V, Scott A 1999 Bangor Longitudinal Study of Ageing: Final Report to the Wales Office of Research and Development for Health and Social Care. National Assembly, Cardiff

Chapter 26

Triangulation

Seamus Cowman

Introduction and background

Triangulation aims to enhance the process of empirical research by using multiple approaches to address research problems. It is claimed that the strengths of one approach will compensate for the weaknesses of another. Multiple approaches may involve, either singularly or combined, more than one method, investigator, data collection sources or multiple theoretical perspectives. Nurse researchers, for example, in identifying the need to incorporate quantitative and qualitative approaches in providing a comprehensive insight into a research problem, have adopted a triangulation of methods as a research approach.

Experienced nurse researchers have generally become polarised in their approach to research through the exclusive use of either a quantitative or qualitative paradigm, one type of data or one theoretical perspective. Within the literature there is general support for the separateness of research approaches, for example qualitative and quantitative paradigms (Duffy 1987). However, in accepting the differences between the approaches, there has been concern among nurse researchers that neither approach in isolation will provide an understanding of human beings and of their health-related needs and nursing care. For more than 20 years there has been an increasing range of nursing literature highlighting the merits of triangulation and demonstrating its use in a wide variety of nursing and midwifery situations (Carin 2005, Carr 1994, Cowman 1993, Shih 1998, Williamson 2005).

Origin and description of triangulation

Triangulation is a term originally used in navigation as a strategy for taking multiple reference points to locate an unknown position. Triangulation was first described as research by Campbell (1956); Campbell and Fiske (1959) are acknowledged as the first researchers to apply triangulation when they promoted a multiple methods approach. One of the earliest and most recognised authorities on the use of triangulation was Norman Denzin. His first book laid down the earliest understandings and definitions of triangulation; Denzin (1970) discussed triangulation as the combination of multiple methods in a study of the same object or event to depict more accurately the phenomenon being investigated.

However, Denzin (1989) later extended his definition from the measurement of discrete concepts to the level of research design, an approach he terms multiple triangulation. Denzin believed that the purpose of multiple triangulation is to overcome the intrinsic bias of single method, single observer, single theory studies, thus confirming the researcher's results and conclusions. Similarly Polit and Hungler (1999) presented a more embracing description of triangulation as the use of multiple methods or perspectives for the collection and interpretation of data about a phenomenon to obtain an accurate representation of reality.

Types of triangulation

In terms of understanding and application Denzin (1970) identified four main types of triangulation (Table 26.1) which were subsequently discussed by Duffy (1987), Mitchell (1986) and Sohier (1988). There have been attempts to distinguish other types of triangulation, such as interdisciplinary triangulation (Janesick 1994) and conceptual triangulation (Foster 1997).

Data triangulation

Data triangulation, or source triangulation, involves the collection of data from multiple sources for

Table 26.1 – *Triangulation summary*

Type of triangulation	Characteristic features
Data triangulation	Uses many different data collection sources in the same study. Time; space; person
Investigator triangulation	Uses more than one researcher to collect and analyse data
Theory triangulation	Use of multiple theoretical perspectives and hypotheses to draw inferences from the data collected in a study
Methodological triangulation	Within-method: involves the combination of approaches from the same research tradition/paradigm in the same study to measure the same variable(s)
	Between-method: involves the combination of approaches from both quantitative and qualitative research traditions. Dissimilar but complementary methods are used with across-method phenomena to try and achieve convergent validity

analysis in the same study with each source focused upon the phenomenon of interest. The characteristic features of data triangulation are that it permits the researcher to discover which dimensions of the phenomenon are similar and which dissimilar across settings and which change over time and which differ by group membership (Mitchell 1986). Such an approach facilitates the researcher's attempts to maximise the range of data which might contribute to a complete understanding of the topic being investigated (Knafl & Breitmayer 1989). Denzin (1989) described three subtypes of data triangulation:

- time;
- space;
- person.

Time triangulation represents the collection of data on the same phenomenon at different points in time (e.g. hours, days, weeks), with a purpose of validating the congruence of the phenomenon across time.

Space triangulation is the collection of data on the same phenomenon at different sites (two or more settings) to test multiple-site consistency and rule out across-site variation.

Person triangulation refers to data collection from more than one level of persons (groups or families), or collectives (communities or organisations). Given the broad range of individual background and experience, Knafl and Breitmayer (1989) highlighted the importance of varying data sources by persons. The socialisation process and the experiences and interactions of these individuals are also important.

Investigator triangulation

Investigator triangulation involves the use of multiple observers, interviewers and coders. Instead of employing more than one method, the researcher makes use of more than one researcher with an underlying aim of counteracting the potential shortcomings of one investigator. Investigator triangulation, therefore, introduces greater reliability in data collection, analysis and interpretation of results.

Theory triangulation

Theory triangulation involves the use of multiple theoretical perspectives and hypotheses to draw inferences from data. It may involve the use of multiple professional perspectives to interpret a single set of data. This method may characteristically entail using professionals outside of the researcher's field of study. Theory triangulation may also incorporate the use of rival hypotheses, testing existing theories and proposing new theories. Denzin (1989) claimed that setting alternate theories against the same body of data is an efficient means of criticism and it conforms to the scientific method.

Methodological triangulation

Methodological triangulation, which predominates in the nursing literature, involves the use of more than one research method in one study, which may occur at the level of design or data collection technique (e.g. structured instrument, observation and interviews).

One of the main strengths of methodological triangulation is to serve as a means of overcoming the methodological divide between quantitative and qualitative paradigms. The polarisation in the use of nursing research methods which has arisen is based on the disparate nature of the principles constituting the two paradigms and has created a separatist versus a combinationist debate. Leininger (1985) described the separatist as a nurse researcher who remains purely committed to either the qualitative or quantitative research perspective. Such nurse researchers want each perspective to remain separate so that neither will be contaminated. In contrast, combinationists believe that they must combine two methods. In defining qualitative research as theory developing, hypothesis generating and quantitative research as modifying, hypothesis testing, Field and Morse (1985) have identified the complementary nature of both.

The nursing literature, in particular, contains discourse on the application of methodological triangulation and its appropriateness as a means of reconciling the use of quantitative and qualitative methods in nursing research (Begley 1996, Bradley 1995, Carr 1994, Cowman 1993, Foss & Ellefsen 2002, Kimchi et al 1991, Redfern & Norman 1994, Sim & Sharp 1998). The primary purpose of methodological triangulation in research is the investigation of a different dimension of the research question being studied. Jick (1979) suggests that this type of triangulation is ideally used when studying complex concepts that contain many dimensions and triangulation facilitates a search for a logical pattern in results. Jick portrays the researcher using triangulation as a 'builder and creator, piecing together many elements of a complex puzzle into a coherent whole' (p. 144).

One of the original tenets of triangulation was validation of results through confirmation (Denzin 1970). The critical factor is that methodological triangulation attempts to overcome the deficiencies inherent in a single method through the use of multiple methods which counterbalance each other, thereby overcoming threats to the validity of findings. To promote validity through methodological triangulation, Denzin (1978) identified two approaches:

- within-method;
- between-method.

Within-method involves the combination of approaches from the same research paradigm in the same study to measure the same variable(s) (Kimchi et al 1991). For example, a qualitative researcher may use interviews and the maintenance of a journal to provide personal data which are then subjected to content analysis to identify recurrent themes or concepts arising from the data. The within-method has been the subject of criticism, even from Denzin (1978), when he suggested that, in many cases, the researcher is still only applying one method (e.g. the use of survey instruments) and the weaknesses of the method still remains.

Between-method, sometimes referred to as across-method, is the most popular type of triangulation. It involves combining approaches from both quantitative and qualitative research traditions. Dissimilar but complementary methods are used with across-method phenomena to achieve convergent validity. It allows for the combination of both qualitative and quantitative methods of data collection within the same study. Denzin (1978) claimed that, by combining methods, observers can achieve the best of each while overcoming their unique deficiencies. The chronology of application of either qualitative or quantitative approaches is raised by Morse (1991) as being either simultaneous or sequential. Morse's distinction is determined by the nature of the theoretical framework and research question/s underpinning the research. In research where theory is inductive, then, ideally qualitative methods should predominate, supported by quantitative methods, and vice versa in research with a deductive theoretical framework.

Multiple triangulation

Multiple triangulation refers to the use of a combination of two or more of the forms of triangulation including data triangulation, investigator triangulation, theory triangulation and methodological triangulation. It is suggested that combining different types of triangulation allows a comparative framework to emerge from the data.

Epistemology of triangulation

There are several arguments in favour of using triangulation in nursing research, such as the complexity of health services, understanding of which calls for multiple methods and perspectives (Foss & Ellefson 2002). Triangulation, by reconciling the paradigmatic assumptions inherent to qualitative and quantitative methods, can provide rich data whilst limiting the propensity to make oversimplified conclusions. Different types of knowledge are gained through different methods; however, the danger is that a researcher may lose sight of the differences underlying the chosen methods. The epistemology of triangulation should not be portrayed as a mix of two different epistemological positions but, rather, be seen as an epistemological position in its own right. Sim and Sharp (1998) discussed an epistemological paradox involved in seeking to use triangulation as a means of validation in qualitative research. The concept of validation assumes a single objective reality whereas qualitative research is founded on the notion of multiple realities. Denzin and Lincoln (1994) claim that triangulation is not a tool or a strategy of validation, but an alternative to validation.

Strengths and weaknesses of triangulation

There are strengths and weaknesses to triangulation (Table 26.2); Bradley (1995) identified that it

Table 26.2 – *Main strengths and weaknesses of triangulation in nursing research*

Main strengths	Main weaknesses
Attempts to reconcile paradigmatic assumptions inherent to quantitative and qualitative research approaches	May lose sight of the differences underlying various methods
Aims for congruence between different types of data	Differentiation of different types of data
Potential to produce rich and productive data	Can produce large volumes of data
Facilitates a process of validation of results	Can result in superficial treatment of some data
Increases completeness in a study	Potential for discrepant findings
Facilitates holistic interpretation and discovery in research	Can be time-consuming and expensive

was initially introduced as a technique to overcome some of the weaknesses of qualitative research in the 1950s and 1960s. I suggest that, by reconciling the paradigmatic assumptions inherent to qualitative and quantitative methods, triangulation has the potential to provide rich and productive data (Cowman 1993).

Generally, both quantitative and qualitative methods have their appropriate areas of application where research questions can be successfully investigated. Triangulation affords the opportunity to combine the advantages of both approaches, through building qualitative and quantitative methods on each other. For example, the results of a qualitative analysis can be used to design a more quantitative study; in particular, the construction of questionnaires and measurement approaches consistent with research objectives. Alternatively,

qualitative approaches can be built on quantitative results. In terms of data collection, Duffy (1987) notes that certain benefits may accrue through the use of triangulation:

- By using qualitative methods prior to quantitative methods, replies to surveys can provide leads for subsequent interviews and observations. Also the requirement to ask background information during an interview could be eliminated should these questions have been answered by the respondents in a previously administered questionnaire;
- Quantitative data can provide information about informants or subjects initially;
- The use of a survey instrument that collects data from all respondents may serve to correct the qualitative research problem of collecting data from only an elite group within the system.

Triangulation, through building qualitative data on quantitative data, has the advantage of enriching the findings though, not alone providing discrete results from quantitative data, and of providing insightful understandings which explain the statistical results.

Triangulation may also facilitate a process of validation of results when results from one part of a study are confirmed by congruent results from other parts of the study. Triangulation can also increase completeness (Shih 1998) when one part of a study presents results which have not been found in other parts of the study. The new information can be complementary to other results, or it may present divergent information.

Wendler (2001) promotes meta-matrix as a construction for second level analysis in triangulation following traditional quantitative and qualitative data analyses. The process of meta-matrix analysis includes the creation of the matrix itself, transcription of data into the matrix, coding data and noting reflections, seeking common phrases and isolating patterns and processes. By using meta-matrix, spontaneous comments and naturalistic events may be obtained and used. This approach, with a focus on capturing the unfolding of the natural and ordinary life and world under study, ensures that the research is embedded in its context.

Triangulation has inherent limitations. In the first instance a researcher may lose sight of the differences underlying the chosen methods. There is a danger of collecting large volumes of data which cannot be analysed or which could be treated superficially. Fielding and Fielding (1986) stressed the danger of multiple methods without simultaneously using the bias checking procedures. Ammenwerth et al (2003) argue that different types of data (e.g. words, figures) obtained by different sources cannot really validate each other, as they present different perspectives and can, therefore, not really be congruent.

The use of different methods in a single study can result in an increase in the amount of resources required due to the number of data collectors needed to gather the different types of data, to analyse the copious data obtained. The use of multiple methods in triangulation requires that the researcher(s) have a wide range of knowledge and expertise on complex designs, methods, analysis and interpretation. Mitchell (1986) discusses this aspect in terms of numerical data (quantitative) and linguistic or contextual (qualitative) data being combined and interpreted; managing overlapping yet divergent concepts arising from the data that are not clearly differentiated; should each data source be weighted? Finally, should each method be considered equally valid and thus weighted equally?

Validity

Complementary results obtained from quantitative and qualitative data can provide some modified type of validation; however, triangulation should not be used as an approach to address the problems of bias, error, invalidity that may be inherent to research work. On the other hand, Silverman (2001), in terms of validity of interpretation, suggests that drawing data from different contexts allows a true 'state' of affairs to emerge, increasing the study's validity. Jick (1979) discusses a

completing, as well as a confirming function to triangulation. He goes on to argue that triangulation can be something more than simply scaling, reliability, and convergent validation; it will ensure a more complete holistic and contextual portrayal of the unit(s) under study.

DePoy and Gitlin (1994) highlighted the alternative role of triangulation in measurement validity by making a distinction between 'triangulation for confirmation' (i.e., to achieve criterion related validity) and 'confirmation for completeness' (i.e., to secure content validity). Having described the completeness function, Shih (1998) described triangulation not as a guarantee of the validity of research, but as a strategy for deepening the analysis in studies and, consequently, as Bradley (1985) suggested, it provides the researcher with greater confidence in the validity of the results. Williamson (2005) agues that the 'convergent function' of triangulation is potentially valuable for quantitative researchers trying to develop measurement instruments. This contrasts with the 'completeness' function of triangulation, which is more likely to be useful to qualitative researchers.

Measurement and criterion related validity are debated by Sim and Sharp (1998) and they suggest that, in triangulation, one of the methods must be granted some form of prior, privileged status as a criterion measure. This may require the researcher to decide in advance of conducting the study that one method is intrinsically more valid than another. As Sim and Sharp (1998) point out, this is not straightforward. A situation of discrepant findings may occur where, for example, the results of a questionnaire and interview may produce different findings and this will require a decision as to which set of results are valid and it may be tempting for the researcher to grant the data from one method some sort of preference. Robson (1993) highlights the situation where the two methods may also lead to similar findings and one of the methods may be taken as a criterion measure to confirm the validity of the other. Therefore, it is important to specify and declare the method used as the criterion measure in the interest of claiming validation.

It has been argued by Fielding and Fielding (1986) that triangulation does not necessarily increase the validity of a study or minimise bias. They conclude that the researcher should combine theories and methods carefully and purposefully with the intention of adding breadth or depth to analysis but not for the purposes of pursuing objective truth.

Case study – using triangulation

The following case study provides an overview of the use of triangulation in a student of student nurse learning (Cowman 1994).

Background to the study

The study essentially aimed to provide an understanding of student nurse learning through the identification of significant factors influencing student nurse learning approaches, preferences and experiences. The literature review on nursing education was wide-ranging and comprehensive and highlighted many and varied factors influencing the learning environments of students in classrooms and clinical environments. The complexity of learning and the multiplicity of factors contributing to an educational exchange were also noted by Beckwith (1991) and it was suggested that numerous elements interact together in the teaching/learning process, including approaches adopted by teachers and learners, the nature of the material to be learned, pre-existing knowledge of relevant material and the nature of assessment.

Consistent with the complexity of the phenomenon under investigation, i.e. learning, the research objectives and hypothesis called for a study the scope of which by necessity had to be wide-ranging in order to capture the myriad factors influencing learning. Therefore, I believed that a single research approach or method would not truly provide a total understanding of student nurse learning, and selected triangulation as the research approach. Cohen and Mannion (1984) in terms of educational research, pointed out that by using and drawing from mutually

exclusive categories of research design, contrasting perspectives can be disclosed. As Jick (1979) pointed out, methodological triangulation is ideally used when studying complex concepts that contain many dimensions.

Study design

The study included all student nurse entrants to programmes of education in Northern Ireland ($N = 408$) and the Republic of Ireland ($N = 714$). At the time of the study (1991) student nurses in Northern Ireland entered the Project 2000 Programme and in the Republic of Ireland student nurses were receiving their education through the traditional apprenticeship system with the student nurse occupying a dual role as learner and employee.

The selected triangulation research approach for the study incorporated quantitative and qualitative approaches including methodological triangulation, with a between-methods approach and data triangulation with time triangulation (Table 26.3).

Table 26.3 – *Outline of data collection approach*

Year 1	Year 2	Year 3
Quantitative data collection	Quantitative data collection	Qualitative data collection
Over 3 months	Over 3 months	Over 3 months
Measurement Questionnaire	Measurement Questionnaire	Measurement Semi-structured interviews
(1) Approaches to learning (2) Teaching/ learning preferences	Course experience	

The application of methodological triangulation (between methods) involved the use of complementary methods from both the quantitative and qualitative research traditions in the form of questionnaires and semi-structured interviews. Data triangulation involved the collection of data from multiple sources focused on the phenomenon of interest – learning. Questionnaire measures included Approaches to Learning, Teaching and Learning Preferences and Course Experiences. A semi-structured interview was used to collect qualitative data. Time triangulation involved the collection of data on learning at different points in time, with data collected from students during the first year, second year and third year of the programme. The quantitative research measures were granted privileged status as a criterion measure. The results of the quantitative data analysis provided the basis for the development of the interview schedule for the semi-structured interviews.

Evaluation of the use of triangulation

Learning is a complex phenomenon and required more than one research approach. The comparative study of learning involved two countries with contrasting educational philosophies, objectives and practices arising from two different models of education. Consequently a single method research approach would have provided data of limited value in that it would not have reflected the more subtle, less tangible features distinguishing student learning inherent to the two models of education. The selected research design of triangulation for a study of student nurse learning was extremely effective as the results of the study provided a comprehensive understanding of the factors influencing student nurse learning (Cowman (1994, 1995, 1996, 1998)). In accepting the inherent differences between the quantitative and qualitative research paradigms, the application of either paradigm in isolation of the other would not have provided a true understanding of learning.

The triangulation design produced rich and productive data and the range of measures resulted in a process of validation of results and facilitated an holistic interpretation and understanding of the difference between the two models of student nurse education and training. The context dependency of student learning was highlighted and this finding was facilitated through the use of data triangulation and time triangulation.

The research approach of using the semi-structured interviews following the collection of quantitative data allowed opportunity for clarification and enriching of quantitative data. The triangulation approach of using the findings from quantitative data as a basis for developing the interview schedule for the semi-structured interviews ensured a sense of completeness to the results of the study.

In the study a number of challenges were inherent to the use of triangulation. The study was time-consuming and expensive owing to the different approaches to data collection including the collection of data across the two jurisdictions. The unit of analysis in the study was student nurse learning and the approach to data collection and analysis maintained a consistent and direct focus on the unit of analysis. Determining a common unit of analysis to ensure that the different methods were examining similar elements provided a challenge to me. Fulfilling the underlying assumption of the two paradigms was also important. For example, in quantitative research the power of the sample and the distribution of data were important elements in determining the data analysis approach. The research in selecting a population study overcame any deficiencies that might have occurred in making decisions about statistical techniques and generalisability.

Conclusion

The use of triangulation by some researchers is perceived as an acceptable answer to the paradox of the division between paradigms. It is claimed that through the use of triangulation the deficiencies intrinsic to a single method, investigator or data collection approach may be overcome. The potential of triangulation to minimise the researcher's personal bias and strengthen the validity of findings is an important feature of its use. Triangulation is not an end in itself, and careful and knowledgeable application of this research method can provide insightful research outcomes beyond what is possible in the traditional single methods/investigator or data collection approach.

EXERCISE

Identify an appropriate research question and present a plan for a between-methods triangulation research design.

References

Ammenwerth E, Iller C, Mansmann U 2003 Can evaluation studies benefit from triangulation? A case study. International Journal of Medical Informatics 70: 237–248

Beckwith J B 1991 Approaches to learning: their context and their relationship to assessment performance. Higher Education. 22: 17–30

Begley C 1996 Using triangulation in nursing research. Journal of Advanced Nursing 24: 122–128

Bradley S 1995 Methodological triangulation in healthcare research. Nurse Researcher 3: 81–89

Campbell D T 1956 Leadership and its Effects upon the Group. Ohio State University, Columbus, OH

Campbell D T, Fiske D W 1959 Convergent and discriminant validation by the multitrait-multimethod matrix. Psychological Bulletin. 56: 81–105

Carin M 2005 Methodological triangulation in midwifery education research. Nurse Researcher 12(4): 30–41

Carr L T 1994 The strengths and weaknesses of quantitative and qualitative research: what method for nursing. Journal of Advanced Nursing 20: 716–721

Cohen L, Mannion L 1984 Research Methods in Education. Croom Helm, Beckenham: 209

Cowman S 1993 Triangulation a means of reconciliation in nursing research. Journal of Advanced Nursing 18: 788–793

Cowman S 1994 Understanding student nurse learning. Unpublished PhD thesis, Dublin City University, Dublin

Cowman S 1995 The learning/teaching preferences of student nurses in the Republic of Ireland: issues and a study. International Journal of Nursing Studies 32(2): 126–136

Cowman S 1996 Student evaluation: a performance indicator of quality in nurse education. Journal of Advanced Nursing 24: 625–632

Cowman S 1998 The approaches to learning of student nurses, the Republic of Ireland & Northern Ireland. Journal of Advanced Nursing 28: 899–910

Denzin N 1970 Strategies of multiple triangulation. In: Denzin N (ed) The Research Act. McGraw Hill, New York: 297–331

Denzin N 1978 The Research Act: A Theoretical Introduction to Sociological Methods, 2nd edn. McGraw Hill, New York

Denzin N 1989 The Research Act: A Theoretical Introduction to Sociological Methods, 3rd edn. McGraw Hill, New York

Denzin N K, Lincoln Y S 1994 Major paradigms and perspectives. In: Denzin N K, Lincoln Y S (eds) A Handbook of Qualitative Research. Sage, Newbury Park, CA

DePoy E, Gitlin L N 1994 Introduction to Research: Multiple Strategies for Health and Human Services. Mosby, St Louis

Duffy M E 1987 Methodological triangulation; a vehicle merging qualitative and quantitative research methods. Image: Journal of Nursing Scholarship 19: 130–133

Field P A, Morse J M 1985 In: Nursing Research: The Application of Qualitative Approaches, Croom Helm, Beckenham, Kent: 1–17

Fielding N G, Fielding J L 1986 Linking Data (Sage University Paper Series on Qualitative Research Methods, vol, 4). Sage, Beverly Hills

Foss C, Ellefsen B 2002 The value of combining qualitative and quantitative approaches in nursing research by means of methodological triangulation. Journal of Advanced Nursing 40: 242–248

Foster R 1997 Addressing epistemological and practical issues in multi-method research: a procedure for conceptual triangulation. Advances in Nursing Science 20: 1–12

Janesick V J 1994 The dance of qualitative research design: metaphor, methodolatry and meaning. In: Denzin N K, Lincoln Y S (eds) Handbook of Qualitative Research. Sage, Thousand Oaks, CA: 209–219

Jick T D 1979 Mixing qualitative and quantitative methods: triangulation in action. Administration Science Quarterly 24: 602–611

Kimchi J, Polivka B, Stevenson J S 1991 Triangulation: operational definitions. Nursing Research 40: 364–366

Knafl K A, Breitmayer B J 1989 Triangulation in qualitative research: issues of conceptual clarity and purpose. In: Morse J M (ed) Qualitative Nursing Research as Contemporary Dialogue. Aspen, Rockville, MD: 226–239

Leininger M M 1985 Nature, rationale and importance of qualitative research methods in nursing. In: Leininger M M (ed) Qualitative Research Methods in Nursing. Grune & Stratton, New York: 1–25

Mitchell E S 1986 Multiple triangulation: a methodology for nursing science. Advances in Nursing Science 8(3): 18–26

Morse J 1991 Approaches to qualitative–quantitative methodological triangulation. Nursing Research 40: 120–123

Polit D F, Hungler B P 1999 Nursing Research; Principles and Methods, 6th edn. Lippincott, New York

Redfern S J, Norman I J 1994 Validity through triangulation. Nurse Researcher 2: 41–56

Robson C 1993 Real World Research: A Resource for Social Scientists and Practitioner-Researchers. Blackwell, Oxford

Shih F J 1998 Triangulation in nursing research: issues of conceptual clarity and purpose. Journal of Advanced Nursing 28: 631–641

Silverman D 2001 Interpreting Qualitative Data, 2nd edn. Sage, London

Sim J, Sharp K 1998 A critical appraisal of the role of triangulation in nursing research. International Journal of Nursing Research. 35: 23–31

Sohier R 1988 Multiple triangulation and contemporary nursing research. Western Journal of Nursing Research 10: 732–742

Wendler M C 2001 Triangulation using a meta-matrix. Journal of Advanced Nursing 35: 521–525

Williamson G 2005 Illustrating triangulation in mixed-methods nursing research. Nursing Research 12: 7–18

Section 4

Data Collection and Analysis

Chapter 27

Interviews

Debra Jackson, John Daly and Patricia Davidson

Introduction

An 'interview' may be defined as a 'meeting of persons face to face, esp. for the purpose of consultation; oral examination of candidate for employment etc.; meeting or conversation between journalist and person whose views are being sought for publication; similar meeting as part of radio or television programme' (*Australian Concise Oxford Dictionary* 1982, p. 526). Questions are framed and asked and if carefully constructed and understood they should elicit the information being sought by the interviewer. Although this approach appears straightforward, there are complexities inherent in interviewing that need to be identified, understood and managed in an optimal way. Fontana and Frey note that:

> *Asking questions and getting answers is a much harder task than it may at first seem. The spoken or written word always has a residue of ambiguity, no matter how carefully we word the questions and how carefully we report or code the answers. Yet interviewing is one of the most common and powerful ways in which we try to understand our fellow humans. (2005, pp. 697–698)*

This chapter includes a broad discussion of the use of interviews in research. It is introductory and designed to cover some basic principles and approaches. Further reading will be necessary to build knowledge and understanding of specific approaches in research design and methodology (Denzin & Lincoln 2005, Minichiello et al 2004).

Why interviews?

A number of factors need to be considered in designing and conducting interviews. The interview involves some degree of verbal (oral or written) exchange and discussion between the interviewer and the participant.

Research interviews are generally audiotaped, meaning that the researcher has a lasting record of the meeting with which to work. Interview data are transcribed, frequently into text for purposes of analysis, and the decision and method of transcription is dependent on the research question(s) and method (Halcomb & Davidson 2006).

Interview: method and methodology

Researchers have various methodologies available to them, and each has a philosophical basis that influences profoundly the conceptualisation of a study (Price 2002). The structure and nature of the questioning will be informed by the theoretical framework that underpins the study.

The theoretical framework of a study will also shape how both interviewer and participant are positioned in relation to the text (and ultimately the knowledge) that is generated from the interview. For example, researchers adopting a Heideggerian stance consider both participant and interviewer to be engaged in a dialogue, through which understanding and knowledge are co-created (Donalek 2005, Lowes & Prowse 2001).

The qualitative research interview is designed to gather narrative which can be used to develop knowledge and understanding of the phenomenon under investigation in a research study. This is derived through analytical processes based on theory and research methodology. When undertaking a qualitative interview the researcher aims to gather a rich, deep description of the research participant's experience (Denzin & Lincoln 2005), from the participant's perspective. Britten (1995) stated that:

In a qualitative research interview the aim is to discover the interviewee's own framework of

meanings and the research task is to avoid imposing the researcher's structures and assumptions as far as possible' (p. 251).

In this context, the researcher is often referred to as the research instrument (Britten 1995, Tollefson et al 2001).

Types of interview

The type of interview chosen will depend on the purpose of the interview. Phenomenological interviews are used to explore the lived experience (Hasty & Shattell 2005) while narrative interviewing is conversational in style. Narrative interviewing allows participants to bring in anything they consider relevant and allows them to articulate their knowledge and experience though storied accounts (Bates 2004).

The more structured an interview is, the greater the standardisation of the questions and the questioning. Structured interviews are sometimes called quantitative interviews and generally involve the administration of structured interview schedules, such as a questionnaire. Interviewers using structured questionnaires are required to ask a predetermined sequence of questions in a consistent manner. Most often the questions are close-ended and require a fixed-choice response (Britten 1995), meaning that the range of possible responses is predetermined. Semi-structured interviews involve the use of topics or broad questions (Polit & Beck 2006), and are not as controlled or fixed as the structured interview. Interviewers normally have a list of trigger or guide questions; there is space for dialogue and for the participant to offer responses that are not predetermined.

Unstructured interviews are also referred to as in-depth or qualitative interviews. The questions are open-ended and there are no predetermined responses presented to participants. As with the semi-structured interview, researchers employing unstructured interviews also have a guide to cover the major areas which will be explored (Wimpenny & Gass 2000). Unlike the structured interview, the unstructured interview is characterised by a participant guided approach. The nature and order of questioning will vary between participants and will be dependent on the issues that they raise in relation to the phenomenon being studied.

Interviews can occur between a researcher and individual participants, or between a researcher and two or more participants simultaneously. Group interviews are more commonly referred to as 'focus groups' and were first used in market research (Sofaer 2002). Focus groups usually comprise people who may be unknown to one another but who share a common characteristic that is of interest to the researcher. An increasing number of studies demonstrate the utility of the focus group in conducting health-related research in culturally and linguistically diverse populations. Other types of group interviewing can include friend or partner dyads (Highet 2003), or family interviewing in which members of a family group are interviewed together (Astedt-Kurki et al 2001).

Many interviews are conducted face-to-face but with advances in technology they can also be conducted by telephone, videolink or online. Use of email, private chat rooms and instant messaging is becoming increasingly common and these methods have definite advantages, especially in relation to cost. Interviews conducted using these technologies can generate cost savings associated with transcriptions, travel and time. They can also open participation up to people from distant locations who would otherwise be unable to participate in interviews because of distance. Davis et al (2004) described using online methods to interview men on their experiences of using the internet to find sexual partners and how safe sex is negotiated in these situations. Use of this technology meant that men who might not otherwise have been willing to present for a face-to-face interview, due to the sensitive nature of the subject matter, were willing to participate.

Despite the perceived advantages of lower costs, greater convenience and perception of greater anonymity, the use of telephone and online technologies can make it more difficult to establish rapport and trust and may ultimately influence the quality of the data obtained (Pridemore et al 2005). Furthermore, Davis et al (2004) noted difficulties with the flow, amount and quality of conversation obtained online, pointing out that a 120-minute online interview generated seven pages of text while a 90-minute face-to-face interview resulted in 30–40 pages.

Ethical considerations when conducting interviews

As in any research process, obtaining informed consent is an essential element of the research interview. When nurses and other health workers conduct research interviews with patients/clients, there is room for confusion with the clinical role (Britten 1995). For this reason, Britten (1995) advised against researchers interviewing their own patients/clients, but should this occur, it is very important that informed consent is obtained. As a part of this process, potential participants need to be informed that they do not have to participate, and that they have the right to withdraw at any time, and that they can stop the interview with no negative consequences to them or their relationship with their health care provider.

Participants have the right to privacy and security of data. Interviewers need to ensure that the site and product of the interview remains private and confidential, and that any reports or papers arising from the study are presented in such a way as to maintain participant confidentiality. To ensure maintenance of privacy and confidentiality, and to ensure that the data are not misused, most institutional ethics committees have strict rules about secure storage and effective destruction of interview data.

The issue of power is one that features largely in the discourses around research interviews. While research participants maintain significant power in that they get to decide what and how much they will disclose, Donalek (2005) pointed out that there is power in being positioned as an expert, and that power has the potential to be abused. The power dynamic is further complicated if there is a pre-existing power relationship between the interviewer and participant, such as may occur when academics are interviewing students, or hospital staff are interviewing patients for research purposes. In situations such as these, people may feel compelled to participate in research interviews and may aim to please the interviewer by providing the responses they think are desired.

Conducting an interview

Because of the way that nurses use interviewing in their normal daily practice, it can be assumed that they will be able to engage easily in research interviews. Indeed, as Donalek (2005, p. 124) noted, it appears 'deceptively simple'. However, in describing their experiences of collecting interview data, Tollefson et al (2001, p. 259) stated: 'interviewing for the purpose of gathering qualitative information for research purposes is different from interviewing for any other purpose'. They go on to highlight the importance of interview preparation, and recognition of factors such as power relationships that will impact on the nature and quality of data that can be collected (Tollefson et al 2001).

Skills needed to conduct an interview

The process of interviewing is complex and requires understanding, training and skill. Sofaer (2002) advised that having novices attend interviews with experienced interviewers can help meet their training needs; however, this could be problematic for the participant, particularly if the subject matter is highly sensitive. Britten (1995, p. 251) commented:

> The novice research interviewer needs to notice how directive he or she is being, whether leading questions are being asked, whether cues are being picked up or ignored, and whether participants are given enough time to explain what they mean.

Though many texts refer to the importance of listening in communication, the style of listening in research interviews is more accurately described as 'listening with analytic intent' (Tollefson et al 2001, p. 263), meaning that we are listening with a different intent to the listening we do in other contexts. Bates (2004) suggested that language can be used to facilitate or impede the flow of information. Thus, it is very important to use language appropriately and to avoid the use of jargon or terminology that may hamper clear understanding.

Clarity is important, and interview questions should be clear, able to be easily understood, open-ended, and unbiased (Britten 1995). Skills such as rephrasing questions or statements and paraphrasing responses are necessary to ensure common understandings and can also be valuable as prompts (Tollefson et al 2001). The use of open-ended clarifying questions assists participants in articulating and describing their experiences (Streubert & Carpenter 1995).

Being comfortable with silence is important; it may be tempting to fill a silence, but these periods of silence can be useful as they give time for a participant to reflect, gather their thoughts and construct a considered response (Tollefson, et al 2001). It is also important to recognise that the interviewer can find the interview a stressful situation. For example, issues related to child abuse and sexual assault may be raised by the participant and this may place the researcher in a difficult situation with regard to protecting confidentiality and recognising their professional responsibilities. This situation underscores the importance of research teams with senior researchers and opportunities for debriefing and supervision.

Preparing for the interview

There are several areas to be considered when preparing to conduct an interview including deciding on a venue to conduct the interviews. The main objective is to ensure a relatively quiet and private space where the participant can talk freely without the risk of being overheard by others. Because of the need to record the encounter it is always good to have an electrical power source nearby, though many devices will function equally well on batteries.

'Ownership' of the space or room in which the interview will take place is also an issue for consideration. While interviews can take place in the homes of participants, this is increasingly being seen as problematic. When considering student work, educational institutions may not be happy to let students go into private homes alone for health and safety reasons. Furthermore, when conducting interviews in private homes it may be difficult to ensure the necessary privacy due to the presence of other people. It is also more difficult to control unplanned interruptions, such as telephone calls, other visitors arriving etc. For these reasons it is preferable to find a suitable neutral space in which to conduct interviews. Suitable sites for interviews can include use of rooms in hospitals or health settings, university campuses, town libraries or similar.

Establishing relationships or rapport in interviewing

The ability to establish a respectful and trusting relationship and create a sense of personal safety in which participants can tell their stories safely is crucial to successful interviewing (Murray 2003, Tollefson et al 2001). If the purpose of the research interview is to gather authentic and rich narrative accounts of phenomena, then the ability to achieve this outcome is very much dependent on a rapport being established between the participant and the interviewer. Participation in research frequently requires people to recall and give voice to traumatic life events. They are asked to disclose freely their thoughts and feelings about lived experiences or phenomena that may be very sensitive and may arouse uncomfortable, distressing feelings for them, such as shame and embarrassment.

To achieve the level of disclosure necessary to gain a quality text from each participant, it is vital that interviewers create an appropriate milieu within the interview context. It is important to be friendly, respectful and culturally aware. Simple strategies such as asking people how they wish to be addressed can convey respect to participants.

There are four main issues, or phases, involved with creating a milieu that will increase the chance of being able to obtain a quality narrative. These are: contact prior to the meeting, the day of the interview, breaking the ice, and creating an accepting, trusting and non-judgemental milieu. Each of these will be discussed briefly.

Contact prior to the meeting: once ethical approval is granted and the recruitment phase of a study begins, there will be some contact between potential participants and interviewer. Potential participants will make contact for further information, clarification of issues, and to make arrangements to participate in the study. Participants may want to know how long the interview will last, and they may ask what type of questions will be asked. It is important at this time to maintain a respectful stance, and to be approachable, courteous, flexible and prepared to answer any questions that might arise.

The day of the interview: it is important to be well prepared so as to minimise the risk of unnecessary interruptions that could destroy or damage rapport. Effective preparation requires that all equipment that could be necessary during the interview is available, including items such as a supply of tissues, refreshments such as a cup of tea, or some water for participants, spare batteries and a spare audiotape for the recording device.

Though participants will have given informed consent to have the interview recorded, it can nevertheless be daunting when they are confronted with the sight of the recording equipment. It can help put people at their ease if the recording equipment is placed in a less obtrusive position. By using distraction techniques, interviewers can adopt strategies to help minimise the effect of the recording equipment; for example, offering a cup of tea or coffee, commenting on the weather and chatting about the study and thanking them for giving their time to participate. In our experience, strategies to help put people at their ease include showing them a copy of the list of trigger, or guiding questions, and providing the opportunity to indicate if there are any questions that they would rather not discuss. Providing assurance that the interviewer will not address these questions is helpful. Though participants seldom have any problems with the questions, giving them this opportunity for clarification helps to redress the power imbalance that exists between researchers and participants, and also indicates a respect for their right to retain control during the interview. It is useful to start the interview with background or demographic questions and only move to more sensitive areas when the participant is relaxed and a flow of dialogue is established.

Creating an accepting, trusting and non-judgemental milieu: it is important to aim for a friendly, informal milieu to put people at their ease and enhance the exchange of information. When interviewing people, particularly about sensitive topics, it is very important to adopt an open stance and convey empathy, support and an air of acceptance (Murray 2003, Price 2004). Any sense of negative judgement will almost certainly affect the quality of the narrative to its detriment and could also jeopardise the trust between the interviewer and the participant (Murray 2003). Murray (2003) described working with vulnerable adolescents and was able to establish trust with these young people by allowing them to 'tell their stories, which were accepted in a non-judgmental, non-blaming, and non-threatening way' (p. 233).

Self-disclosure can sometimes be used to enhance the sense of acceptance when interviewing about sensitive matters, and this also lends some mutuality to the interview encounter (Murray 2003, Reinharz 1992). Britten (1995) asserted that being interactive, rather than expecting the dialogue to all go one way, will enhance the encounter and suggested that interviewers should be prepared to be questioned by participants as to their own views and opinions on the subject matter. This can pose a problem because in providing responses to these questions, researchers could sway the opinions and thoughts of the participant. However, failure to respond to the questions posed by participants, may have a negative effect on the flow of the interview. This problem could be avoided by telling participants at the outset that it will be possible to ask questions of this nature after the interview has concluded (Britten 1995).

Terminating the interview appropriately is very important; the literature suggests that abrupt termination, with no time for small talk or refreshments, can leave people feeling 'used' (Donalek 2005). When the interview reaches a conclusion, some time should be allowed to relax and unwind (Donalek 2005). This is an opportunity to thank the participant for giving their time and sharing their experience, and to ensure that they are satisfied from participating in the interview process.

Some benefits and challenges associated with the use of interviews

Benefits

Participants often report positive effects from participating in qualitative interviews (Donalek 2005, Murray 2003). Murray (2003) suggested that the therapeutic benefit of the qualitative interview is also associated with participants being able to give voice to aspects of their lives that may have been previously kept secret because of shame or fear. Telling their stories may help participants arrive at new understandings about themselves and their experiences (Murray 2003). Furthermore, participating in a research project can create a sense of helping others, and so bring something positive to an experience that may have been sad or traumatic (Donalek 2005).

Challenges

There are several impediments to unstructured interviews – participants need to be able to articulate and reflect on their experiences. There is a paucity of literature regarding the long-term effects of participating in unstructured interviews on sensitive subjects. Britten (1995) identified several pitfalls that can beset the qualitative interviewer. These include: interruptions, distractions, anxiety associated with participating in the interview, the possibility of embarrassment or awkwardness, the interview becoming a teaching or counselling session, superficiality, and difficulties with common language. Most of these difficulties can be overcome with careful planning and experience.

Data management and analysis

A well-developed research proposal is critical before beginning your research project (Price

2002). This proposal and philosophical underpinnings will guide your analysis method. Data management and analysis can be aided by a range of computer software packages but is not mandatory. What is critical is devotion of time to become immersed in the data so that the voices of the participants are heard and appropriately represented.

EXERCISES

Working with a learning partner (either a student peer or work colleague), or in a small group, try the following exercises:

1. Consider the issues raised in this chapter, reflect on some of the problems with interviewing, and what groups of people could be maginalised by this method of data collection? Make a list and have a brainstorming session to develop strategies that a researcher could use to try to problem solve these issues.
2. Working with a student or colleague partner, set up an interview space, obtain tape recording equipment and practise interviewing one another on your experiences of a specific topic. Remember to:

   - develop a list of guiding questions or topics for discussion before you begin the encounter
   - focus on actual experiences, rather than opinions
   - have a turn at being both interviewer and interviewee.

3. Following Exercise 2 above, listen closely to the audiotapes. Reflect on your skills and make note of how you used communication. Pay particular attention to the following questions:

   - Did you use questioning appropriately?
   - Did you allow the participant to respond fully?
   - Did you talk over the participant?
   - Did you clarify anything that was ambiguous?
   - Did you finish sentences for the participant?
   - Did you respond appropriately to the participant's emotional cues?
   - Did you allow the participant to raise issues of concern in relation to the topic?
   - Did you end the encounter appropriately?

4. Write a reflection on your thoughts and feelings about participating in a qualitative interview. In writing your reflection, consider the following points:

   - your feelings in relation to speaking while being audiotaped
   - your feelings in relation to asking a series of questions
   - your feelings in relation to asking questions that could possibly be considered intrusive
   - your feelings in relation to being asked a series of questions
   - your feelings in relation to being asked questions that could possibly be considered intrusive.

5. Following Exercises 3 and 4 above, arrange to meet with your interview partner and debrief one another about the experience and share your reflections on the interview experience. Think about how perceptions might differ between being an interviewer and interviewee.

Conclusion

As demonstrated above, the interview is a powerful research tool to reveal information, values, attitudes and beliefs from a range of respondents. In many ways, interviews are an ideal method for nurses and other workers in the health and welfare sectors. This is because these professionals use interviews in their everyday working lives and rely on the development of trusting and therapeutic relationships in order to achieve their goals. In spite of these existing skills, it is important that careful planning occurs to ensure that meaningful data are derived from the interview process and the welfare of the interviewer and participant are protected.

References

Astedt-Kurki P, Paavilainen E, Lehti K 2001 Methodological issues in interviewing families in family nursing research. Journal of Advanced Nursing 35: 288–293

Australian Concise Oxford Dictionary. 1982 Oxford University Press, Oxford

Bates J A 2004 Use of narrative interviewing in everyday information behavior research. Library and Information Science Research 26: 15–28

Britten N 1995 Qualitative research: Qualitative interviews in medical research. British Medical Journal 311: 251–253

Davis M, Bolding G, Hart G, et al 2004 Reflecting on the experience of interviewing online: perspectives from the Internet and HIV study in London. AIDS Care 16: 944–952

Denzin N K, Lincoln Y S. 2005 The Sage Handbook of Qualitative Research, 3rd edn. Sage, Thousand Oaks, CA

Donalek J 2005 The interview in qualitative research. Urologic Nursing 25: 124–125

Fontana A, Frey J H 2005 The interview: From neutral stance to political involvement. In: Denzin N K, Lincoln Y S (eds) The Sage Handbook of Qualitative Research, 3rd edn. Sage, Thousand Oaks, CA

Halcomb E J, Davidson P 2006 Is verbatim transcription of interview data always necessary? Applied Nursing Research 19: 38–42

Hasty C, Shattell M 2005 'Putting feet to what we pray about': The experience of caring by faith-based care team members. Journal of Hospice and Palliative Nursing 7: 255–262

Highet G 2003 Cannabis and smoking research: interviewing young people in self selected friendship pairs. Health Education Research 18: 108–118

Lowes L, Prowse M 2001 Standing outside the interview process? The illusion of objectivity in phenomenological data collection. International Journal of Nursing Studies 38: 471–480

Minichiello V, Madison J, Hays T, et al 2004 Doing qualitative in-depth interviews. In: Minichiello V, Sullivan G, Greenwood K, Axford R (eds) Handbook of Research Methods for Nursing and Health Science. Pearson/Prentice Hall, Melbourne: 411–446

Murray B L 2003 Qualitative research interviews. Journal of Psychiatric and Mental Health Nursing 10: 231–238

Polit D F, Beck C T 2006 Essentials of Nursing Research: Methods, Appraisal and Utilization, 6th edn. Lippincott, Williams & Wilkins, Philadelphia

Price B 2002 Laddered questions and qualitative data research interviews. Journal of Advanced Nursing 37: 273–281

Price B 2004 Conducting sensitive patient interviews. Nursing Standard 18(38): 45–52

Pridemore W A, Damphouse K R, Moore R K 2005 Obtaining sensitive information from a wary population: a comparison of telephone and face-to-face surveys of welfare recipients in the United States. Social Science and Medicine 61: 976–984

Reinharz S 1992 Feminist Methods in Social Research. Oxford University Press, New York

Sofaer S 2002 Qualitative research methods. International Journal for Quality in Health Care 14: 329–336

Streubert H, Carpenter D 1995 Qualitative Research in Nursing: Advancing the Humanistic Imperative. Lippincott, Philadelphia

Tollefson J, Usher K, Francis D, et al 2001 What you ask is what you get: learning from interviewing in qualitative research. Contemporary Nurse 10: 258–264

Wimpenny P, Gass J 2000 Interviewing in phenomenology and grounded theory: is there a difference? Journal of Advanced Nursing 31: 1485–1492

Chapter 28

Focus Groups

Pauline Joyce

Introduction

In the previous chapter focus groups were defined. Another simple definition of focus group interviewing is: 'a group of individuals selected and assembled by researchers to discuss and comment on, from personal experience, the topic that is the subject of the research' (Powell & Single 1996, p. 499). The use of focus groups has grown in nursing (Webb & Kevern 2001). It is accepted that using 'focus groups' implies the researcher is actively encouraging of, and attentive to, group interaction (Kitzinger & Barbour 1999). The main advantage of focus groups is the opportunity to observe a large amount of interaction and discussion on a topic in a limited period of time. The person facilitating the focus group is called the moderator. Sometimes an assistant moderator is present to take notes and observe interactions.

Collecting data by focus groups

Focus group interviewing has been used as a sole method of data collection in some studies (Bulmer 1998, Hodges et al 2001, Verpeet et al 2005) and as one of a number of qualitative data collection methods in others (McCutcheon & Pincombe 2001). Focus groups have also been employed in the initial phase of studies as a means of developing items for inclusion in later surveys (McLeod et al 2000, Sim & Snell 1996), or to pursue poorly understood survey results, thus serving as a source of follow-up data to assist the primary method (Hodges et al 2001, McCutcheon & Pincombe 2001, Morgan 1997).

The advantage of collecting data by focus group is the ability to observe group interaction on a

Box 28.1 – *When to use focus group interviews*

Focus group interviews should be considered when:

- You are looking for a range of ideas or feelings that people have about something
- You are trying to understand differences in perspectives between groups or categories of people
- The purpose is to uncover factors that influence opinions, behaviour, or motivation, e.g. under what conditions should a health worker admit a mistake?
- You want ideas to emerge from the group
- You want to pilot test ideas, plans or policies
- The researcher needs information to design a large-scale quantitative study
- The researcher needs information to help shed light on quantitative data already collected

Box 28.2 – *When not to use focus group interviews*

Focus group interviews should not be considered when:

- You are asking for sensitive information that should not be shared in a group or could be harmful to someone if it is shared in a group
- The environment is emotionally charged, and a group discussion is likely to intensify the conflict
- Other methodologies can produce better quality information
- You cannot ensure the confidentiality of sensitive information

topic. It provides evidence about similarities and differences in the participants' opinions and experiences as opposed to the researcher reaching these conclusions from analyses of separate statements from individual interviews. Nonetheless, the individual interview has clear advantages over the focus group with regard to the amount of control that the researcher has and the greater amount of information that each participant has time to share. Boxes 28.1 and 28.2 provide some considerations (modified from Kreuger & Casey 2000) for when to use, and not to use, focus groups.

Preparation for the focus group interview

The literature varies on the optimum size of a focus group. Generally, between four and eight participants are recommended. Fewer than four is not considered a focus group. It is difficult to predict accurately the precise number of participants. Interviewees can cancel for a variety of reasons as the date approaches. Morgan (1997) suggested over-recruiting by 20%. However, it has been highlighted

that this figure should be closer to 50–100% for nurses (Macleod Clark et al 1996) because nurses may be difficult to recruit due to shift patterns and workload. The optimum size of the group may also reflect the characteristics of participants as well as the topic being discussed (Bloor et al 2001). Focus groups in Michell's (1999) study on teenage lifestyles consisted typically of three or four pupils and were made up of friends and peers who were comfortable about attending the sessions together. However, this study used 76 one-to-one interviews and 21 focus groups. Larger groups can also present problems. Groups that are too large can become difficult to moderate and participants can feel frustrated if they have inadequate time to express their views or opinions. The more outgoing participants can dominate the interaction so that everyone present may not be contributing to the discussion. The number of participants can also have significant implications for recording and transcribing the group discussion.

Purposive sampling is frequently used for focus groups where the participants are recruited. Purposive sampling is based on the belief that a researcher's knowledge about the population can be used to hand-pick the cases to be included in the sample (Polit & Hungler 1995). Random sampling is seldom used because of the small number of participants involved in focus groups. In addition, a randomly sampled group from the general population may be unlikely to hold a shared perspective on the research topic and may not be able to generate meaningful discussions (Jennings et al 2005). In terms of group composition it has been suggested that different hierarchical levels within a group should be avoided (Kreuger & Casey 2000, Macleod Clark et al 1996). If a power differential exists, some participants may be reluctant to participate in the discussion (Mansell et al 2004). Another consideration is to decide whether to include people who are complete strangers or to access pre-existing groups (Barbour 2005).

Once you have selected participants it is important to set locations, meeting dates and times that do not conflict with popular activities and functions. Select a location that is easy to travel to, safe, has refreshments and with adequate transportation and parking. The location will need to be free from visual or audible distractions. Comfortable chairs and a table should be available for writing notes and holding a microphone (Kreuger & Casey 2000). A round table may be better than a rectangular one so that moderators can be placed in a position equal to the participants (Fig. 28.1).

Contact with potential participants should be direct and personalised (Lane et al 2001). The first contact can be two weeks before the interview and usually takes the form of a letter (Fig 28.2). It is a good idea to build a convincing case in your letter to include the benefits of carrying out this study and how the results will be used. When the participant agrees to take part in the focus group, follow up with a personalised letter, approximately one week before the session. This letter can provide additional details about the session, location and topic. It is worthwhile providing some refreshments prior to the interview. This time can act as a warm-up for participants to introduce themselves to each other and to the researcher. In seeking informed consent from participants to take part in the interview, the researcher should be clear that note-taking and recording facilities will be employed (Powell & Single 1996).

A focus group moderator has been defined as 'a facilitator or discussion leader, not a discussion participant' (Fern 2001, p. 73). Likewise Morgan (1997) suggested that the title 'moderator' reflects an orientation towards 'helping out someone else's

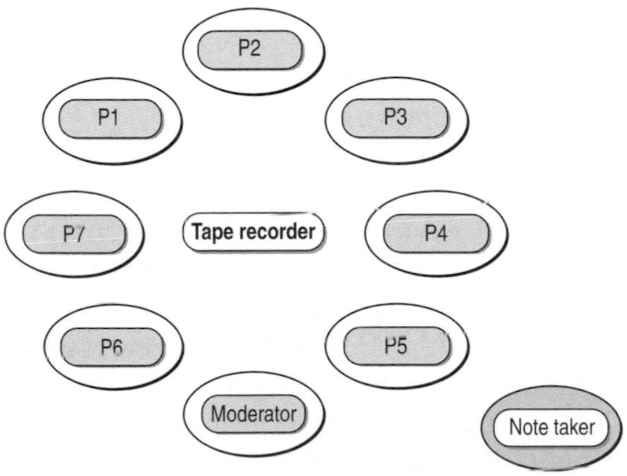

Figure 28.1 – *Group layout.*

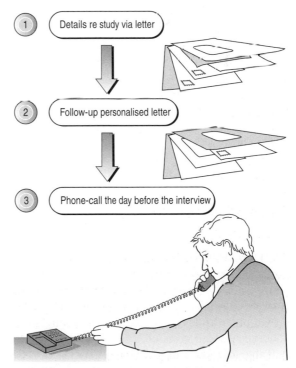

Figure 28.2 – *Contact with participants.*

Box 28.3 – *Moderator skills*

- Know key questions
- Respect
- Ability to listen
- Be aware of timing

Table 28.1 – *Preparation checklist*

Preparation checklist	Considerations
Determining the size of the group	4–8 participants
Deciding on the number of groups	More than 1 if sole method
Selecting and recruiting participants	Purposive sampling
Set meeting dates, time, location	Any conflicting functions?
Personalise contacts	3 contacts
Develop appropriate questions	Not too many

discussion' (p. 48). The underlying message from much of the literature on moderating focus groups is that the participants must feel comfortable with the moderator (McLeod et al 2000, Nyamanthi & Shuler 1990, Sim 1998). The participants need to feel that the moderator has no vested interest in the outcome of the focus group. Equally, the most influential factor affecting the quality of the focus group is the moderator's respect for the participants (Kreuger & Casey 2000) (Box 28.3). This includes the ability to listen and the self-discipline to withhold personal viewpoints. The moderator facilitates the discussion and, as such, is a background rather than a foreground figure. Too much control may do the study a disservice, but the moderator must apply skilful facilitation if there is over-domination of the group by particular participants. Likewise, the moderator must encourage contributions from the more reticent members of the group.

Developing appropriate questions for a focus group is as important as for a one-to-one interview. Too many questions will not give the participants enough time to talk about each issue. One suggestion is to begin with questions that will generate discussions among the participants. Even though these opening questions are not the core of the researcher's interest, they will help promote a lively interview (Morgan 1995). Pre-testing the interview guide can be undertaken through individual interviews, as these are easier and cheaper to organise than focus groups. However, Webb (2002) carried out a pilot focus group and made changes for subsequent focus groups.

Table 28.1 provides a preparation checklist for the focus group interview.

Conducting the focus group interview

A pre-group self-completion questionnaire seeking demographic information may be used and participants should be asked to sign a consent form. These can be collected immediately before the group starts and can be a convenient time-filler in these awkward minutes waiting for people to arrive. Bloor et al (2001) suggested using the pre-group questionnaire to check for possible differences of viewpoints on the study topic within the group. Knowledge of these underlying issues can be advantageous to the researcher in interpreting the focus group data.

Flip charts and notes are used to collect data from the focus group but audio recording is now common. Equipment that is suitable for recording one-to-one interviews may not always produce a recording of sufficient quality when used with groups. Tape recorders with microphones which contain an automatic volume control should be avoided as they will adjust the volume to cope with a loud speaker so that you can miss some data from a quieter speaker who follows (Bloor et al 2001). Where an external microphone is used, it is important to check that both the cassette recorder and the microphone attachment are switched on. It is a good idea to start the group interview by asking members to identify themselves. This can serve a dual purpose. You can play back the recording and check audibility. The recording of names can also help the transcriber to identify the individual voices but this may have the disadvantage of making some participants self-conscious. You need to assure the participants of confidentiality and that you will use pseudonyms when presenting the data from the study.

The moderator should provide a brief overview of the study and encourage the participants to take an active role in the group. It should be explained that the session will be in the form of a discussion and that the group members should not wait to be invited before they contribute to the discussion. The moderator can stress that there are no right or wrong answers, that all views are of interest, and that the aim is to hear as many different viewpoints or experiences as possible. The moderator can add that the participants can agree or disagree with other viewpoints and are free to say what they think. It is important to ask the participants to treat what others say as confidential and not to repeat the viewpoints and experiences outside the session.

Kreuger and Casey (2000) stated that there is often the tendency for novice researchers to move too quickly from one topic to another when there is a pause in the discussion. They believe that this pause can prompt additional points of view, especially when coupled with eye contact from the moderator. However, the moderator may need to probe for additional information when participants make vague comments or say 'I agree'. Probing can involve such questions or comments (Finch & Lewis 2003, Kreuger & Casey 2000), as listed in Box 28.4.

Throughout the discussion it is important to be alert to group participants' body language (Finch

Box 28.4 – *Probing questions and comments*

- Would you explain further?
- How do other people feel?
- Would you give me an example of what you mean?
- Can you say a bit more about that?
- Is there anything else?
- Please describe what you mean.

& Lewis 2003). Nodding, or shaking of heads, or utterances that may not be picked up by the audio recorder, may demonstrate agreement or disagreement with viewpoints. The participants need to be encouraged to speak these views, otherwise these will be lost.

While it is unlikely that all participants will contribute equally to the discussion, the moderator needs to encourage a flow of contributions (Finch & Lewis 2003). Dominant participants may sometimes see themselves as experts. It may be necessary to restrain their contributions, especially if they are always first to answer a question and other participants become increasingly silent. Non-verbal attempts to deal with this type of participant include withdrawing eye contact, leaning away, looking at others and gesturing to others to speak (Finch & Lewis 2003). If this strategy is unsuccessful a more direct tactic may be needed. For example, 'Thank you Joan. Are there others who wish to comment?' or 'Does anyone feel differently?' or 'That's one point of view' (Kreuger & Casey 2000). To avoid confrontation, the moderator will want to endeavour to emphasise the value of the dominant person's contribution but also the importance of hearing from all participants.

Shy respondents and reflective thinkers often say little and think carefully before speaking. Eye contact might be enough to encourage them to speak as it would be counterproductive to pressurise a participant to contribute. To encourage their participation the moderator may say 'Martin, I don't want to leave you out of the conversation, do you want to add to that?' If the person decides to remain uncommunicative, the moderator may not wish to probe further and focus instead on the other participants. The study below illustrates the practicalities of a study using focus groups.

An example of a focus group study

The focus group study by Webb (2002) addressed many of the issues highlighted in this chapter. Five focus groups were used to explore, from the perspectives of enrolled nurses, what prevented them coming forward for conversion to registered nurse status. Webb selected this approach because the interactions within the focus group can be significant. In addition, individuals do not always form an opinion in isolation and can be influenced by listening to and sharing views with others (Webb 2002). Enrolled nurses ($n = 43$) were invited to participate. Recruitment involved personal letters and follow-up telephone calls. However, there was a low level of attendance. The first focus group interview was used as a pilot and resulted in minor changes. The focus groups were completed within four months. Each interview ran for one hour and 15 minutes. A central venue was chosen to facilitate participants' travel to the venue. The moderator was a colleague of the researcher and took no part in the interview. The researcher acted as the facilitator of the interview. A focus group discussion guide consisted of open-ended questions which moved from general to challenging. The discussion was audiotaped and written notes were taken contemporaneously. Prior to closure of the interview, the researcher made a summary of the main discussion points, allowing an opportunity for final questions or comments. The research provided an understanding of where the local strategy to persuade enrolled nurses to convert to registered nurse status had succeeded, in terms of positive experiences. It also identified pitfalls for pursuing this strategy in the absence of organisation-wide support, especially from managers and enrolled nurses themselves. Webb concluded that focus groups play a valuable role in both research and the involvement of people in organisational change.

Virtual focus groups

A virtual focus group (VFG) is a computer-mediated group interview technique. This internet-based focus group is becoming more popular as the use of the internet has grown, and as people's lives and work schedules become busier and more complicated (Moloney et al 2003). A VFG has been described as 'an asynchronous (not live) group discussion of topics in which participants have had similar experiences' (Dickerson 2004, p. 159). Generally, a password-protected web page is set up which participants can access. The web page will have a discussion board where participants are free to log on at any time, read others' postings (responses) and post their own thoughts and opinions. The website will usually be available for a specified period of time, e.g. four weeks, to allow participants time to respond to others' comments. However, these discussions can last longer. 'Threaded discussion' is the term used to refer to the organisation of postings on a web page (Nyamanthi & Shuler 1990). The moderator may post new 'threads' as starting points of the discussion and may add questions and probes throughout to clarify discussion points. The initial posting may start as 'Please tell us about your everyday experiences living with ...' Participants can also initiate questions they wish to post to other participants or to the moderator. Reminder emails can be sent to participants when new questions are posted (Dickerson 2004). The complete narrative is saved on the web for the specified time frame of the VFG so participants can scroll up and down to see what has transpired over the life of the group.

As with actual focus groups, there are advantages and challenges in using VFGs. The convenience for participants is a principal advantage of using a VFG. As with recruitment for 'offline' focus groups, it is recommended that more individuals are approached than required due to the possibility of non-responses (Stewart & Williams 2005). The web page can be accessed intermittently when convenient for the participant. Furthermore, the internet format provides participants with a 'safe' forum, since they do not feel it necessary to answer every question (Moloney et al 2003). Balanced against this may be limited access to a computer or poor computer skills. Following the initial costs of establishing a website and purchasing computer equipment, the logistical costs of VFGs can be much lower than with actual focus groups. Once established, the technology can be reused. Data entry and analysis are quicker and cheaper as narratives can be transferred directly to software (Moloney et al 2003).

Maximising the participation of group members in the discussion and controlling the direction of the group's conversation is challenging in the VFG. The moderator cannot address the shy or dominant participant directly. Equally, the observation of non-verbal expressions and tones of voices are not available to the moderator and participants (Hewson et al 2003). The location of the focus group interview is an important consideration in preparing for the face-to-face interview. However, there is no control over the locations of the participants in a VFG. Each participant can enter their comments on the internet in different locations; for example, a quiet room at home or a noisy office at work (Stanton 1998). The variation of context may have some influences on the responses given to the discussion. Despite these challenges Bloor et al (2001) asserted that 'virtual focus groups are ... a new dimension of an established method, offering new opportunities in focus group research' (p. 86).

Ethical considerations

Ethical approval should be sought. When recruiting participants, researchers must ensure that full information about the purpose and uses of participants' contributions is given (Homan 1991). Being honest with participants and keeping them informed about the expectations of the group and topic, and not pressurising them to speak, is important (Gibbs 2005). The participants should be guaranteed that the tapes recording the discussion will be subject to rigorous safeguards and formal assurances of confidentiality and anonymity (Powell & Single 1996). Where some people find it easier to discuss issues in a group setting, e.g. for sensitive issues, others may prefer the private nature of a one-to-one interview (Michell 1999). When facilitating sensitive discussions it is important to be aware of the comfort level of the group and to be alert to verbal and non-verbal cues of discomfort. Farquhar (1999) suggested acknowledging embarrassment, allowing

tension-releasing jokes without avoiding the topic at hand. It is important to recognise and respect personal boundaries so that individuals do not feel pressurised to pursue uncomfortable areas. The experience of taking part in the interview may be distressing in itself for some participants as some painful experiences and memories may be revisited. Some debriefing after the focus group, or referral to counselling services, may be necessary. Group members should also be reminded that participation is entirely voluntary and that they can withdraw from the study at any time.

Benefits of focus groups

The benefits of focus groups can be summarised as follows:

- The opportunity to observe a large amount of participant interaction about a topic in a short space of time (Kreuger & Casey 2000, Morgan 1997).
- They may encourage a greater degree of spontaneity in the expression of opinions than alternative methods of data collection (Butler 1996).
- They can provide a 'safe' forum for the expression of views as respondents do not feel obliged to respond to every question (Vaughn et al 1996).
- They facilitate natural quality controls on data collection, e.g. participants tend to provide checks and balances on each other and extreme views tend to be 'weeded out' (Robinson 1999).
- The debates between group participants allow the researcher to explore how people 'make up their minds' about differing perspectives (Carter & Henderson 2005).

Limitations of focus groups

Many of the potential limitations of focus groups can be avoided by careful planning. However, there are a number of limitations recognised despite good planning, which can be summarised as follows:

- The number of questions covered in the discussion may be limited as the response time will vary between participants (Robinson 1999).

- The researcher/moderator is less in control than in one-to-one interviewing (Jackson 1998).
- Individual characteristics of participants may present challenges for the moderator, e.g. the dominant talker who prevents other shyer participants from getting their viewpoint across (Kreuger & Casey 2000). Thus they may not be seen as empowering for all participants and conflicts may arise.

Conclusion

This chapter has addressed the key issues for collecting data using focus group interviewing. Whether used as a sole method of data collection, or as one of a number of methods, preparation for the interview is vital to its success. The justification for using focus groups should come from the purpose of the study and the data you are seeking. Planning is crucial and should involve the use of a preparation checklist to ensure you have a good attendance and relevant discussion. The moderator skills cannot be underestimated for this type of research approach. Finally, the preparation of probing questions and comments will ensure that you collect data that are rich and will provide you with in-depth information on the topic under discussion.

EXERCISES

1. Without referring back on the text, can you list five main practicalities of organising a focus group interview?
2. Write down a research question, which could be explored by collecting data via focus group interviews. Plan out exactly how you will recruit participants for these groups using the checklist in Table 28.1.
3. You have decided to act as moderator of one of the focus group interviews above. Make a plan of the layout of the group, and list the particular skills you will need to demonstrate, taking into account the mix of power bases and personalities for the group.

References

Barbour R S 2005 Making sense of focus groups. Medical Education 39: 742–750

Bloor M, Frankland J, Thomas M, et al 2001 Focus Groups in Social Research. Sage, London

Bulmer C 1998 Clinical decisions: defining meaning through focus groups. Nursing Standard 12(20): 4–10

Butler S 1996 Child protection or professional self-preservation by the baby nurses? Public health nurses and child protection in Ireland. Social Science and Medicine 43: 303–314

Carter S, Henderson L 2005 Approaches to qualitative data collection in social science. In: Bowling A, Ebrahim S (eds) Handbook of Health Research Methods; Investigation, Measurement and Analysis. Open University Press, Milton Keynes

Dickerson S S 2004 Technology–patient interactions: internet use for gaining a healthy context for living with an implantable cardioverter defibrillator. Heart and Lung 34: 157–168

Farquhar C 1999 Are focus groups suitable for 'sensitive' topics? In: Barbour R S, Kitzinger J (eds) Developing Focus Group Research, Politics, Theory and Practice. Sage, London: 36–46

Fern E F 2001 Advanced focus group research. Sage, London

Finch H, Lewis J 2003 In: Richie J, Lewis J (eds) Qualitative Research Practice: A Guide for Social Science Students and Researchers. Sage, London

Gibbs A 2005 Focus Groups, Social Research Update. Online. Available: www.soc.surrey.ac.uk/sru/SRU19.html 24 Aug 2005

Hewson C, Yule P, Laurent D, et al 2003 Internet Research Methods, a Practical Guide for the Social and Behavioural Sciences. Sage, London

Hodges H, Keeley A C, Grier E 2001 Masterworks of art and chronic illness experiences in the elderly. Journal of Advanced Nursing 36: 389–398

Homan R 1991 Ethics in social Research. Longman, Harlow

Jackson P 1998 Focus group interviews as a methodology. Nurse Researcher 6(1): 72–84

Jennings B M, Heiner S L, Loan L A, et al 2005 What really matters to healthcare consumers. Journal of Nursing Administration 35(4): 173–180

Kitzinger J, Barbour S 1999 Introduction: the challenge and promise of focus groups. In: Barbour R S, Kitzinger J (eds) Developing Focus Group Research, Politics, Theory and Practice. Sage, London: 1–20

Kreuger R A, Casey M A 2000 Focus Groups: A Practical Guide for Applied Research, 3rd edn. Sage, Newbury Park CA

Lane D, McKenna H, Ryan A 2001 Focus group methodology. Nurse Researcher 8(3): 45–59

McCutcheon H, Pincombe J 2001 Intuition: an important tool in the practice of nursing. Journal of Advanced Nursing 35: 342–348

McLeod P J, Meagher T W, Steinert Y, et al 2000 Using focus groups to design a valid questionnaire. Academic Medicine 75: 671

Macleod Clark J, Maben J, Jones K 1996 The use of focus group interviews in nursing research: issues and challenges. Nursing Times Research 1: 144–153

Mansell I, Bennett G, Northway R, et al 2004 The learning curve: the advantages and disadvantages in the use of focus groups as a method of data collection. Nurse Researcher 11(4): 79–88

Michell L 1999 Combining focus groups and interviews: telling how it is; telling how it feels. In: Barbour R S, Kitzinger J (eds) Developing Focus Group Research, Politics, Theory and Practice. Sage, London: 36–46

Moloney M F, Dietrich A S, Strickland O, et al 2003 Using internet discussion boards as virtual focus groups, Advances in Nursing Science 14: 274–286

Morgan D L 1995 Why things (sometimes) go wrong in focus groups. Qualitative Health Research 5: 516–523

Morgan D L 1997 Focus Groups as Qualitative Research, 2nd edn. Sage, London

Nyamanthi A, Shuler P 1990 Focus group interview: a research technique for informed nursing practice. Journal of Advanced Nursing 15: 1281–1288

Polit D F, Hungler B P 1995 Nursing Research. Principles and Method, 5th edn. Lippincott, Philadelphia

Powell R A, Single H M 1996 Methodology matters – V: focus groups. International Journal for Quality in Health Care 8: 499–504

Robinson N 1999 The use of focus group methodology – with selected examples from sexual health research. Journal of Advanced Nursing 29: 905–913

Sim J 1998 Collecting and analyzing qualitative data: issues raised by the focus group. Journal of Advanced Nursing 28: 345–352

Sim J, Snell J 1996 Focus group in physiotherapy evaluation and research. Physiotherapy 82: 189–198

Stanton J M 1998 An empirical assessment of data collection using the Internet. Personal Psychology 51: 709–725

Stewart K, Williams M 2005 Researching online populations: the use of online focus groups for social research. Qualitative Research 5: 395–416

Vaughn S, Schumm J S, Sinagub J 1996 Focus Group Interviews in Education and Psychology. Sage, Thousand Oaks, CA

Verpeet E, Dierckx B, Van der Arend A, et al 2005 Nurses' views on ethical codes: a focus group study. Journal of Advanced Nursing 51: 188–195

Webb B 2002 Using focus groups as a research method: a personal experience. Journal of Nursing Management 10(1): 27–35

Webb C, Kevern J 2001 Focus groups as a research method: a critique of some aspects of their use in nursing research. Journal of Advanced Nursing 33(6): 798–805

Chapter 29

Questionnaires

Kader Parahoo

- Introduction: what is a questionnaire?
- The purpose of questionnaires
- Developing and planning questionnaires
- Constructing questionnaires
- Ethical implications
- Advantages and limitations of questionnaires
- An example of a questionnaire
- Conclusion

Introduction: what is a questionnaire?

A questionnaire is a research instrument consisting of a list of questions with instructions on how to record the answers. It is mostly designed to be completed by respondents themselves (self-administered). Respondents complete the answers and return the questionnaire to the researcher. Alternatively, researchers can, face-to-face or by telephone, ask the questions and record the responses. Web-based and email questionnaires, which are becoming increasingly popular, require participants to respond electronically.

The purpose of questionnaires

Questionnaires are often used to collect data on attributes (e.g. demographic details or personality traits), attitudes, beliefs, experience (including perceptions and feelings), behaviour (past, present and future) and activities (e.g. bed occupancy or use of resources). Questionnaires can be used to examine patterns, trends and statistical correlations (relationships) between variables (e.g. between alcohol consumption and occupation). The type of data required by questionnaires is mostly quantifiable. They offer the possibility for respondents to remain anonymous and they are suitable for sensitive topics which people may be reluctant to talk about.

Questionnaires are valuable in providing data to inform policy, practice and education. On page 300 are some examples of the use of questionnaires in nursing research:

Policy: District and practice nurses' public health practice and training needs (Newby et al 2005).

Practice: Asthma treatment needs: a comparison of patients' and health care professionals' perceptions (Hyland & Stahl 2004).

Education: Are mentors ready to make a difference? A survey of mentors' attitudes towards nurse education (Pulsford et al 2002).

Developing and planning questionnaires

Developing questionnaires is systematic, time-consuming and laborious, requiring much preparation before the first question is phrased. Research questions should be clear and realistic. An example of research questions for a study which used a questionnaire can be found in Ahlberg et al (2004, pp. 207–208). The aim of the study was to provide knowledge about predictors of cancer-related fatigue. The research questions were:

- How do patients diagnosed with uterine cancer describe their experience of fatigue, psychological distress (anxiety and depression), coping resources and quality of life?
- What are the correlations among general fatigue, psychological distress, coping resources and quality of life in patients with uterine cancer?
- Does the degree of psychological distress (anxiety and depression) or coping resources predict the degree of general fatigue in patients with uterine cancer?

Research questions, or objectives, have to be feasible and realistic bearing in mind the resources available, including time. The length of the questionnaire and the degree of burden on respondents should also be considered.

The research questions may indicate whether there is a need to 'reinvent the wheel' or whether existing questionnaires, or scales, can be used (with permission from the originator/s). At the planning stage, researchers should take into account who the 'audience' for the questionnaire is (e.g. children, older people, professionals or lay persons) and how they will be accessed. Preliminary enquiry about the feasibility of obtaining an adequate sample for the study should be made. The sample size should be kept in mind at this stage.

In summary, serious consideration should be given to the research topic and questions, the nature and size of sample, the role and tasks of team members and the resources available for the study before the questions can be formulated.

Constructing questionnaires
Layout and structure

The questionnaire should be structured in such a way that it is user-friendly, easy to understand and to answer. The research questions or objectives provide a guide to how the questionnaire is structured and how many questions are asked. For example, if a questionnaire examines nurses' knowledge of and attitudes to research, and their research activities, then each of these key concepts or variables (knowledge, attitude and behaviour) should be allocated a number of questions to address these issues adequately. These key variables could form different sections in the questionnaire. It could start with demographic questions followed in turn by sections on knowledge, attitudes and activities. Such a structure will provide a logical sequence of questions.

Question wording

One underlying principle of question wording is to keep questions short. This should, however, be balanced with the need to be specific about what is being asked. An example of a short question is:

	Yes	No
Do you smoke?	☐	☐

This question, however, lacks specificity. It is not clear whether smoking in this case refers to cigars, cigarettes, a pipe or cannabis. It also does not specify the period of smoking. A clear and specific question could be:

Yes No

Do you currently smoke cigarettes? ☐ ☐

A simple question such as: What is your current income? can be interpreted differently by respondents. Some may think it refers to income before tax and others, after tax. It is also not clear whether they should give monthly or annual figures, nor if it is their own or their household's income. Words like 'sometimes', 'regularly', 'frequently', 'average' or 'majority' can be vague and can mean different things to different people. Where possible ask questions that respondents can quantify. Words like 'access', 'priority', 'perceptions' can be difficult for people to understand. It is better to ask them if they use (instead of 'access') health services, or what their views (instead of perceptions) are. Question wording should also reflect the vocabulary and the reading age of potential respondents.

Leading questions

Avoid these: they are worded in such a way that they encourage respondents to give the answer the researcher wants. An example of a leading question is:

Eating fatty food can be harmful to health. Do you agree that all food products should be labelled?

Yes No

☐ ☐

It would be hard for people to answer 'no' to such a question.

Double-barrelled question

Sometimes two questions are merged into one and it is difficult to give one answer to them. For example:

Were you satisfied with the service and the price?

Yes No

☐ ☐

The respondent may have been satisfied with the service but not with the price.

Hypothetical question

Researchers should avoid asking hypothetical questions as they are not real enough for people to seriously give their views on them. For example:

Do you think there should be more ambulances?

Yes No

☐ ☐

Few people will reply 'no' to this question.

Questions about other people

Questionnaires should be about respondents' own views, attitudes, knowledge or behaviour, not about other people's. A question such as:

Do you think people are in favour of capital punishment?

Yes No

☐ ☐

is asking respondents to guess an answer, because it is not possible for them to know whether people are in favour or not.

Questions which can be obtained more easily from other sources

If a researcher wants to know the visiting times for relatives on a particular ward, there is no point in asking this question to all nurses on the same ward. They may, however, be asked about their views on whether the visiting times are helpful or not to visitors.

Slang

Slang words, professional terminologies, abbreviations (even well-known ones) should be avoided.

Questions which strain the memory of respondents

Asking respondents how many times they went to a supermarket in the last six months may not be easy for some to answer. The time frame is too long and respondents would not be able to give exact figures even if the time frame was reduced to three months. In this case, the researcher can offer 'frequency bands' as shown below:

> In the last 3 months, how many times did you go into a supermarket?
>
> None ☐
> 1–5 ☐
> 6–10 ☐
> 11–20 ☐

Care should be taken to avoid overlapping categories.

Finally, it is important to test the questionnaire (discussed later in the chapter) before it is administered.

Question format

Questions can be asked in a variety of formats or styles, but the choice of format depends on the type of data which the researcher requires. Questions can be closed or open-ended. For example, if the question is 'What sources do you access when seeking information about blood pressure?', the researcher can provide a list of answers which the respondent can choose from (closed). Alternatively they can be asked to list as many sources as they can (open-ended). The common formats used for questions are described below.

Multi-choice questions

Apart from questions requiring a 'yes' or 'no' answer, researchers can offer participants a list of items which they can choose from to indicate their response. For example, respondents could be asked to indicate their mode of travel from home to work, from the following:

> Car ☐
> Bus ☐
> Train ☐
> Bicycle ☐

With multi-choice questions, the researcher must ensure that all the possible options are provided. Even then, an additional box for 'other' should be included in case the respondent in the above example travels by a mode of transport that the researcher had not thought of (e.g. by motorbike). Clear instructions as to whether respondents should 'tick' one or more boxes should be given. In the above example it may be that some people may travel by bus or car before catching a train.

Ranking questions

Some researchers want respondents to rank a list of items in order of priority, preference, importance or frequency.

Rank order questions can pose difficulties to participants as it is not easy to choose from two or more items which are of equal importance. For ranking questions, the number of items should be kept low.

Rating scales

There are three main types of rating scales: verbal, numeric and analogue.

Verbal rating scales use words to indicate the degree or frequency of a behaviour or experience. For example:

> Please indicate your level of satisfaction with your job by selecting one of the options below:
>
> Very high ☐
> High ☐
> Average ☐
> Low ☐
> Very low ☐

One of the disadvantages of using words is that they can mean different things to different people. What is 'average' for some may be 'high' for others.

Attitude scales are another form of verbal scale. The most popular one, the Likert scale (Likert 1932), consists of a series of statements and respondents are asked to indicate whether they 'strongly agree', 'agree', 'neither agree nor disagree', 'disagree' or 'strongly disagree' with each of them. Each response is given a score from 1 to 5 and the total score represents the intensity of the attitudes.

A numeric rating scale consists of a line with an adjective at one end and its opposite at the other. The line is divided into equal steps (5, 7, 9 or 11) and respondents are asked to select a number to indicate, for example, the usefulness of a particular source of information on the scale below:

Completely   Extremely
useless   useful

|____|____|____|____|____|____|____|
   1   2   3   4   5   6   7

The number of steps varies according to individual researchers, although they normally consist of an odd number of steps (5, 7 or 9) so that the middle number can be interpreted as 'neutral' or average. Care should be taken to use adjectives that are polar opposites to avoid confusing respondents.

Sometimes the scale is divided into steps but the numbers do not appear on them, as shown below:

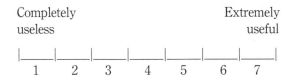

Completely   Extremely
useless   useful

This type of scale is similar to the Semantic Differential (SD) scale developed by Osgood et al (1957) who used it to explore dimensions of meaning of concepts relating to objects, situations and people. For example, the SD can be used in course evaluation. Students are given a statement (stem) and asked to indicate their views by putting an 'X' between the adjectives at each end related to the statement, as in the following example.

The 'Introduction to Research' module was

Boring   Stimulating
|____|____|____|____|____|____|____|

Useless   Useful
|____|____|____|____|____|____|____|

Waste of time   Worthwhile
|____|____|____|____|____|____|____|

The bipolar adjectives at the end of each statement have to be chosen carefully. Bowles (1986) selected the bipolar adjectives for an SD scale in her study of the attitude toward menopause from several sources including the literature and two other existing scales. The adjectives must reflect the participants' experience and usual expressions.

Visual scales are similar to the SD scale in that respondents are asked to respond by putting a mark on a line with a verbal description at each end. The difference between them is that in visual scales (also called visual analogue scales, VAS) there are no marked or numbered steps on the line. The respondent has to 'visualise' where their response would fit on the scale. The length of the line (which can be horizontal or vertical) can vary from 10 to 20 cm; longer lines can make it difficult for respondents to decide where to put their mark. VAS are used frequently in measuring patients' perception of their pain (see e.g. Lin & Wang 2005) but can be used to measure other concepts such as anxiety, hope, or fatigue, as in the example below:

Please indicate your feeling of fatigue by putting an 'X' on the line:

No fatigue   Extreme fatigue
|_____|

Open-ended questions

The purpose of structuring questions and answers is to facilitate the collection and analysis of data in a standard form. For example, if a researcher wanted to know if patients are satisfied with a service, they can be given a series of statements relating to aspects of the service and be asked to rate them. These 'aspects' of the service are selected by the researcher not the respondent. There are times when the researcher may want respondents to identify 'aspects' of the service which they (respondents) find satisfactory or not. In this case instead of giving them 'statements' or 'clues', they can be asked an open-ended question such as:

Which aspects of the Out of Hours service are you satisfied with?

_____

_____

_____

_____

This type of question is described as open-ended because respondents are free to write the answers in their own words. It is useful for obtaining respondents' views. While they may appreciate being asked to express themselves, they may also feel burdened if too many of these type of questions are asked.

The problem with open-ended questions is that the amount and quality of responses can vary between individuals. There is also a high non-response rate to those questions and this can affect the generalisability of the findings. The analysis of data can be very time-consuming, especially if there are many respondents. Nonetheless, it is a question format which can provide useful data from respondents' perspectives and in their own words. One way to impose some control or structure in open-ended questions is to ask them specific questions, such as:

Please list 3 aspects of the service which could be improved?

1. _____

2. _____

3. _____

These are only some of the main formats in which questions can be designed. The choice depends on the type of data required, the population who will answer the questions, and the type of data analysis that will be carried out.

Instructions

Instructions should be clear and unambiguous. Respondents should be made aware if they are to select one or more items. The choice of whether to ask respondents to put an 'X' in, or tick '✓' a box, or circle an answer, is up to the researcher. Sometimes words or phrases are printed in 'bold' or 'italics' or are underlined to emphasise their importance. While these may be helpful in focusing respondents' attention, they should be kept to a minimum, otherwise the effects they are expected to achieve may be weakened.

Filter questions are sometimes inevitable. These questions are used to screen participants who do not have to answer all the questions because some may not be applicable to them. An example of a filter question is given below:

                                                     Yes   No

1.   Do you eat dairy products?   ☐   ☐
If no, please go to question 3.

2.   Which of the following dairy products do you consume daily?

Yoghurt   ☐
Milk   ☐
Cheese   ☐
Butter   ☐

(please tick more than one box, if appropriate)

	Yes	No
3, Are you allergic to nuts?	☐	☐

Filter questions can facilitate respondents to address only the questions relevant to them and thereby avoid potential frustrations of being faced with questions which do not apply to them. However, too many filter questions may also 'frustrate' respondents who may feel they are negotiating a maze of questions.

Testing the questionnaire

An important part in the process of constructing a questionnaire is to ensure that the data collected are valid and reliable. Validity depends on the extent to which the questionnaire, as a whole, addresses the study's objectives. Reliability refers to the consistency with which participants of similar characteristics and outlook understand and respond to the questions. In quantitative research if the tools are considered valid and reliable, then it is assumed that the data which they collect should also be valid and reliable. Piloting the questionnaire and submitting it to peer review can enhance its validity and reliability.

The above strategies can help to enhance the validity of questionnaires. Their reliability can be assessed by administering the questionnaire to the same group of respondents (five to 10) on two occasions (with at least a week's interval). The responses can then be compared to find out the degree of congruence between them; the higher the congruence, the higher the reliability. This is referred to as the test–retest method.

Peer review, on the other hand, consists of giving the questionnaire to people who have research experience to comment on the extent to which the questionnaire meets the research objectives. The main purpose of peer review is to assess (and comment on) the face and content validity of the questionnaire.

Face validity refers to the extent to which the questionnaire appears to fulfil its objectives. It is a quick review rather than an in-depth examination. Although it is a weak form of validity, it serves the function of giving a 'second opinion' on the questionnaire. Content validity, on the other hand, requires the expert judgement of other researchers and of experts on the topic being investigated. A systematic way of ensuring the content validity of the questionnaire is to ask each expert (three or four) to rate each question in terms of clarity and relevance. The responses from each expert can then be compared, followed by changes if appropriate. For an explanation of how content validity was assessed in one study see Lynn (1986). Other forms of validity, which are mainly associated with standardised scales, are discussed in Parahoo (2006).

Covering letter

The covering letter or sheet explains what the research is about, whose research it is, how it is funded, what potential contribution it can make (e.g. in terms of informing policy and/or practice), the incentives or rewards offered and the implications for the participant if he or she decides to take part in the study. Assurances of confidentiality and anonymity (if appropriate), and the address to contact the researcher, should also be given. The covering letter should not coerce people into taking part, but it should be informative enough to help them to make up their own mind to participate or not. It should be written without jargon or obtuse terminology and at the appropriate reading level of prospective participants. Researchers should not make unrealistic claims about the benefits of the study or make promises that cannot be fulfilled.

Enhancing response rate

Two main strategies to enhance response rates at the disposal of researchers are: incentives and reminders. Incentives range from small sums of money (e.g. to cover time taken to respond), vouchers, sample products or gifts. The inclusion of stamped addressed envelopes is standard practice in questionnaire studies.

Reminding people to complete and send back questionnaires is useful in increasing responses. These reminders are often in the form of postcards, telephone calls or an additional copy of the questionnaire. If a coding system is used (i.e. participants are identified by a number), then only those who did not respond are sent a reminder; otherwise reminders should go to everyone in a sample, regardless of whether they have responded or not (with a note to ask them not to respond again, if they have already done so). Sometimes two or three reminders are sent. However, researchers find that there are diminishing returns after the first reminder. The timing for the first reminder is usually three to four weeks after the questionnaire is expected to have been received by the participant. The other reminders could be at two- or three-week intervals.

The finished product

Presentation, length, paper quality, colour, structure, wording and tone can affect participants' decisions to give their precious time to it or not. The increasing facilities offered by the internet have opened up vast possibilities to use this medium in questionnaire design, data collection and analysis (Couper et al 2004).

Ethical implications

Questionnaires can be intrusive as they can seek personal beliefs and details that one would hesitate to ask in interviews. It can make people uncomfortable about revealing their views, behaviours or attitudes. They should be informed in the covering letter that they do not have to answer the questions if they find them intrusive.

In some cases, questionnaires can bring back unhappy memories. For example, a questionnaire on child abuse may make respondents reflect on their own treatment as children and thus could trigger new thoughts and actions which would not necessarily have occurred without the questionnaire. Researchers must reflect on the study topic and decide whether to use other methods, such as face-to-face interviews.

Questionnaires can raise concerns about health issues which, in turn, can cause respondents to worry about their own health. It could motivate them to taking steps to become more healthy, but they can also become alarmed. This is why it is important to provide a contact address which they can access if they have any queries.

These ethical implications show that questionnaires may have the potential to cause harm. However, the principle of beneficence (the potential benefit of the study to the individual/society) should be balanced against that of non-maleficence (research should cause no harm to participants). Clearance from a Research Ethical Committee should be obtained prior to the starting the study.

Advantages and limitations of questionnaires

Questionnaires are most appropriate for providing data on prevalence, trends, incidence and patterns in relation to attitudes, beliefs, experience and behaviour. One of the main purposes of questionnaires is to collect data from a random sample of people which can be generalisable to similar populations. Questionnaires are useful for evaluative and comparative purposes. Data can be collected from people spread around the world and in a short time. Online, email and telephone administered questionnaires can reach people in remote areas quicker than postal questionnaires. Questionnaires developed for one study can also be made available to other researchers, thus saving resources. Compared with face-to-face interviewing, the questionnaire is relatively cheap and quick, it demands less time and participants can answer them in their own time and at their own pace.

Questionnaires can potentially guarantee anonymity and this may encourage some respondents to reveal details of beliefs or behaviour which they may not do in interviews. However, not all questionnaires are anonymous. For the purpose of follow-up, a serial number may be allocated in order to identify those who have responded or not.

One of the main limitations of questionnaires is that they provide little scope for probing and clarifying respondents' answers. However, they are not designed for this. The structure and wording of questions and response categories can reflect the researcher's bias.

Low response and uncompleted questions can affect the quality and generalisability of data. Not everyone has access to telephone and online facilities, including emails, and not everyone can read or write sufficiently to be able to respond to questionnaires.

Since questionnaires rely heavily on self-reports, it is difficult to ascertain whether respondents themselves completed the questionnaire or if their responses were influenced by others.

While, some of these limitations are inherent in the method, properly constructed and tested questionnaires can overcome most of them.

An example of a questionnaire

Chen et al (2005) used a questionnaire (see pp. 268–270 of their article) to collect data in their study of 'nursing models and self-concept in patients with spinal cord injury (SCI)'. The research questions were:

1. Are rehabilitation nurses in SCI nursing aware of the importance of developing positive self-concept among their patients?
2. How do rehabilitation nurses assess a patient's self-concept following SCI and do they experience difficulty?
3. What nursing interventions are used in helping the patient with SCI to reshape positive self-concept?
4. Are the current nursing models relevant to the development of positive self-concept among patients with SCI?

This was a descriptive, comparative study of nurses in Taiwan and the United Kingdom; therefore, a questionnaire was deemed to be appropriate by the research team.

As this was the first study of its kind, and no previous questionnaire was available, the researchers developed their own questionnaire. Items were drawn from the literature and the researchers' experience. The questionnaire was structured in seven parts, as explained below:

The questionnaire consisted of seven main areas: (1) demographic data; (2) nurses' understanding of self-concept; (3) nurses' awareness of changes in self-concept; (4) nurses' difficulties in assessing self-concept; (5) nursing interventions; (6) needs of nurses; and (7) nurses' perceptions of current nursing models used in SCI care.

EXERCISE

Suppose you are asked to:

a. Evaluate nursing care in your clinical area from the perspective of patients/clients
or
b. Evaluate teaching and learning on a course from the perspective of students.

Here are some of the activities you can do which can help you to learn how to develop a questionnaire:

1. Formulate three or four objectives or research questions for one of the above studies.
2. Make a list of the different aspects of nursing care or the course which the questionnaire should cover.
3. Formulate a multi-choice, ranking and open-ended question, as well as a visual analogue scale and semantic differential scale.
4. Discuss the advantages and limitations of the questionnaire for your selected study.
5. List the ethical implications of using a questionnaire in this study and discuss how you would address them.

This exercise can be carried out individually or in groups of three or four.

Conclusion

Questionnaires are valuable for collecting quantitative data, which can show trends and patterns of phenomena as well as correlation between variables. They are used routinely to obtain data on people's views, attitudes and behaviour. Constructing them requires particular attention to the structure and layout as well as to the format and wording of questions. Strategies such as piloting and expert review can help to enhance the validity and reliability of questionnaires. Finally, questionnaires have ethical implications which should be carefully considered.

References

Ahlberg K, Ekman T, Wallgren A, et al 2004 Fatigue, psychological distress, coping and quality of life in patients with uterine cancer. Journal of Advanced Nursing 45: 205–213

Bowles C 1986 Measure of attitude toward menopause using the semantic differential model. Nursing Research 35: 81–85

Chen H-Y, Boore J R P, Mullan F D 2005 Nursing models and self-concept in patients with spinal cord injury – a comparison between UK and Taiwan. International Journal of Nursing Studies 42: 255–272

Couper M P, Tourangeau R, Kenyon K 2004 Picture this: Exploring visual effects in web survey. Pubic Opinion Quarterly 68: 255–266

Hyland M E, Stahl E 2004 Asthma treatment needs: a comparison of patients' and health care professionals' perceptions. Clinical Therapeutics 26: 2141–2152

Likert R 1932 A Technique for the Measurement of Attitudes. McGraw Hill, New York

Lin L-Y, Wang R-H 2005 Abdominal surgery, pain and anxiety: preoperative nursing intervention. Journal of Advanced Nursing 51: 252–260

Lynn M R 1986 Determination and qualification of content validity. Nursing Research 35: 382–385

Newby K, Wallace L, Wareing H 2005 District and practice nurses' public health practice and training needs. British Journal of Community Nursing 10: 214, 216–218, 220

Osgood C, Suci G, Tannenbaum P 1957 The Measurement of Meaning. University of Illinois Press, Urbana, IL

Parahoo K 2006 Nursing Research: Principles, Process and Issues. Palgrave, Basingstoke

Pulsford D, Boit K, Owen S 2002 Are mentors ready to make a difference? A survey of mentors' attitudes towards nurse education. Education Today 22: 439–446

Chapter 30

Observation

Sonja McIlfatrick

Introduction

Parahoo (1997) noted that observation could be considered invaluable for studying human behaviour, either on its own or in conjunction with other research methods. This is because the directness of watching what people do and listening to what they say is fundamentally important to real world research (Robson 1993). This chapter will seek to explore the use of observation as a method of data collection, examining the strengths and weaknesses of using observation as well as some of the ethical and practical considerations. The main types of observation, structured and unstructured, will be discussed along with an exploration of the role of the researcher in observation. Finally, this chapter will detail an example of a study of observation as part of a larger study.

What is observation?

The term observation has been described in the *Concise Oxford English Dictionary* as 'the action or process of closely observing or monitoring, and the ability to notice significant details'. Observation is not unique to research and can be considered as part of everyday life. Adler and Adler (1994) noted:

> For as long as people have been interested in studying the social and natural world around them, observation has served as the bedrock source of human knowledge. (p. 377)

As a research method, observation involves the researcher watching, listening and recording phenomena systematically (Bowling 2002). Silverman

(1993, p. 42) noted that researchers need to recognise the value of using all their senses and the importance of 'using our ears as well as our eyes during observational work'. An early classic example of this distinct research method was Goffman's (1961) study of the total institution, where he obtained employment in a psychiatric institution in order to observe it.

Observation can be used in surveys, case studies and experiments, either in isolation or alongside other methods, such as questionnaires and interviews. Observation epitomises the idea of the researcher as the research instrument and involves 'going into the field', describing and analysing what has been observed (Mays & Pope 1995). However, it can be argued that observation is a relatively underused research method in nursing (Kennedy 1999). According to Parahoo (1997) this is surprising given the practice base of nursing and the fact that nurses rely heavily on observation during their clinical work.

Why use observation as a method of data collection?

Often the key objective for using observation is to check whether what people say they do is the same as what they actually do. As Hammersley (1990) suggested:

To rely on what people say about what they believe and do, without also observing what they do, is to neglect the complex relationship between attitudes and behaviour. (p. 597)

Other reasons for using observation as a method of data collection may include:

- providing insight into interactions;
- helping to illustrate the whole picture;
- capturing a sense of the context and whole social setting in which people function;
- helping to inform about the influence of the physical environment (Mulhall 2003).

Some phenomena lend themselves well to observation (Polit & Hungler 1995), including characteristics and conditions of individuals, verbal and non-verbal communication behaviours, activities, skill attainment and performance and the characteristics of an environment. Some examples of phenomena that have been studied by observation include: 'home care for people with dementia' (Briggs et al 2003); 'children's participation in decision-making' (Runeson et al 2002); 'men's experiences of chest pain' (White & Johnson 2000); 'social support in nursing homes' (Patterson 1995); 'patient dignity in intensive care settings' (Turnock & Gibson 2001); 'district nursing decision-making' (Kennedy 1999); 'nurses' role in an operating department' (McGarvey et al 1999); and 'interaction between nurses, parents and children in intensive care' (Endacott 1994).

Structured observational methods

Structured observation can be considered as an approach in which the aspects of the phenomenon to be observed are operationally defined and decided in advance. Structured observations describe behaviours accurately and reliably, remove subjectivity as far as possible (Pretzlik 1994) and set the boundaries of what is to be observed prior to data collection. According to Parahoo (1997), structured observations usually involve quantifying the specific aspects of a phenomenon such as the presence or absence of a particular behaviour and the frequency and intensity with which it happened. Therefore, the development of an observation 'schedule' or 'checklist' (Box 30.1) is important to define exactly what it is you are trying to observe and the terms to be investigated. For example, in a study of patient exposure in an intensive care unit, Turnock and Gibson (2001) developed an observation proforma to provide information specifically on the following: who was involved in each incident; the areas of the body exposed (such as chest; front genitalia; legs; buttocks); the nature of the intervention (examination; hygiene; elimination); timing of any explanation; length of exposure and the use of screens. This type of proforma can prove useful in avoiding situations

Box 30.1 – *Observational checklist*

WHERE? The setting: this relates to the actual physical environment. What does it look like? What is the context?
WHO? The participants: description of who is in the setting; the number of people and their roles. How do they behave, dress?
WHAT? Activities and interactions: a description of the daily process of activities. What is actually going on? Is there a clearly defined sequence of activities?
WHEN? Frequency and duration: when did the situation observed begin? How long does it last? Is the situation recurring and if so how often?
WHY? Personal reflection: includes researcher's thoughts and feelings about what is going on and personal reflections.

when different observers use different terms to describe the same site of exposure.

Some possible ways to assist the development of an observation framework include: a review of the literature for tried and tested tools, using expert opinion, concept definition and analysis and translating the concept into items or indicators. For example, Barlow (1994), exploring the quality of nursing care provided for sick children, was able to use established quality assurance tools to help provide a focus for some of the elements in the development of a schedule. Some of the categories included:

- individualised care/parental involvement;
- physical well-being of the child:
  safety
  infection control
  observations;
- psychological well-being of the child and family:
  comfort and rest
  communication.

Polit and Hungler (1995) noted that each category needs to be explained in detail, with an operational definition, to enable observers to have clear criteria for assessing the occurrence of the phenomenon

under investigation. To develop recording and subsequent analysis further, categories can then be given codes. For example, Booth et al (2001) carried out a non-participant structured observation study to compare the interventions of qualified nurses with those of occupational therapists during morning care with stroke patients. This involved developing an observational instrument (based on previous work) for categorising interaction styles (Fig. 30.1).

Observational instruments need to be assessed for content validity and reliability. For structured observations to have validity, this means the

Nature of contact interaction	Code
No contact	0
Supervision	1
Prompting/instructing	2
Providing articles	3
Facilitation	4
Giving physical assistance	5
Doing for	6

Explanation for categories
0 No contacts: no contact with helper and patient
1 Supervision: Observing the patient and his/her activities with the purpose of ensuring the rehabilitative effects of each action in maintaining safety.
2 Prompting/instructing: Any communication (non-physical) between the helper and the patient that is intended to assist the patient in completing the activity attempted.
3 Providing articles: This includes providing washing and grooming equipment, preparation of clothing and any other necessary equipment. The actual activities are carried out by the patient using equipment provided.
4 Facilitation: Calculated use of equipment or activity to facilitate the patient's movement, e.g. putting a limb through a natural movement sequence prior to the patient attempting the activity.
5 Giving physical assistance: Actually helping the patient to carry out an activity. The actions of the helper must be rehabilitative in nature, e.g. helping somebody stand up and providing physical support while the patient pulls up his trousers.
6 Doing for: All actions which are 'done to' or 'on' the patient by a member of staff. The patient is passive and makes no active contribution.

Figure 30.1 – *Structured observational instrument: categories of interaction styles. (From Booth et al 2001, with permission of Blackwell Publishing.)*

observer must observe what they were supposed to observe. It is important that the operational definitions are clear and that the categories employed represent the phenomenon under investigation. One way of assessing content validity of the observation schedule is to give the schedule to a panel of experts for review. Reliability relates to the consistency with which the observer matches a behaviour or activity with the category on the observation schedule, and the consistency of recording it each time it happens (Parahoo 1997). This can involve both intra-observer (one observer at different times) and inter-observer (more than one observer) reliability. The data can then be used to calculate an index of agreement, with values ranging from 0.00 to 1.00, with the higher values indicating more agreement and thereby more reliability. The training of observers has been identified as a crucial aspect in helping to improve validity and reliability (Turnock & Gibson 2001).

The role of the observer in structured observation is non-participative where the observer stands 'outside' of what is being observed and tries not to exert any influence on the situation (discussed in a later section). Structured observations adopt mostly a deductive approach when the behaviour or activity is observed against predetermined units of observation. As it is not always possible to observe every behaviour or activity continuously, sampling is required including time sampling or event sampling. Time sampling is where the observer selects time periods when the observations will take place (e.g. an hour at four-hourly intervals over a specified time). For example, suppose a researcher wanted to observe the behaviour of patients and nurses during chemotherapy treatment. During a one-hour observation period they could decide to sample behaviours rather than observe the entire hour. An approach could be to sample randomly 10-minute periods from the total of six periods over the hour. However, it is important that the decisions around the length and number of observations are informed by the aims of the research. Event sampling is where the observer selects pre-specified events for observation (e.g.

shift changes in a ward or cardiac arrests). Event sampling usually requires that the researcher has some prior knowledge regarding the occurrence of events. This type of approach is usually preferable to time-sampling when the events of interest for the study are infrequent throughout a day and are at risk of being missed if specific time-sampling frames are selected.

Unstructured observational methods

Unstructured observations are useful for situations where little is known about the phenomenon under investigation or when the existing knowledge is lacking. Mulhall (2003) maintained that the use of the term 'unstructured' can be misleading. Observation is unstructured in that it lacks a list of predetermined behaviours. Therefore, unstructured observation can be considered as an inductive, naturalistic approach that is qualitative and flexible in nature. The advantage of the unstructured approach relates to the idea that the more structured quantitative methods can be considered as too 'mechanistic' and 'superficial' to 'render a meaningful account of the intricate nature of human behaviour' (Polit & Hungler 1995, p. 307). According to Adler and Adler (1994), the unstructured type of observation:

> ... occurs in the natural context of occurrence, among actors who would naturally be participating in the interaction, and follows the natural stream of everyday life. (p. 378)

The unstructured method can be used to look at single cases (case studies) or complex social organisations (ethnographic approach) (Pretzlik 1994). Using this approach, the researcher is considered as the main tool for data collection and analysis, with the purpose of arriving at as complete an understanding of the phenomenon as possible (Parahoo 1997). Pretzlik (1994) noted that unstructured observation allows the observer to take notes about their observations on an ad hoc basis, with the process being left to the observer to determine. A problem with this is that the researcher may be selective in what to focus on, reflecting their personal interest. It is possible that researchers will omit a whole range of data to confirm their own pre-established beliefs, leaving the method open to the charge of bias.

When using an unstructured observational approach, data are recorded in the form of field notes and logs. Field notes can be considered as descriptions and accounts of people, tasks, events, behaviour and conversations and are useful in recording events 'as they happen' (Pretzlik 1994). In maintaining field notes it is vital that raw behaviour is recorded alongside the researcher's interpretation of the meaning of the behaviour. Barber-Parker (2002), exploring patient teaching in an oncology unit, provided an example of keeping observational (teaching activities), theoretical (attempts to derive meaning) and methodological notes (reflecting research questions and self-critique of research procedures) as recommended by Schatzman and Strauss (1973).

Observations can be recorded using audio or video. Atkinson and Hammersley (1994) commented that the use of such technology allows the researcher to assume a 'privileged gaze', in which the relationships with the participants become less relevant to the collection of data. However, establishing relationships with participants is important in gaining their agreement to being observed and videotaped. Paterson et al (2003) suggested that the use of video recording can add depth and breadth to observations by providing data that the researcher was not able to access in participant observation, and by supplementing field notes through a retrospective review. Latvala et al (2000) provided an analysis of some of the potential advantages and disadvantages of using videotape recording as a method of observation in psychiatric nursing research. They found that one of the essential advantages of videotaping was the ability to capture many varied, detailed, precise interactions and behaviours. Other advantages included the ability to review situations repeatedly – helping in the analysis of data; a reduction in self-report fatigue and subjectivity; and the inclusion of both verbal and non-verbal information. Some of the

limitations relate to mechanical problems with equipment, the influence of the videotape on behaviour and ethical considerations concerning personal privacy, informed consent and respect for the self-determination of psychiatric patients.

The analysis of the data for unstructured observations is similar to that for qualitative interviews and can include the use of phenomenological or grounded theory methods (White & Johnson 2000). It is important to note that qualitative work derives its validity not from the representativeness of its sample but from the thoroughness of its analysis (Silverman 1993). Ashworth (1994) noted that there can be difficulties associated with data analysis for both structured and unstructured observations, with the need to present observation data in a clear, accurate, comprehensive and credible way. Similar to most qualitative research the sampling approach adopted is likely to be purposive. Purposive sampling is based on the belief that a researcher's knowledge about the population can be used to hand-pick the cases to be included in the sample (Polit & Hungler 1995).

Role of the observer

One of the major considerations for researchers using observation as a method of data collection is what role they should adopt and their level of participation. These will vary according to the nature of the research setting and the aim of the research project (as discussed previously). A distinction is commonly made between participant and non-participant observation. A participant observer is someone who participates in the event he or she is observing whilst a non-participant observer maintains a more detached and passive role during data collection (Pretzlik 1994). Gold's (1958) classic typology identified four roles in observation (Table 30.1). These roles are.

- the complete participant who interacts covertly with the situation;
- the participant-as-observer, who interacts and spends most of the time participating in a group's activities, gaining an insider's perspective;

Table 30.1 – *Observational research roles*

Observational role	Activities of the role
Complete participant	Involves participating in a group whilst concealing observer's role
Participant as observer	Most of time spent on participating. Overt observation; undertakes prolonged observation
Observer as participant	Most of time spent observing with small proportion of time spend participating. Overt observation
Complete observer	No participation, maintains distance, no interaction, role concealed

- the observer-as-participant, who observes participants overtly for brief periods, alongside conducting interviews;
- the complete observer, who is detached from the setting and whose role is concealed.

These roles can be considered on a continuum ranging from complete participation with the setting and activities being observed to complete detachment.

As a complete participant, the researcher would undertake the observation covertly with the participants not being aware of the researcher's purpose. It is very unusual for nurses to adopt a complete participant role as this involves an element of deception with the concealment of their observer status. The rationale for the covert observation is to reduce the risk of the observed altering their behaviour and has been used to investigate sensitive topics and behaviours that may have otherwise remained hidden (Mays & Pope 1995). The argument against covert observation relates to the right to privacy and informed consent, the right for participants to know they are part of a study. There are obvious ethical considerations required in the use of covert observation and some justifications have been made in studies involving sensitive

areas. For example, Field (1989) described some early covert work investigating the care of dying patients, with researchers working as health care assistants in order to collect data. Johnson (1992, p. 222), in discussing some of the ethical implications of Field's study, concluded that it is 'impossible to say whether Field's approach is absolutely right or wrong'. Moreover, Clarke (1996) provided a thorough discussion on the merits of covert observation in his study of a secure (forensic) unit. These questions associated with adopting particular roles and issues between covert and overt studies are indicative of much wider ethical and methodological considerations for observational studies.

Demarcation between these positions is often not clear and may not always fit neatly into the two categories of participant or non-participant observation (Sarankos 1998). Rather, the observer may combine elements of these roles and the proportion of time spent observing and participating may vary (Pretzlik 1994). Merrell and Williams (1994) noted that researchers will often have to make tactical decisions about their role in response to the opportunities and restrictions that they encounter as the study proceeds, despite their original intentions. Kite (1999) provided a personal account of some of the difficulties when conducting research as a participant observer in an intensive care unit. In addition, based on their experiences of using a semi-covert study for observing patient care in intensive care settings, Turnock and Gibson (2001) consider that it may not be possible to categorise the observer role within existing definitions and that it may be better merely to summarise the role as a way of illustrating validity.

'Entering the field': access, rapport and practical considerations

Alongside the potential dilemmas associated with the role to adopt, there are other important considerations for researchers 'entering the field'. These relate to issues of access and obtaining a balance between establishing rapport whilst remaining a sufficient distance for the purposes of data collection. Bonner and Tolhurst (2002) noted that when the researcher is considered as an 'insider', this can assist the exploration of practice and deepen an understanding of the phenomenon being studied. The need to develop trust and rapport between researchers and study participants is vital in assisting the researcher to 'get back stage' and learn more about the group's experiences and behaviours (Polit & Hungler 1995). However, Gerrish (1997) noted that overfamiliarisation with a setting could lead to assumptions about what was being observed without seeking clarification for the rationale underpinning particular actions.

Other issues include obtaining consent and practical considerations over behaviour, dress and the recording of data. Briggs et al (2003), exploring the care at home for people with dementia, provided a useful discussion on some of these process issues including gaining and maintaining access to the research setting, disengaging, what can or cannot be observed and the validity of data and analysis. They found that having a first interview prior to observation helped to build up rapport and enabled the researchers to be accepted into the household and thus undertake the periods of observation. They also found that participants could only tolerate the observation for a limited time (three hours). Another practical problem related to the difficulty in disengaging from the participants as there were issues with emotional dependence and social contact.

Some of these ethical and practical considerations are also be elucidated through a research study I undertook in 2005. This was a qualitative study that was undertaken to explore the role of the respiratory nurse specialist (RNS) and was part of a larger study exploring innovative nursing and midwifery roles in Northern Ireland (McKenna et al 2005) (Box 30.2). Through this example I have sought to highlight some of the real considerations that need to be addressed when 'entering the field'.

Evaluating observations

To help evaluate observational methods the researcher should examine both the strengths and limitations of this approach. Some possible strengths include:

- Observation is useful in situations where informants are unable to provide the information or can only give inexact answers during interviews. For example, Runeson et al (2002) noted that observation is particularly useful for research with children as their verbal ability may be limited.
- Observation can be considered as an ongoing dynamic activity and a wealth of knowledge can be derived from observing nursing practice where it happens; therefore observational methods can uncover and describe the activity rather than depend on self-report data.
- Observation is useful in helping to ensure rigour when combined with other methods.
- Unstructured observational approaches are useful for exploratory research.

Some limitations include:

- It has been noted that observational methods are time-consuming and impractical over prolonged time.
- This can result in a sense of 'observer fatigue' and the observer can be distracted.
- The effect of the observer on the 'observed'. It can be argued that when people know they are being observed, they become self-conscious and potentially change their behaviour. This type of observer effect is commonly known as the 'Hawthorne effect'. Morse (2001) highlighted the importance of a period of acclimatisation to allow those working in the field to get used to the presence of the researcher. It is also important to value the explanations prior to the observation. Endacott (1994) noted that the way the researcher explains the purpose of the observation may in itself cause bias by consciously or unconsciously making the observed participants act in a different manner.

Box 30.2 – *Research example: unstructured observation*

McIlfatrick et al (2007): Exploring an innovative role in respiratory nursing practice

The aim of this study was to explore the role of the respiratory nurse specialist (RNS) with the specific objectives of examining the organisational infrastructure, working relationships, career paths, perceived benefits and enablers and barriers to making this role successful. A naturalistic case study methodology was adopted, with a variety of data collection approaches including semi-structured interviews, non-participant observation of practice and a review of job description and other relevant documentation relating to the post.

Observation was undertaken using an unstructured non-participative approach and involved the researcher shadowing the post holder while the latter was going about her usual duties. Two distinct aspects of the participant's role were observed: a nurse-led assessment clinic (4 hours) and a pulmonary rehabilitation programme (3 hours). Data were recorded in detailed field notes and included the following: a description of the activity; the post holder's approach to the activity; an outline of how this practice was innovative; potential benefits to patients; and any thoughts/perceptions of the interaction/activity.

See example of field notes maintained during one observation:

WHERE: Nurse-led assessment clinic, in a small room in local hospital. There was a variety of equipment present including inhalers, nebulisers, spirometry; blood pressure monitoring equipment. No other medical staff present, they can be accessed by telephone.

WHO: A patient enters the room extremely distressed and breathless, and starts to recount a story of how he had attended the local A&E department the previous night owing to his breathlessness.

WHAT: This story involved him spending 3 hours in casualty to then be sent home and he expressed his anger at this situation. At the end of this story the patient started to get upset and stated that he could no longer go on like this and he wanted the nurse to do 'anything, something for him'. The nurse then commenced a variety of investigations and assessment, alongside immediate treatment to relieve the man's distress and breathlessness. Following this, some discussion took place regarding longer care options.

WHEN: The consultation with this patient took 45 minutes in total.

WHY: [personal reflection]: the researcher noted a complete physical and emotional transformation in the patient. The end of the consultation included a discussion with the patient and his wife about future treatment plans and the possibility of pulmonary rehabilitation (something he had previously refused), with the patient stating that he felt so much better physically and psychologically as he felt something could be done for him.

Comments:

1. The researcher found that it was beneficial to undertake interview prior to observation as this allowed them to develop rapport and get to know the post holder in advance of the observation.
2. The researcher also found it useful to develop some guidance for the observation within an overall unstructured approach. This helped to give some focus and direction.
3. The researcher experienced difficulty in maintaining the non-participant role. Rather she would suggest that her role changed on occasions to more of an 'observer as participant'. For example, a particular patient asked questions and sought reassurance from researcher (who was also identified as a nurse) whenever the post holder left the room.
4. The researcher found that it was difficult to take detailed field notes that are not merely descriptive but also interpretive.

- There are various ethical and practical difficulties associated with the use of observation. These can include issues such as informed consent and covert research. For example, Mulhall (2003) noted that there is a practical problem of how, especially in large and busy social settings, to inform and obtain consent from everyone who might 'enter' the field of observation. Mulhall (2003) also expressed concerns about participants' understanding of consent and questioned that if nurses agree to being observed while delivering patient care, does this consent include being observed when talking to colleagues? These problems are compounded by the unpredictability of observational work.

Other ethical dilemmas relate to conflict between the role of the researcher and that of the nurse. Nurse researchers could face an ethical dilemma whether to intervene in cases where they observe bad practice or when asked questions by participants. This can lead to problems associated with being distracted from the focus of the study and the observation of practice, as well as causing tension between their role as a nurse and as a researcher. *The Code of Professional Conduct for Nurses and Midwives* (NMC 2002) clearly indicates the need to intervene if patient care or safety is compromised. Such an intervention has an implication for the role of the researcher as an observer. In a study of nursing practices in intensive care settings, Turnock and Gibson (2001) experienced difficulty in maintaining their role as non-participant observers. Rather, they were viewed as 'quasi insiders' as they were known to the staff as having knowledge of intensive care nursing, which meant they were asked by staff to 'keep an eye on the patient for a minute', while the nurses were engaged in other activities. The researchers found this request difficult to refuse as they were aware of the pressure on staff but it did result in a change of role to 'observer as-participant'.

Conclusion

Observation is a method of gathering data through direct observation of a phenomenon and is a valuable data collection tool in nursing research. The techniques used vary according to the aims of the study, the role adopted during the observation, awareness of the role and the level of structure imposed on the observation. Structured observational methods, often used within quantitative studies, involve the use of observation schedules and are based on the development of categories or pre-existing criteria. Sampling may include either event or time sampling for selecting the behaviours, events, conditions or interactions to be observed. Qualitative studies usually involve more unstructured observations with the aim of gaining more understanding of the phenomena of interest. The main methods of recording data are field notes and logs of events and activities. Observational methods, similar to other methods of data collection, have many strengths, limitations and ethical considerations.

EXERCISES

1. Examine the positive and negative aspects of an experienced intensive care nurse undertaking participant observation on the behaviour of intensive care nurses.
2. Imagine you are waiting in a doctor's surgery and wish to explore the waiting behaviour of patients. How would you start to develop an observation tool? What factors would you need to consider?
3. Formulate a research question from practice and consider whether this problem is amenable to observation. Specify whether an unstructured or structured approach would be preferable and provide reasons for your answer.

4. Read Booth et al's (2001) observation study comparing nurses and occupational therapists washing and dressing stroke patients. Review this paper in light of the following criteria:

- phenomenon under observation
- observation tool (construction, validity and reliability)
- strategies and sampling for observation
- data analysis.

References

Adler P A, Adler P 1994 Observational techniques. In: Denzin N K, Lincoln Y S (eds) Handbook of Qualitative Research. Sage, Thousand Oaks, CA

Ashworth P 1994 Analysis of observed data. Nurse Researcher 2(2): 56–66

Atkinson P, Hammersley M 1994 Ethnography and participant observation. In: Denzin N K, Lincoln Y S (eds) Handbook of Qualitative Research. Sage, Thousand Oaks, CA: 248–261

Barber-Parker E D 2002 Integrating patient teaching into bedside patient care: a participant observation study of hospital nurses. Patient Education and Counselling 48: 107–113

Barlow S 1994 Drawing up a schedule for observation. Nurse Researcher 2(2): 23–29

Bonner A, Tolhurst G 2002 Insider–outsider perspectives of participant observation. Journal of Advanced Nursing 9: 7–19

Booth J, Davidson I, Winstanley J, et al 2001 Observing washing and dressing of stroke patients: nursing interventions compared with occupational therapists. What is the difference? Journal of Advanced Nursing 33: 98–105

Bowling A 2002 Unstructured and structured observational studies. Research Methods in Health. Open University Press, Buckingham: Ch. 15

Briggs K, Askham K, Norman I, et al 2003 Accomplishing care at home for people with dementia: using observational methodology. Qualitative Health Research 13: 268–280

Clarke L 1996 Participant observation in a secure unit: care, conflict and control. NT Research 1: 431–440

Endacott R 1994 Objectivity in observation. Nurse Researcher 2(2): 30–40

Field D 1989 Nursing the Dying. Routledge, Tavistock

Gerrish K 1997 Being a 'marginal native': dilemmas of the participant observer. Nurse Researcher 5: 25–34

Goffman E 1961 Asylums. Penguin, Harmondsworth

Gold R 1958 Roles in sociological field investigation. Social Forces 36: 217–223

Hammersley M 1990 What's wrong with ethnography? The myth of theoretical description. Sociology 24: 597–615

Johnson M 1992 A silent conspiracy?: some ethical considerations of participant observation in nursing research, International Journal of Nursing Studies, 29: 213–223

Kennedy C 1999 Participant observation as a research tool in a practice based profession. Nurse Researcher 7(1): 56–65

Kite K 1999 Participant observation, peripheral observation or aparticipant observation? Nurse Researcher 7(1): 44–55

Latvala E, Vuoikila-Oikkonen P, Janhonen S 2000 Videotaped recording as a method of participant observation in psychiatric nursing research. Journal of Advanced Nursing 31: 1252–1257

McGarvey H E, Chambers M, Boore J R P 1999 Collecting data in the operating department: issues in observational methodology. Intensive and Critical Care Nursing 15: 288–297

McIlfatrick S, McKenna H, Keeney S, et al 2007 Exploring an innovative role in respiratory nursing practice: A case study approach. Primary Health Care Research and Development (in press)

McKenna H, Richey R, Sinclair M, et al 2005 An exploration of innovative nursing and midwifery roles within the Northern Ireland HPSS. Unpublished Report

Mays N, Pope C 1995 Qualitative research: observational methods in health care settings. British Medical Journal 311: 182–184

Merrell J, Williams A 1994 Participant observation and informed consent: relationships and tactical decision making in nursing research. Nursing Ethics 1: 163–172

Morse J 2001 Qualitative Nursing Research: A Contemporary Dialogue. Sage, Beverly Hills, CA

Morse J 2003, Perspectives of the observer and the observed. Qualitative Health Research 13: 155–157

Mulhall A 2003 In the field: notes on observation in qualitative research. Journal of Advanced Nursing 41: 306–313

Nursing and Midwifery Council 2002 Code of Professional Conduct. NMC, London

Parahoo K 1997 Nursing Research, Principles, Process and Issues. Macmillan, Houndmills

Paterson B L, Bottoroff J, Hewatt R 2003 Blending observational methods: possibilities, strategies and challenges. International Journal of Qualitative Methods 2(1), Article 3. Online. Available: http://www.ualberta.ca/~iiqm/backissues/2_1/html/patersonetal.html4 Dec 2005

Patterson B J 1995 The process of social support: adjusting to life in a nursing home. Journal of Advanced Nursing 21: 682–689

Polit D F, Hungler B P 1995 Nursing Research: Principles and Method, 5th edn. Lippincott, Philadelphia

Pretzlik U 1994 Observational methods and strategies. Nurse Researcher, 2: 4–124

Robson C 1993 Real World Research. Blackwell, Oxford

Runeson I, Hallstrom I, Elander G, et al 2002 Children's participation in the decision making process during hospitalization: an observational study. Nursing Ethics 9: 583–598

Sarankos S 1998 Social Research 2nd edn. Macmillan, Basingstoke

Schatzman L, Strauss A L 1973 Field Research. Prentice Hall, Englewood Cliffs, NJ

Silverman D 1993 Interpreting Qualitative Data. Sage, London

Turnock C, Gibson V 2001 Validity in action research: a discussion on theoretical and practice issues encountered whilst using observation to collect data. Journal of Advanced Nursing 36: 471–477

White A, Johnson M 2000 Men making sense of their chest pain – niggles, doubts and denial. Journal of Clinical Nursing 9: 534–537

Chapter 31

Q Methodology in Nursing Research

Carl Thompson and Rachel Baker

- Introduction
- Research questions suitable for Q methodological enquiry
- Q methodology – a walkthrough
- Strengths of Q methodology
- The limitations of Q methodology
- An example of a Q sort study
- Conclusion
- Resources

Introduction

The chapter is structured into three sections. First, we will outline the kinds of research questions that Q methodology is designed to answer and provide some examples of its use. Then we will outline the main stages of any Q methodological enquiry before highlighting the differences between Q and (more conventional) R methodological statistical enquiry. Finally, the relative strengths and limitations of Q methodology as an approach to understanding the meaning that people bring to the social construction of phenomena will be explored.

Research questions suitable for Q methodological enquiry

As with any research approach, the choice of method should be determined by the kinds of research questions that the methodology is designed to answer. Q is designed to answer research questions that focus on self-referent subjectivity – either individual or shared within groups. Self-referent subjectivity in this regard means communication of one's point of view (Brown 1980). Subjectivity is present in such remarks as 'it seems to me . . .', or, 'in my opinion . . .'. When such phrases accompany behaviour they usually indicate that someone has attempted to make sense of the meaning associated with personal experience and cognition. Q methodology has at its core the ability to access such frames of reference and to reveal their structures and forms. Q is used to study matters of taste, values and beliefs about which limited varieties of alternative stances are taken (Stainton Rogers 1995).

Examples of research questions and areas to which Q has been applied include:

■ exploring economic rationality, health and life-style choices in people with diabetes (Baker 2003);
■ the social construction of the meaning of 'quality' in the National Health Service (Thompson 1997);
■ the meaning of health and illness (Stainton Rogers 1991);
■ concepts of 'accessibility and usefulness' associated with research information sources (Thompson et al 2001);
■ the social construction of barriers to research utilisation in health care (McCaughan et al 2002);
■ lay perceptions of mental health (Herron 2000);
■ the ethics of end-of-life decision making (Wong et al 2004);
■ patients' understanding of irritable bowel syndrome. (Stenner et al 2000).

In sum, Q methodology is most useful when the phenomenon under investigation (health beliefs, service quality, accessibility etc.) can be seen as socially constructed. According to this view:

People communicate to interpret events and to share those with others. For this reason it is believed that reality is constructed socially as a product of communication. Our meanings and understandings arise from our communication with others. How we understand objects and how we behave towards them depend in large measure on the social reality in force. (Littlejohn 1992, p. 190)

In seeking to understand the communication of beliefs on a phenomenon, Q methodologists reveal the structures of meaning surrounding a construct for the purposes of observation and study.

Q methodology – a walkthrough (See Box 31.1)
Selecting the Q set

The concourse is the starting point of every Q study. It comprises the set of views, opinions and beliefs (rather than facts) about a particular topic

Box 31.1 – *The main stages of a Q method study*

■ Construction of a Q sample as a means of representing the possible characteristics of the phenomenon under investigation. The Q sample contains stimuli that will trigger reflection on views and beliefs on the part of the respondent.
■ Construction of a P (or person) sample. The P sample is made up of people most likely to inform understanding of the phenomenon being investigated (as with purposive sampling in qualitative enquiry) The respondent systematically rank orders the Q sample stimuli into a Q sort according to a condition of instruction, such as 'sort the following according to those that most represent my views to those that least represent my views'.
■ The first stage of analysis consists of transposing or 'flipping' the data set so that individuals (cases) become variables and variables (Q sorts) become the cases. Bivariate correlation coefficients of the $N \times N$ Q sorts are generated and then factor analysed. So similar Q sorts, not traits or Q sample items, are revealed. The association of each individual with the underlying factor (or perspective) is indicated by the factor loading.
■ Scrutinising factor scores reveals the relative weighting for each of the Q sample items for each of the Q-sort-based perspectives. Each perspective has a factor array (or composite Q sort for all the people who define that factor) and also the statistically different items (i.e. those that make its perspective distinctive) can be examined through a series of pairwise comparisons.
■ The final stage involves looking at where the perspectives converge and diverge and how this relates to extant theory and/or *a priori* assumptions or propositions.

of concern. The Q set is a sample of items (usually statements but other items, such as pictures, can also be sorted) drawn from the concourse. The selection of statements to be sorted by respondents can be either *unstructured* or *structured*. In the former, items are chosen which are presumed to be of relevance to the study but where the emphasis is on representation. In the latter, sample items are chosen to represent points in a theoretical matrix. Here, the use of structured samples is akin to semi-structured schedules for interviews. The structure ensures specific dimensions of an argument or set of propositions are included. However, it is important to note that due to the immense number of possible permutations contained in a Q sort, the researcher is able to exert little influence over the factors that emerge. For example, a simple 10-item Q sort contains 1 209 600 (10 factorial) potentially unique sorts.

Regardless of whether a structured or unstructured Q set is used it should, as far as possible, represent the 'communication concourse' of potential value sets. The number of items in the Q set varies between studies, but usually lies between 20 and 100 statements (Barbosa et al 1998).

Person sample (the P set)

In Q, individuals are selected purposefully according to their personal attributes depending on the research topic and not on the basis of statistical power. P set sizes vary between studies. 'Intensive' studies focus on small numbers of individuals who each undertake several Q sorts under different *conditions of instruction*. Brown (1996) described an example of such an intensive study in health research: a single respondent was asked to reflect on the quality of care received from his surgeon and to sort the Q set from, 'most like the care given by my surgeon' to 'most unlike'. He was then asked to repeat the sort with respect to the care received from each of three nurses, the care provided by his mother during childhood illnesses and his care during another hospitalisation. The Q sorts produced by this individual were then subject to

factor analysis to identify the factors associated with the different care experiences.

'Extensive' studies, in contrast, sample a larger P set in order to obtain Q sorts from a wide range of different people. The preferred size of the P set is related ultimately to the number of factors yielded and the way in which individual Q sorts 'load' on them and hence cannot be established firmly until data are collected. As a guide to the size of the P set, Brown (1996) suggested that 40–60 persons is more than likely adequate.

The power of purposive sampling lies in the ability to select information-rich cases and individuals likely to either strengthen or challenge emerging theory. The relationship between the individuals selected, the sampling frame used, and the type of generalisability is the same as in most qualitative techniques: i.e. the factors (points of view) that emerge provide the structure and form of shared views – rather than predicting the percentage of individuals subscribing to them in the population.

The Q sort

Data for factor analysis arise from individuals rank-ordering Q set items according to a 'condition of instruction' – a process known as Q sorting. Examples of typical conditions of instruction are:

Sort the items according to those with which you most agree (+5) to those with which you most disagree (−5).

Sort the items according to those that are most like object/person X (+5) to those most unlike that object/ person (−5)

As a first basic sort and means of familiarisation, respondents are asked to place the cards in three roughly equal piles, for example 'agree', 'disagree', and 'neutral'. The Q sort then follows, using a grid or scale marked, for example, from −5 to +5 and the number of cards permitted in each 'pile' or 'column' stated. An example of a sorting grid for a structured sort is shown in Figure 31.1.

Each space in the grid indicates the positioning of an item on the continuum from −5 to +5. Two

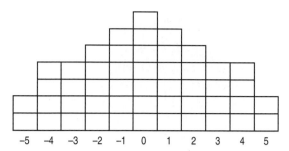

Figure 31.1 – *Q sort response grid.*

items are placed in the '+/−5' positions, four items in the '4' and '3' positions and so on. Making use of these three piles, respondents are then asked to consider the cards in their 'agree' pile, select two cards that are, for example, 'most like me' and place these in the +5 column. Next, selecting from the cards that they disagree with, respondents are asked to select the two cards that are 'most unlike me', placing those cards in the −5 column. This process is repeated until all cards are placed (49 in this example), finishing at the centre of the distribution.

The example above is a 'forced' Q sort in which respondents are obliged to sort statements into a quasi-normal distribution. 'Forcing' the sort in this way is merely a convention allowing respondents to sort statements in a systematic manner. Whether distributions are skewed, flattened, inverted or rectangular the impact on the factors that emerge is minimal, and certainly not statistically (or theoretically) significant (McKeowan & Thomas 1988). Even with forced distributions, respondents are free to place items where they wish. Although the range and number of statements are predetermined, the respondent alone decides where each statement is placed. This contrasts with traditional rating scales where items are scored serially and contextual information excluded. Q sorters control the rank and therefore the contextual significance of each item. The distribution does not represent an index of predefined meaning as in a scale but rather the sorter's attributed meaning of the scale. This process therefore taps into far richer subjective strata of data than conventional rating scales.

The positioning of items is then recorded by transcribing numbers associated with each statement onto a data sheet that usually incorporates a similar scale or grid ready for data entry. Often qualitative interview or open-ended questionnaire data are collected after the Q sorting procedure as a further means of elaboration. These qualitative data are used to aid interpretation of the factors.

Data analysis

Once the items have been sorted by respondents, correlation and factor analysis is performed. The first step is the calculation of a correlation matrix, which represents the degree of similarity between individuals' Q sorts. Correlations (r) are calculated using the following formula:

$$r = 1 - (\text{sum Diff}^2/\text{sum indiv}^2)$$

where Diff represents the difference between the 'rank score' (e.g. −5 to +5) given to each item between two respondents in question, and indiv represents the rank score given by each individual. The correlation matrix is thus derived by repeating this calculation for each respondent compared with every other respondent to produce a table for n respondents of $n \times n$. Correlations range from −1 to 1, a negative correlation indicating that Q sorters have ranked the items differently. In the unlikely event that two Q sorts were identical the sum of the differences would be 0 and r would be equal to 1, representing a perfect correlation.

Factor analysis

Factor analysis is a method of reducing a large number of test scores to a smaller number of factors that lend themselves more readily to interpretation (Pett et al 2003). Whilst the convention is to factor analyse *by item,* (questionnaire items/ test scores as the variables of interest), Q methodology uses *by-person* factor analysis, focusing on the patterns *between* respondents – represented by their Q sorts. To achieve such an analysis it is necessary to transpose or 'flip' the data set (rows or cases become columns or variables).

Two main approaches are taken in the factor analysis of Q sort data: *varimax* rotation and *judgemental* rotation. Often analysts will consult both solutions. By selecting a technique such as varimax rotation – commonly used alongside principal components analysis (PCA) in factor analysis – the statistical sophistication of the method results in higher levels of explained variance and a simple structure which maximises the similarities within factors and the differences between them (orthogonality). Judgement is still required in the selection of how many factors to retain, although rules of thumb such as eigenvalues exceeding 1, or scree plot cut-offs are often used (Fig. 31.2).

Many Q experts recommend judgemental (or theoretical) rotation (Brown 1993). Judgemental rotation allows the analyst to view the factors from different angles before arriving at a factor solution. For example, specific individuals can be defined as reference variates and factors rotated around them. For example, suppose that a group of nurses, including the chief nurse, have provided sorts. Rotating to maximise the chief of nursing's sort may reveal relationships hitherto unrecognised. Since it is the researcher who decides to rotate in this way, it is called 'judgmental rotation'.

To understand judgemental factor rotation, think of two factors plotted in a kind of space. In the example shown in Figures 31.3 and 31.4, Factor 1 is a horizontal line on a plane. Factor 2 is derived

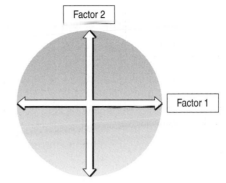

Figure 31.3 – *Factors, factor space and planes.*

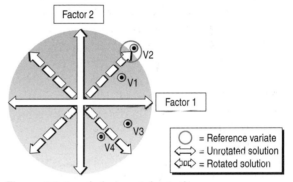

Figure 31.4 – *Judgemental rotation.*

(or extracted) from the variance that Factor 1 cannot account for. You can see that both factors are perpendicular (or orthogonal) to each other because they do not share any variance. Because of this, think of Factor 2 as a vertical line perpendicular to Factor 1.

Each person's Q sort lies somewhere in the plane that these two factors now form. The factor loadings, which represent the correlation between the underlying perspective and the person, can also be thought of as the person's coordinates on this plane.

When the unrotated factor solution is first generated, factor 'axes' may not align well with the pattern of individuals and the loadings may show no clear pattern and so distinguishing between perspectives is difficult. In judgemental rotation we can choose a reference variate and rotate the 'axes' round so that loadings more closely correspond to the people and so become more meaningful.

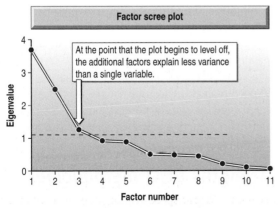

Figure 31.2 – *An eigenvalue scree plot.*

Factor scree plot

At the point that the plot begins to level off, the additional factors explain less variance than a single variable.

Intuitively this may seem wrong (and not very statistical or 'scientific'), but the relative relationships between individual's Q sorts will be preserved.

Whilst the analyst has more control over the solution using this method, factors cannot be forced into particular solutions. The value of judgemental rotation is illustrated by Brown in his description of a Q study based in a psychiatric ward. Of the four factors retained for rotation, the fourth had an eigenvalue less than 1 and only one Q sort defining it (Brown 1980). Examining the non-statistical information, however, it was clear this factor represented the viewpoint of the most senior decision maker in the team. To exclude this factor would have resulted in the loss of important data. The ability to rotate the factors with respect to local context or theoretical concepts (such as power relations) is a valuable one. Judgemental rotation enables exploratory hypothesising about patterns of data. Proponents of judgemental rotation highlight the potential lack of sensitivity (contextual or theoretical) of statistically driven factor solutions (such as varimax) (McKeowan & Thomas 1988).

Factor loadings, factor arrays and factor scores

Factors are represented by the factor array. This is a composite Q sort derived from the weighted averages associated with individual sorts with the resultant meaning revealed by calculated factor scores. Factor scores are the calculated 'rank score' (e.g. -5 to $+5$) for each item in the factor array. In this way, each factor can be represented using the original scoring grid by placing statements on the spaces on the grid.

Factor loadings represent the degree of concordance between an individual's Q sort and the factor $- 2$ to 2.5 times standard error (SE) is used as a guide (McKeowan & Thomas 1988) to establish whether or not such a correlation is high enough to be considered significant, where SE is calculated by $SE = 1/\sqrt{N}$ and N is the number of statements. In the grid shown in Figure 31.1, for example, $N = 49$ and so the correlations are considered substantial where $r > 2$ to 2.5 times $1/\sqrt{49}$: i.e. where r falls in or above the range 0.29–0.36.

Interpretation

The aim of the interpretive phase is to tease out the separate accounts underpinning the patterns of Q sorts, according to their similarities and differences.

The interpretation of factors in Q methodology is iterative in nature, requiring reflection on the structure of the concourse, and reference to theoretical frameworks, as well as the specific features delineating and binding the factors.

Factor arrays are central to the interpretation of each factor. Unlike conventional factor analysis, it is the factor scores (rather than factor loadings) associated with each factor and Q sort items that are compared. Important sources of information in the interpretation of factors are the items placed at each end of the spectrum; neutral items; items which distinguish or represent common views between factors; any apparent discrepancies within the factor array and apparent differences between item interpretations across factors. Laying out the factor arrays on full size grids is a useful aid to the interpretation of factors, as are the qualitative accounts collected during and after the Q sorts.

The factors

The resulting factors represent the different accounts around the topic of interest. Factors vary in number, although typically there will be fewer factors using judgemental rotation than using statistical rotations and eigenvalue cut-off rules (usually an eigenvalue of less than 1 is dropped from analysis). Descriptive labels are usually attached to each factor and factors are usually presented together with a description and the statistical information conveyed by factor loadings and scores.

Strengths of Q methodology

Q methodology has strengths that qualitative research lacks. Stainton Rogers has criticised the analysis of interview data because of 'the mystery of the classification' (Stainton Rogers 1991, p. 122). The key challenge of qualitative analysis is to interpret and classify rich and complex data sets such that they can be presented in a useful way. One of the difficulties in meeting that challenge lies in the ability to articulate precisely what the analysis 'was'. Qualitative analysis is clearly an intellectual process and a technical one – using coding, themes and so forth – but this process is often difficult to express completely. Reflexivity, triangulation and other techniques are often used to present 'trustworthy' accounts that acknowledge the input of the researcher and the researched in the production of findings, but ultimately the researcher may harbour concerns that their analysis is to some extent an artefact structured by their expectations. Q allows unexpected or counterintuitive accounts to emerge. This is possible because, whilst the concourse and Q sampling depend on the researcher and their epistemological 'baggage', the Q sort is ultimately self-referent. In Q, respondents control the classification process (Stainton Rogers 1991).

A further strength of Q methodology is its suitability for topics where respondents do not necessarily have a readily constructed story. Qualitative researchers have developed ways to tackle unfamiliar areas, using repeated interviews with the same respondents, for example, or allowing subjects extended time to reflect on the topic under investigation. Q methods do not rely on respondents' ability to articulate a consistent or coherent rationale; rather, the shared accounts between respondents emerge through the factors, leading Brown to comment, 'Q methodology reveals dimensions which are intrinsic, or inherent, in a concourse, i.e. which emerge from it naturally' (Brown 2001).

At an ontological and epistemological level, Q is more easily combined with qualitative methods than other quantitative approaches (see Thompson et al 2001). Hence, Q goes some way to bridging the much noted chasm between qualitative and quantitative techniques. Q combines the ability to elicit a simple structure from complex data whilst remaining mindful of subjectivity and personal interpretation. Such a reasoned combination is alien to (or at least suppressed in) most quantitative methods. It is this combination of the subjective with explicit and structured analytic techniques that makes it such a distinctive approach.

The limitations of Q methodology

Q is not a technique for large-scale generalisable research along logical-positivistic lines where the proportion of individuals subscribing to a point of view is deemed important. The analytic focus of Q remains squarely on the point of view causing the group to 'cluster'. Q also breaks the assumption of independence central to the logic of statistical enquiry. When one places a Q sample statement somewhere in a continuum it *does* affect the placing of the next statement. However, some authors have questioned whether this violation is significant and suggested that an adequately sized Q sample and the raising of the required probability from 0.05 to 0.01 for significance in factor loadings can combat this (Kerlinger 1986).

Aside from these methodological considerations, Q has some significant practical limitations: undertaking a Q sort as a respondent is time-consuming. The method (if poorly explained) also has the potential for poor completion and high error rates in recording the locations of the Q set items. Whilst postal completion is possible (indeed, one of the authors – Thompson – has used this method in two large research projects), attention to detail at the instructional stage is vital.

An example of a Q sort study

McCaughan et al (2002, available free from http://eprints.whiterose.ac.uk/archive/00000050/) and colleagues were interested in the shared subjectivities of acute care nurses with respect to those barriers that prevent them using research findings in their clinical decision making.

Aim. To examine the barriers that nurses feel prevent them from using research in the decisions they make.

Background. The research literature on research utilisation in nursing has developed significantly over the past 20 years. However, this literature is characterised by a number of weaknesses: self-reported utilisation behaviour; poor response rates and small, non-random sampling strategies. Surveys of barriers to research use in practice are very prone to social desirability bias in that nurses may simply say what they think the researcher wants to hear.

Design. McCaughan and colleagues nested a Q methodological study inside a bigger case study of three large acute hospitals and their relationships with research information. The mixed method study collected and analysed anonymised qualitative interviews, observation, and documentary audits. These data formed the basis of the 'concourse' around barriers to research use in the three sites and the consequent Q sample. Q methodological modelling of shared subjectivities amongst nurses was undertaken in the nurses' workplace. One hundred and eight nurses were interviewed, 61 of whom were also observed for a total of 180 hours, and 122 nurses were involved in the Q modelling exercise (representing a response rate of 64%).

Results. Four perspectives were isolated that encompassed the characteristics associated with barriers to research use. These related to the individual, organisation, nature of research information itself and environment. Nurses clustered around four main perspectives on the barriers to research use:

1. Problems in interpreting and using research products, which were seen as too complex, 'academic' and overly statistical.
2. Nurses who felt confident with research-based information perceived a lack of organisational support as a significant block.
3. Many nurses felt that researchers and research products lack clinical credibility and that they fail to offer the desired level of clinical direction.

4. Some nurses lacked the skills and, to a lesser degree, the motivation to use research themselves. These individuals liked research messages passed on to them by a third party and sought to foster others' involvement in research-based practice, rather than becoming directly involved themselves.

Conclusions. Rejection of research knowledge is not a barrier to its application. Rather, the presentation and management of research knowledge in the workplace represent significant challenges for clinicians, policy-makers and the research community.

Conclusion

Q is a technique that should be part of any nurse researcher's methodological toolkit. It offers transparency and demonstrable rigour that is often missing from 'pure' qualitative approaches to similar research problems and yet also possesses much of the contextual and reflexive benefits associated with qualitative research techniques. Its ideographic focus means that issues of power, language and setting can be incorporated into designs, whilst simultaneously allowing for between-person comparisons. Whilst a basic knowledge of factor analysis is required, Q is relatively easy to operationalise and yields rich, theoretically informed, findings. As a method of illustrating the structures and forms that exist in the social world it has real utility.

Resources

- http://www.lrz-muenchen.de/~schmolck/ qmethod/ This is the Q method home page. It offers a fantastic set of resources including scanned versions of classic texts and software downloads for handing Q analysis.
- http://www.pcqsoft.com/ This is a commercial package for handling Q analysis which some people find easier than the free PQMETHOD software available from Peter Schmolk's Q homepage.

EXERCISES

Point your web browser to http://www.lrz-muenchen.de/~schmolck/qmethod/webq/sexatt/index.html
and have a go at web-based Q sorting for the sexual attractiveness study of Peter Schmolck. How did you
find it? Was it easy or hard? How long did it take you? Did you pay more attention to the images than if
you had undertaken a simple Likert scale based survey?

Try and come up with five research questions you could answer using a Q methodological approach.
Now explain to a friend why you would use Q.

Glossary

Term	Definition
Concourse	The universe of subjective viewpoints on a subject.
Q set	The set of items/statements, usually transcribed onto cards, which respondents are asked to sort according to the condition of instruction.
P set	Sample of persons selected (usually on theoretical grounds) to sort the Q sample.
Condition of instruction	All Q sorts are conducted according to some condition of instruction, i.e. direction to sort with reference to some specification such as sorting the cards representing your own point of view, from those 'most like me' to those 'least like me'.
Q sort	The arrangement of items or statements by respondents according to the condition of instruction. Can be forced or unforced and administered by the researcher or self-administered.
Rotation	Rotation is a statistical technique in which the relation between Q sorts as they are represented in factor space can be examined from different angles.
Factors	Factors are analytic constructs calculated using correlations to reduce a large number of variables to a small number of underlying dimensions. In Q methodology each factor is seen as a distinct account relating to the topic studies, constructed from the correlations between individuals' Q sorts.
Factor array	The composite Q sort representing a factor derived from the weighted averages of individual Q sorts.
Factor loadings	Factor loadings represent the degree of concordance between an individual Q sort and a factor.
Factor scores	Scores given to statements in the composite Q sort corresponding to the original values used in the Q sort (e.g. -5 to $+5$).

References

Baker R 2003 Economic rationality, health and lifestyle choices. PhD, University of Newcastle.

Barbosa J C, Willoughby P, Rosenberg C A, et al 1998 Statistical methodology: VII. Q-Methodology, a structural analytic approach to medical subjectivity. Academic Emergency Medicine 5: 1032–1040

Brown S R 1980 Political Subjectivity. Yale University Press, New Haven

Brown S R 1993 A primer on Q methodology. Operant Subjectivity 16: 91–138

Brown S R 1996 Q methodology and qualitative research. Qualitative Health Research 6: 561–567

Brown S R 2001 Narrative vs Q? (25 Jan 2001). Available via the Q method listserv archives at http://www.qmethod.org/Tutorials/qlistarchives.htm (you will need to register first – see web page instructions for getting a password)

Herron S 2000 Lay perspectives of mental health: a Q method study. Journal of Contemporary Health 8: 25–33

Kerlinger F N 1986 Foundations of Behavioural Research, 3rd edn. CBS College Publishers, New York

Littlejohn S W 1992 In: Theories of Human Communication. Wadsworth, London: 190–191

McCaughan D, Thompson C, Cullum N, et al 2002 Acute care nurses' perceptions of barriers to using research information in clinical decision making. Journal of Advanced Nursing 39: 46–60

McKeown B, Thomas D 1988 Q Methodology. Sage, Newbury Park, CA

Pett M A, Lackey N R, Sullivan J J 2003 Making Sense of Factor Analysis in Health Care Research: A Practical Guide. Sage, London

Stainton Rogers R 1991 Explaining Health and Illness: An Exploration of Diversity. Harvester/Wheatsheaf, London

Stainton Rogers R 1995 In: Smith J A, Harre R, Van Langenhove L (eds) Rethinking Methods in Psychology. Sage, London: 178–192

Stenner P H D, Dancey C P, Watts S 2000 The understanding of their illness amongst people with irritable bowel syndrome: a Q methodological study. Social Science and Medicine 51: 439–452

Thompson C 1997 Quality: A multimethod exploration of a contested NHS concept. DPhil thesis, University of York.

Thompson C, McCaughan D, Cullum N 2001 The accessibility of research based knowledge in UK acute settings. Journal of Advanced Nursing 36: 11–22

Wong W, Eiser A, Mrteck R, et al 2004 By-person factor analysis in clinical ethical decision making: Q methodology in end-of-life care decisions. American Journal of Bioethics 4: W8–W22

Chapter 32

Narrative Research and Analysis

Sion Williams and John Keady

Introduction

Narrative equals life; absence of narrative equals death. (*Tzvetan Todorov cited in* Christman 2004, p. 695)

As human beings we portray ourselves through story, and story-making is integral to human consciousness (Bruner 2004). At its most basic level, narrative research and analysis is about asking for people's stories, listening and making sense of them and establishing how individual stories are part of a wider 'storied' narrative of people's lives (Bruner 2004, Roberts 2002). Riessman (1993) highlighted the lack of a precise definition resulting in researchers adopting a variety of stances that use narrative as a metaphor for 'telling about lives' that often includes 'just about anything' (p. 17) or is particularly restrictive. The defining attributes of narratives as research focus on their quality as 'discrete units' that incorporate a beginning and ending (Riessman 1993), and at the heart of the narrative enterprise is the study of lives through the use of biographical research approaches (Roberts 2002). However, the conceptual diversity of narrative approaches, and the lack of a 'binding theory' (Riessman 1993), results in a range of strategies proposed to interpret and represent people's lives based upon their individual accounts.

What is narrative research?

Narrative research has emerged from a range of disciplines, such as anthropology, linguistics, cultural studies and ethnography (Berger 1997, Polkinghorne 1988). The mode of analysis has also evolved and reflects the influence of these different disciplines on the form and function of narrative research, resulting in highly structured analysis or interpretive strategies (Wiles et al 2005). Osatuke et al (2004) asserted that narratives preserve the 'rich complexities of lived experience' and draws listeners to the person's 'complexly textured world' through characterisation, plot and theme (p. 193). There are a number of proposed evaluative criteria for narrative research, such as trustworthiness and authenticity (Mishler 1995) and a process of 'consensual validation' (Lieblich et al 1998).

Narrative research appears as both a separate and an integrated approach. The lack of a 'binding theory' (Riessman 1993) results in the narrative research form emerging, and being located within, an existing philosophical and methodological stream, primarily within the fields of phenomenology and ethnography which are also characterised by diversity. For instance, there are numerous examples of narrative work as part of the emphasis upon meaning elicited through text and discourse based on the phenomenological hermeneutic approach underpinned by the philosophy of Paul Riceour (Cole & Knowles 2001).

A core value of narrative research is that it provides a 'lens' through which to explore the complexities and map out the relationships between selfhood, identity and the social world (Bruner 2004, Lieblich et al 1998, Roberts 2002, Somers 1994, Somers & Gibson 1994). Such an account examines the interplay between past and present construction of self, and at its heart is concerned with uncovering an emic perspective on the lifecourse through the 'performance' of a narrative (Fig. 32.1).

Mishler (1995) provided a three-part typology for classifying narrative studies according to the focal point of the research. Firstly, reference and temporal order identifies relationships between narrated events and 'real-time' events; secondly, textual coherence and structure refers to the linguistic and narrative strategies for the 'construction of

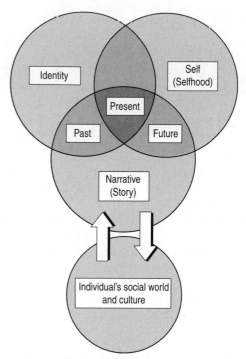

Figure 32.1 – *The narrative lens.*

the story' (p. 7); and thirdly, narrative sets the story in a wider social and cultural context. The typology developed by Mishler (1995) summarises the key features of narrative research as 'process' and establishes the importance of 'form' and 'function' in narrative research.

To develop an understanding over how these core relationships work in practice, Lieblich et al (1998) provided an important heuristic framework that separates the interpretation and analysis of narrative according to what is described as an holistic-to-categorical continuum, clarifying the significance of 'form' and 'function' in narrative research approaches (Box 32.1).

The philosophical and methodological roots of narrative research are rich and varied (Manning & Cullum-Swan 1994, Roberts 2002) and formulate an intriguing and flexible method of qualitative inquiry. Narrative research is not alone in being the subject of multiple variations and interpretations (Denzin & Lincoln 1994, 2000) and the developments in narrative research are driven by a

Box 32.1

- Holistic-content mode embraces the life story as a whole and addresses the meaning from the text in its entirety.
- Holistic-form mode utilises the guide of looking for plots or structure to life stories, seeking meaning as turning points and endings.
- Categorical-content mode is similar to content analysis and involves the separation of textual utterances in order to construct an analysis.
- Categorical-form mode is more linguistic in orientation, the use of metaphors and language to articulate underpinning ideas and thoughts.

Source: Lieblich et al (1998).

renewed interest in 'narrative' and 'story' across a range of disciplines. Moreover, interest is fuelled by a cross-fertilisation of ideas, methods and techniques of data collection and analysis.

Initially grounded in life history research (Lawler 2003, Roberts 2002), narrative research has emerged centre-stage in sociology, particularly in the case of ethnography, as there has been a marked shift away from modernist arguments about the dominance of social structures (Lawler 2003). The scope of narratives as a form has been extended beyond representation (Riessman 1993) and they are now identified as having not only a personal but a public dimension; they 'neither begin nor end with the research setting: they are part of the fabric of the social world' (Lawler 2003, p. 243).

The adoption of particular interpretive strategies reflects social, historical or cultural orientations and involves a dynamic movement in the treatment of narratives. For example, there is an increasing interest in 'textuality' as part of narrative in the social sciences, with a renewed emphasis on written or spoken text as not only reflecting but producing social reality (Lawler 2003). Health care and

nursing retains some diffuse conceptions of 'narrative' and its relationship to 'story' (Paley & Eva 2005) yet also mirrors a shift in the attentiveness to the personal construct of reality and its role in understanding the wider social 'story' of care (McCance et al 2001).

Locating narrative

A narrative account requires two key features to be present: a discourse as the basis for a narration, and the narrative which has to be attentive to time and therefore involves a temporal dimension (Lieblich et al 1998, Roberts 2002). A third feature delineates the architecture of the narrative form, described by Denzin (1989) as a simple scheme consisting of a beginning, a middle and an end that is linear and sequential, has a 'plot' but is also past orientated and 'makes sense' to the narrator.

We would suggest that narrative research and narrative accounts are best understood using a dramaturgical rather than the traditional literary metaphor. Indeed, Goffman (1974) identified storytelling as a 'performance', and Riessman (1993) emphasised the importance of 'performance' in representing experience as narrative. This metaphor highlights the centrality of communication and the purpose of conveying meaning, or what Gubrium and Holstein (1997) describe as 'horizons of meaning' to an audience.

Identity is central to the narrative inquiry (Bruner 2004, Roberts 2002) and the weaving of the past and present elements of identity into a temporal dimension develops a construction of 'self' that can be understood separately – as occurring in the past – and also synthesised into the present in a temporally organised whole (McAdams & Janis 2004). In this sense narratives are constructed and 'authored' by individuals with a purpose and presented as 'unified' (McAdams & Janis 2004). This is developed further by Somers (1994) who highlighted the relational aspects of narratives by mapping out what can be understood as four inter-related narrative 'scripts' that are an inherent part of any performance. These are:

- the person's own 'inner world' (ontological narrativity);
- the social context and its expectations (public narrativity);
- the broad cultural and historical context (master narrativity);
- the researcher's frame of reference (conceptual narrativity).

A key reciprocal relationship exists between ontological and public narrative, informing the formulation of selfhood. For instance, McCreight (2004) identified the 'grief ignored' by male partners following a miscarriage and stillbirth. Previous research and a social (public) narrative focused on the expectation that men were emotionally strong to support their partner. However, McCreight (2004) highlighted how such a perception contrasted with the inner world experience of men and what Somers (1994) characterised as their personal (ontological) narrative. The public narrative of men only having a supportive role ignored the meanings they attached to the loss and their personal emotional tragedy, involving self-blame, loss of identity and the need to hide their feelings of grief and anger.

Not only do narrators provide a structure (Denzin 1989), but researchers impose and seek 'plots' and there is a recognised tendency of narrative work to arrange events and the structure of a life in a coherent order (Plummer 2001). Riessman (1993) identified a number of key elements that provide form in narratives:

1. Structure – the common elements include a starting point or point of departure for researchers, as it unifies form and function: an abstract (summary of the substance of the narrative), orientation (time, place, situation, participants), complicating action (sequence of events), evaluation (significance and meaning of the action, attitude of the narrator), resolution (what finally happened) and coda (returned to the present).
2. Plot – plots frame the narrator's sense of meaning and these vary from tragedy, comedy, romance, satire and so act as archetypes and points of reference for representation.

3. Agency and truth – the degree of 'truth' attached to narrative reflects the researcher's perspective (in essence their conceptual narrative), whether linguistic or phenomenological.

The narrative involves the narrator's performance to the researcher-as-audience and incorporates how the 'performance' is viewed and interpreted. Somers (1994) challenged this paradigm and described it as being 'representational' – in other words, providing 'false order' to the chaos of lived experience. Hence, Somers (1994) presented different layers of narrative that involve the participant and researcher and focus on personal and social dimensions of identity, emphasising the dynamic nature of social interchange (Gergen & Gergen 1984). Furthermore, recognising the importance of conceptual narratives highlights the importance of how researchers approach narratives based on a particular frame of reference. For instance, as Riessman (1993) identified over a decade ago, narrative research drawing on Western traditions tends to emphasise the importance of chronological, rather than episodic sequences in narrative, and the spectrum of approaches are influenced by a range of social science perspectives. Representation of the 'story' in narratives is informed not only by conceptual narrativity but also by the cultural master narrative and public narrative, that provide the 'theatre' of social context for the narrator's performance and underpin the judgements made by the researcher-as-audience, as well as its grounding in their respective biographies (Fig. 32.2).

Narrative methods

McCance et al (2001) highlighted that interviews are the most frequently chosen method when using narratives approaches. The shape and form of the encounter will be determined by the approach adopted to frame the particular narrative study and will require attentiveness to the complexities of 'talk': its multilayered, contextual and aural qualities (Wiles et al 2005). A number of issues need to be borne in mind in considering the narrative interview, such as:

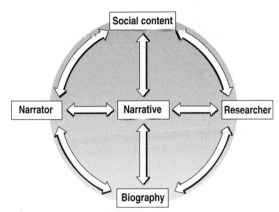

Figure 32.2 – *The dynamics of narrative research: A narrative quadrangle.*

1. Selecting the interview format – in narrative work the preferred format is unstructured (rather than the structured or semi-structured format) in order to enable the personal narrative to emerge (McCance et al 2001) and allowing open questions to be used (Riessman 1993).
2. Asking the right question – the content of the interview questions is also important and Riessman (1993) suggested the use of an interview guide consisting of five to seven broad questions based upon the research question.

The basic form of a narrative interview may also be developed as part of a group and participatory process (Arlanda & Street 2001) and requires equal sensitivity. The central aim of any interview is to facilitate the story to be told and see how respondents make sense of their lives (Riessman 1993) and describe their experience and actions (Polkinghorne 1995).

Narrative analysis

Paley and Eva (2005) noted that although 'story' and 'narrative' are used interchangeably as terms, not all 'story' is narrative but narrative includes story. This was a theme reiterated by Roberts (2002) and important in locating the place of narrative research in the broader area of biographical approaches. Making sense of narratives frequently

refers to the terms 'analysis' and 'interpretation' being used interchangeably (Wiles et al 2005). Some clarity is provided by conceptualising analysis as an activity of making sense of data whilst interpretation is more than analytic explanation. Rather, interpretation involves understanding the meaning of social action and gets 'under the skin' of the complexity described by Somers (1994) as a person's 'ontological narrative'.

The framework detailed earlier by Lieblich et al (1998) in Box 32.1 highlighted the importance of recognising explicitly the framework guiding the researcher and the narrative work, such as reading, interpreting and analysing narrative using one of the four basic strategies. Lieblich et al (1998) provide a useful benchmark for the analysis and interpretation of data produced from narrative research, emphasising the connection between the form (how to approach the narrative) and function (what is the focus of analysis):

1. Holistic-content – involves two approaches to analysis, firstly as an overarching 'case' study drawing on the general themes and emerging foci from the narrative; or secondly, using a specific segment of the text to demonstrate the story as a whole. Both involve reading/listening to the material several times until a pattern emerges focused on the whole story and its context. This results in an initial overview, and any exceptions that challenge it, emerging as a first impression, and in unusual features such as contradictions being noted. A particular focus, or theme, is identified that seems to dominate the text from beginning to end, either spatially, being repetitive or through the depth of description. These are marked and re-read separately. Throughout this process the researcher should keep an analytical trail through careful notation and increasing sensitivity to the text by the re-reading process.
2. Holistic-form – involves a focus on the narrative as a whole but with careful attentiveness to the formal aspects of structure in the narrative as an expression of the perspectives of the

storyteller. A basic series of plots underpin this form of analysis, the progressive narrative advances steadily, the regressive narrative identifies deterioration and decline whereas stable narratives indicates little change. The overarching storylines of tragic, comic, heroic, romantic and satire provide a broad staging for the analysis. An additional strut to the strategy focuses on its cohesiveness as a 'good story'. The analytic process firstly identifies thematic focus of the plot in the narrative, 'in what way does the content lend structure to the plot?' The researcher draws from this the direction taken by the content and provides the basis for the second step that identifies the dynamics of the plot 'inferred from particular forms of speech' (Lieblich et al 1998, p. 91). Again the content provides clues to the underpinning structure of the story, and words or phrases indicate a tragic or heroic plot line. Lieblich et al (1998) mapped these two aspects of this approach as a representational graph.

3. Categorical-content – this approach breaks the text into smaller units of content prior to analysis and follows the principles and techniques of content analysis. The broad parameters for such analysis are the selection of a subtext based on the separation of text that relates to the proposed research question; the definition of content categories provides the means for classifying the units of analysis (words, sentences or phrases), identifying themes that are shared in the subtext, sorting the material into categories based on assigning sentences and so on to the relevant categories and finally drawing conclusions by analysing numerically or descriptively and revisiting the original research question.

4. Categorical-form – this involves a focus on the oral narrative with the aim of analysing the speaker and the narration in order to understand what the dialogue can disclose about the speaker. A focal point for Lieblich et al (1998) was how discourse uncovers cognitive abilities and the articulation of story as well as the emotional underpinning of the content. It requires selection of a set of criteria and classifications in order to understand the deep linguistic structures of the text and is a micro-analysis, such as the use of features in speech, their intensity and frequency. For instance, detailed descriptions of events belie a challenge in expressing difficult emotions, using adverbs like 'suddenly' may indicate the expected or unexpected nature of an event and mental verbs (I thought or I understood) display the extent to which an experience is subject to a conscious form of mental processing.

The 'narrative turn' is seen as the hallmark of narrative analysis and it provides a method of identifying 'life patterns' and understanding, not only personal, but community experience and meanings (Plummer 2001). However, the 'turn' is grounded in a particular approach to the narrative as a research endeavour and linked to a mode of analysis that fits the particular narrative 'form', such as holistic or categorical (Lieblich et al 1998). At its centre narrative methods and analysis pivot upon acknowledging that 'talk' is used strategically as well as to represent ideas and involve social norms, values and power (Wiles et al 2005). It can be seen from the framework presented by Lieblich et al (1998) that narrative methods involve the exploration and articulation of language, without being constrained solely to discourse analysis. As indicated by Somers (1994), the relationship between personal (ontological), social-community (public) and cultural-historical (master) narratives is central. It is not surprising that different approaches and emphases have evolved to manage and interpret these complex interrelationships, using either holistic or categorical methods (Lieblich et al 1998) of accessing and analysing the narratives of people. Narrative involves 'talk' in a variety of forms and Wiles et al (2005) described how narrative methods and analysis in essence involve five basic approaches, whether presented verbally or in written form, these being:

1. The evaluative component of talk. This involves a structured approach to narrative emphasising that a narrative is actively constructed with a

sensitivity to the response and needs of the audience. There is portrayal and internalised self-control to ensure that the narrative 'fits' with prevailing (public) assumptions and values. The aim of analysis is to examine how the story is told within the interview and unfolds, giving clues to the purpose behind the narrative form and the factors motivating the speaker. It allows the researcher and the narrator to be partners in the interpretive process and explore shared personal-public meanings.

2. The multilayered nature of talk. This elaborates on the premise that 'talk' operates on many levels and has many functions and effects. For instance, Riessman (1993) described ideational, interpersonal and textual purposes in language as a means of conveying meaning. The textual content (how things are said) in many ways provides an indication and clues to the relationship between personal and social worlds described in narrative talk. Also, Riessman (1993) highlighted that not all audiences are able to share/access meanings embedded in narratives and a 'multilayered analysis' examines the relational aspects of the narrative, including personal, social and (master) historical contexts and its apparent 'messiness' (Wiles et al 2005).

3. The contextual nature of talk. This focuses on the 'performance' of narrative, particularly in the interview setting. The connection between the narrator and researcher requires greater performance if meaning is not shared and has to be emphasised. It also relates to power relations as part of the process of providing a narrative and the nature of the performance can constrain communication and understanding. A good example is the balance between the uniqueness and the typicality of an event, with a dramatic event being played down in order to prevent it being dismissed by the listener.

4. The ways groups use and interpret talk. Narrative analysis also takes account of how groups 'tell stories' differently and researchers focus on the portrayal of the story using a dramatisation approach (Riessman 1993): identifying the act (what was done), the scene (where or when was it done), the agent (who did it), agency (how the person did it) and purpose (why). Here the focal point is who is narrating as well as how.

5. The aural features of talk. This emphasises the aural and oral nature of narratives and elaborates on interpretation, recognising not only the visual and written context. Some researchers target the 'oral performance' (Wiles et al 2005) by attentiveness to the structure of the discourse and language. The rhythm of the sentences, the pauses and non-verbal expressions are the indicators used as part of the interpretive act.

Evaluating narrative

Denzin (1989) provided a simple scheme consisting of a beginning, a middle and an end that is linear and sequential, has a plot but is also past-orientated and finally makes sense to the narrator. This scheme was echoed in later texts (see: Lawler 2003). Riessman (1993) and Mishler (1995) defined the basic attributes for narrative research and established evaluative criteria. The work by Lieblich et al (1998) constructed an heuristic model that clarified the purpose of the research with the narrative approach and the mode of analysis, paralleled by a continuum by Paley and Eva (2005). Furthermore, Wiles et al (2005) synthesised and fleshed out the complex nature of 'narrative talk' and its analysis and representation in a variety of forms, defined as multilayered, contextual and aural qualities of narrative. However, as Lieblich et al (1998) noted, 'each approach is more suitable for some purposes than for others' (p. 479).

Diversity is an advantage; as Goncalves et al (2004) identified, it is a distinctive feature of human beings that they have the capacity to use language to construct personal (and community) experiences as narratives; indeed, he argued we are 'narrative beings'. Contemporary narrative research through its diversity enables researchers to explore the connections between people's sense of self, identity and their social world, drawing upon the epistemology of linguistics and hermeneutic philosophy (Cole & Knowles 2001). Narratives provide 'meaning bridges' (Osatuke et al 2004) through the construct of the self (and its story) as the storyteller, irrespective of the foci of interpretation, and centred on the 'semiotic glue' constructed of words, symbols and signs that hold our experiences together.

The limitations of narrative research are an inherent part of its focus on accounts of self and its diverse nature resulting in a variety of forms and functions. At the centre of a consideration of problematic issues surrounding narrative is the role of memory. As Freeman (1993) highlighted, any narrative account is a 'rewriting the self' and is itself an interpretive act and results in some 'submerged story threads' (Osatuke et al 2004). In this sense narratives address self-understanding (Freeman 1993) and situate a sense of selfhood in a temporal frame, providing an interpretation of connections, coherence, movement and direction (Gergen & Gergen 1984) as part of what Spivak (1997 cited in Lawler 2003) described as writing a running biography with 'life language' rather than 'word language'. The task of accessing 'life language' requires the use of 'word language' and its careful interpretation and analysis in order to make sense of the storied narrative of individuals and wider communities. Making sense of 'life–word language' requires a variety of approaches to the narrative enterprise and the organisation of stories, such as through emplotment and the use of particular techniques of analysis. Furthermore, the personal is also seen as speaking of the social world with meta-narratives (Lawler 2003), master or meta-narratives (Somers 1994) or macro narratives (Osatuke et al 2004) relating accounts of how personal selfhood and identity is constructed as part of social interchange (Gergen & Gergen 1984). The issue of authorship and unity presents an important tension in narrative research and its analysis. It is important to acknowledge the researcher's or the 'author's voice' in narrative work (Clandinin & Connely 1994) and not seek to overwrite the life language (Spitvak cited in Lawler 2003) evident in the narrative.

The use of narrative in nursing research: a case example

Overcash (2004) argued that nursing is well suited to using narrative research and provides the ideal 'forum' for gaining narrative data as 'the ear for the intimate accounts and personal thoughts' (p. 15). The case of narrative as informing the knowledge that underpins practice has, in recent years, been augmented by an interest in narrative research (Frid et al 2000). In particular, a narrative approach is cited as highly relevant in answering clinical questions and uses techniques that are familiar to nurses, such as interviewing, communicating and listening, in addition to its possible therapeutic implications (Overcash 2004). However, a lack of conceptual and methodological clarity creates a 'fog' around the use of narrative research due to its adoption by a wide range of disciplines, and the use of competing approaches and strategies. Recently, Paley and Eva (2005, p. 83) have highlighted the inconsistent nature and functions of narrative research in health care in the following way:

- narrative as a naïve account of events;
- narrative as the source of 'subjective truth';
- narrative as fiction;
- narrative as a form of explanation.

These challenges are attributed to a lack of clarity over the meaning and usage of 'narrative' and 'story' (Paley & Eva 2005), reflecting their interchangeable use in nursing (Fagermoen 1997, Rittman et al 1997). Frid et al (2000) also identified that 'narrative' as a term has permeated nursing science and is linked to its theoretical underpinnings as part of a consideration of the debates on 'caring' as a concept. Paley and Eva (2005) also suggested that the lack of clarity between 'story' and 'narrative' exacerbates misconceptions and leads to the 'current tendency to romanticize narratives' (p. 84).

As part of the social world of health care and nursing, the term 'narrative' has also been prominent as part of 'illness narratives'. Hyden (1997) characterised three different types of narrative:

illness as narrative, narrative about illness and narrative as illness. In general, narrative has been seen as a vehicle within health and social sciences for exploring patient experiences and suffering and 'giving them a voice' (Hyden 1997). However, as Bury (2001) identified, the renewed interest in 'illness narratives' belies their diverse and complex nature. In brief, the diverse types are:

- 'contingent narratives' that address a person's beliefs regarding the causes and effects of illness on everyday life;
- 'moral narratives' that provide an account and form part of the adjustment in the relationship between the person, their illness, their identity and hence their 'moral status' as an individual in society;
- 'core narratives' that connect the person's experience to the wider sociocultural levels of meaning attributed to the illness and suffering.

These broad narrative types are augmented by the sub-forms of characterisation of narratives based on the archetypes of heroic, tragic, ironic and comic, also regressive or progressive narratives. As an area of interest, narratives are being further used in the field of health care such as the developments in exploring suffering as part of 'trauma narratives' (Eid et al 2005), but also the meaning of suffering in psychiatric patients (Fredriksson & Lindstrom 2002), patients experiencing pain (Carter 2004) and

cancer narratives (Van Der Molen 2000). In the field of dementia studies, there is a growing interest in storytelling and narrative (Cheston et al 2004), building on the work of researchers such as Mills (1998) who wrote a seminal text on narrative identity and dementia.

Conclusion

We have argued in this chapter that narrative research presents challenges and opportunities. Furthermore, the field of narrative is focused on 'opening up' narration and the exploration of biography, identity and people's sense of self and their place in their social world. It is imperative for narrative analysis to be underpinned by a structure that makes explicit the approach being adopted and describes the relationships regarding authorship and the voice of the narrator. This chapter outlined that narrative research and analysis represents a number of approaches that are best understood using frameworks, such as Mishler's (1995) and Lieblich et al's (1998) in order to interpret how narrative and the 'narrative turn' is used in practice as part of a narrative study, and why. Furthermore, we have highlighted the different layers of narrativity that make up a narrative account and identified the dynamic-storied nature of narratives as representations of self, identity, the social world and as complex 'performances'.

EXERCISE

Chaptering your life: a 20 minute-exercise adapted from Gubrium (1993).

1. Students should divide into pairs, respectively adopting the role of a narrator and researcher. The researcher should ask the narrator to give a narrative account of their life by arranging it into 'chapters'. The chapter headings and their content should be documented by the researcher.
2. The researcher should examine the chapter headings and their content and seek to identify a 'plot' that emerges from the narrative account. The researcher should decide how the headings represent the narrator's 'story' and arrange them to provide a storyline with a beginning, middle and end.
3. This storyline should then be shared with the narrator and its authenticity agreed.
4. The narrator and the researcher should then change roles and repeat the exercise.

References

Arlanda S, Street A 2001 From individual to group: use of narratives in a participatory research process. Journal of Advanced Nursing 33: 791–797

Berger A A 1997 Narratives in Popular Culture, Media and Everyday Life. Sage, London

Bruner J 2004 The narrative creation of self. In: Angus L E, McLeod J The Handbook of Narrative and Psychotherapy; Practice, Theory and Research. Sage, London

Bury M 2001 Illness narratives; fact or fiction? Sociology of Health and Illness 23: 263–285

Carter B 2004 Pain narratives and narrative practitioners: a way of working 'in relation' with children experiencing pain. Journal of Nursing Management 12: 210–216

Cheston R, Jones K, Gilliard J 2004 'Falling into a hole': narrative and emotional change in psychotherapy group for people with dementia. Dementia: The International Journal of Social Research and Practice 3: 95–109

Clandinin D J, Connely F M 1994 Personal experience methods. In: Denzin N K, Lincoln Y S (eds) Handbook of Qualitative Research. Sage, London: 413–427

Christman J 2004 Narrative unity as a condition of personhood. Metaphilosophy 35: 695–713

Cole A L, Knowles J G 2001 Lives in context: the art of life history research. AltiMira Press, Oxford

Denzin N K 1989 Interpretive Biography. Sage, London

Denzin N K, Lincoln Y S 1994 Handbook of Qualitative Research. Sage, London

Denzin N K, Lincoln Y S 2000 Handbook of Qualitative Research, 2nd edn. Sage, London

Eid J, Johnsen B H, Saus E 2005 Trauma narratives and emotional processing. Scandinavian Journal of Psychology 46: 503–510

Fagermoen M S 1997 Professional identity: values embedded in meaningful nursing practice. Journal of Advanced Nursing 25: 434–441

Fredriksson L, Lindstrom U A 2002 Caring conversations – psychiatric patients' narratives about suffering. Journal of Advanced Nursing 40: 396–404

Freeman M 1993 Rewriting the Self: History, Memory, Narrative. Routledge, London

Frid I, Ohlen J, Bergbom I 2000 On the use of narratives in nursing research. Journal of Advanced Nursing 32: 695–703

Gergen M M, Gergen K J 1984 The social construction of narrative accounts. In: Gergen K J, Gergen M M (eds) Historical Social psychology. Erlbaum, Hillside, NJ

Goffman I 1974 Frame Analysis. Harper and Row, New York

Goncalves O F, Henriques M R, Machado P P P 2004 Nurturing nature: cognitive narrative strategies. In: Angus L E, McLeod J (eds) The Handbook of Narrative and Psychotherapy; Practice, Theory and Research. Sage, London

Gubrium J R 1993 Speaking of Life: Horizons of Meaning for Nursing Home Residents. Aldine de Gruter, Hawthorne, NY

Gubrium J F, Holstein J A 1997 The New Language of Qualitative Method. Oxford University Press, Oxford

Hyden, L 1997 Illness and narrative. Sociology of Health and Illness 19: 48–69

Lawler S 2003 Narrative in Social Research. In: May T (ed) Qualitative Research in Action. Sage, London

Lieblich A, Tuval-Mashiach R, Zilber T 1998 Narrative Research: reading, analysis and interpretation. Applied Social Research Methods Series, vol 47. Sage, London

McAdams D P, Janis L 2004 Narrative identity and narrative therapy. In: Angus L E, McLeod J. (eds) The Handbook of Narrative and Psychotherapy; Practice, Theory and Research. Sage, London: 159–173

McCance T V, McKenna H P, Boore R P 2001 Exploring caring using narrative methodology: an analysis of the approach. Journal of Advanced Nursing 33: 350–356

McCreight B S 2004 A grief ignored: narratives of pregnancy loss from a male perspective. Sociology of Health and Illness 26: 326–350

Manning P K, Cullum-Swan B 1994 Narrative, content and scientific analysis. In: Denzin N K, Lincoln Y S (eds) Handbook of Qualitative Research. Sage, London: 463–483

Mills M A 1998 Narrative identity and dementia: a study of autobiographical memories and emotions. Ashgate, Aldershot

Mishler E G 1995 Models of narrative analysis: a typology. Journal of Narrative and Life History 5: 87–123

Osatuke K, Glick M J, Gray M A, et al 2004 Assimilation and narrative: stories as meaning bridges. In: Angus L E, McLeod J (eds) The Handbook of Narrative and Psychotherapy; Practice, Theory and Research. Sage, London: 193–210

Overcash J A 2004 Narrative research: a viable methodology for clinical nursing. Nursing Forum 39: 15–22

Paley J, Eva G 2005 Narrative vigilance: the analysis of stories in health care. Nursing Philosophy 6: 83–97

Polkinghorne D E 1988 Narrative Knowing and the Human Sciences. State University of New York Press, Albany

Polkinghorne D E 1995 Narrative configuration in qualitative analysis. In: Hatch J A, Wisniewski R (eds) Life History and Narrative. Falmer Press, London

Plummer K 2001 Documents of Life 2: An Invitation to a Critical Humanism. Sage, London

Roberts B 2002 Biographical Research. Open University Press, Buckingham

Riessman C K 1993 Narrative Analysis. Qualitative Research Methods Series 30. Sage, London

Rittman M, Rivera J, Godown I 1997 Phenomenological study of nurses caring for dying patients. Cancer Nursing 20: 115–119

Somers M R 1994 The narrative constitution of identity: a relational and network approach. Theory and Society 23: 605–649

Somers M R, Gibson G D 1994 Reclaiming the epistemological 'other': narrative and the social constitution of identity. In: Calhoun C (ed) Social Theory and the Politics of Identity. Blackwell, Cambridge, MA: 37–99

Van Der Molen B 2000 Relating information needs to the cancer experience. 1. Jenny's story: a cancer narrative. European Journal of Cancer Care 9: 41–47

Wiles J L, Rosenberg M W, Kearns R A 2005 Narrative analysis as a strategy for understanding interview talk in geographic research. Area 37: 89–99

Chapter 33

Qualitative Data Analysis: Achieving Order out of Chaos

Mike Nolan

- Introduction
- What is qualitative research? What is qualitative analysis?
- Qualitative analysis: underlying principles
- Resolving methodological and conceptual conflict – the views of Janice Morse
- Future challenges for qualitative research in health care: enabling user and carer involvement

Introduction

The title of this chapter highlights succinctly the dilemmas faced when attempting to capture the dimensions of qualitative data analysis. For, as Atkinson and Delamont (2005) noted, the field is extensive, and the full range of methodological debates and practical approaches cannot be adequately covered even in an entire book. Inevitably, therefore, a contribution such as this must be partial and incomplete; indeed there may be some who find it superficial, or even inaccurate. The situation is not helped by 'internal conflicts' amongst qualitative researchers themselves (Morse 1994), which have resulted in qualitative data analysis becoming a 'contested site of multiple practices' (Schwandt 1997), lacking a consensus as to the best approach to adopt (Creswell 1998).

Little wonder then that qualitative analysis has been described as a:

> '... vast and varied enterprise ... (requiring) an immensely diverse set of practices ... (under-pinned by) a great diversity of theoretical approaches, practical problems and local research traditions. (Seale et al 2004, p. 2)

It would therefore appear that neophyte qualitative researchers, hoping to achieve some order from their mass of seemingly 'chaotic' data, are faced with potentially even greater chaos if they consult the methodological literature. Clearly, then, this chapter cannot provide any definitive answers, nor do I intend to give a simplified 'how to' guide to data analysis, although I will provide some pointers as to where such approaches can be found.

Rather, following the advice of Seale et al (2004), I will adopt a more pragmatic stance and highlight some principles that I have found useful in my own research practice and, paraphrasing their words, this chapter will therefore 'recount and reflect on my own research experience as well as that of others from whom I have learned'.

In setting the scene, the chapter begins with a very brief overview of what is meant by qualitative research, before providing a potential definition of qualitative analysis. Subsequently, and despite the variability noted above, I will identify a number of commonalities underlying qualitative analysis prior to highlighting some of the existing 'frameworks' for analysis.

What is qualitative research? What is qualitative analysis?

Denzin and Lincoln (2005b, p. 2) suggested that 'a complex interconnected family of concepts and assumptions surround the terms qualitative research', and whilst most authors argue that the primary purpose of qualitative research is to generate theory (Lathlean 2006, Liamputtong & Ezzy 2005, Morse 1994), agreement is by no means universal. In tracing the evolution of qualitative research over the last several decades, it is suggested that the overall aim has become increasingly more emancipatory and political, so that qualitative research is now seen as 'a democratic project committed to social justice in an age of uncertainty', helping people to move from 'ideas to inquiry, from inquiry to interpretation, and from interpretation to praxis, to action in the world' (Denzin & Lincoln 2005a).

Even if the focus is limited to inquiry and interpretation, the range of potential analytic strategies remains extensive, and in such circumstances it is essential that the 'rationale' for the choice of method adopted is clearly explained (Seale et al 2004). Some degree of informed choice is therefore always necessary and this is, in part, determined

by the interests of the researchers involved. As Denzin and Lincoln (2005a, p. xi) noted, 'the issues and concerns of qualitative researchers in nursing and health care . . . are decidedly different from those of researchers in cultural anthropology'. Moreover, of the several different methods of qualitative analysis available, 'some are appropriate for exploring data, others for making comparisons and then for building and testing models, nothing does it all' (Ryan & Bernard 2000).

With regard to this chapter my choice has been informed by the writing of Ryan and Bernard (2000). They identify two broad 'traditions' in qualitative analysis that they term the 'linguistic' tradition and the 'sociological' tradition. They see qualitative data as comprising mainly text, which itself can take multiple forms:

By qualitative data we mean text: newspapers, movies, sitcoms, email traffic, folktales, life histories. We also mean narratives – narratives about getting divorced, about being sick, about surviving hand-to-hand combat, about selling sex, about trying to quit smoking. In fact most of the archeologically measurable information about human thought and human behaviour is text, the 'good stuff' of social science. (Ryan & Barnard 2000)

In 'making sense' of such 'good stuff' they consider that the 'linguistic' tradition sees the text itself as the object of analysis using techniques such as narrative, conversation and discourse analysis. In contrast, the 'sociological' tradition views text as an account of, or proxy for, experience. It is this latter approach that will be considered in this chapter.

However, qualitative analysis is not a 'magical' process (Morse 1994), and if we are to demystify what it is then some form of definition is required. After considering several definitions, the following by Schwandt (1997) appears to me to be amongst the most helpful:

Broadly conceived, this (data analysis) is the activity of making sense of, interpreting or theorising about data. It is both an art and a science, and is undertaken by means of a variety of procedures that facilitate working back and forth between data and ideas. It involves the processes of orga-nising, reducing and describing the data, drawing conclusions or interpretations from the data, and warranting these interpretations. If data could speak for themselves, analysis would not be neces-sary. (Schwandt 1997, p. 4)

But analysis is necessary and, even operating within a broad 'sociological' tradition, decisions as to the approach to use are still required. Miller and Crabtree (1992) likened this process to taking a photograph in which it is necessary to decide which camera to use, which scene to focus on, and which filter to select. Using this analogy the camera would relate to the broad methodological approach, the scene to the object of inquiry or study, and the filter to the theoretical orientation that is applied.

Qualitative analysis: underlying principles

Compared to quantitative approaches, where data are structured and strategies for analysis are often predetermined, qualitative analysis is more flexible (Donovan & Sander 2005) and is neither linear nor predictable (Liamputtong & Ezzy 2005). Further-more, whereas in quantitative research data collec-tion precedes analysis, the relationship is different in qualitative research. Data collection and analysis proceed in an iterative fashion (Donovan & Sander 2005, Lathlean 2006, Ritchie et al 2003), each informing the other. Therefore, data analysis begins early and guides subsequent data collection (Lathlean 2006).

For example, in my own early research I was interested in the experiences of carers who sup-ported a family member, and who used respite care services (Nolan 1990, Nolan and Grant 1992a, 1992b). Virtually all of the literature at the time described caring as burdensome or difficult and so the focus of my early questioning was about the extent to which respite care provided relief from such burden. However, initial analysis of the data suggested that, whilst caring was often difficult, it was by no means always a problem, and many

carers also gained considerable satisfaction from their role. As a result of this early analysis, the focus of data collection, and indeed the study as a whole, broadened to consider the potential rewards and satisfactions of carers and the impact of respite care on these. Further analysis of the data identified differing sources of satisfaction, and also high-lighted the fact that carers' acceptance of respite care hinged critically on the extent to which the cared-for-person had a positive respite experience. As a result, we proposed a 'mid-range' theory that provided practical ways in which respite care could be made more acceptable to both the carer and the cared-for-person (see Nolan & Grant 1992b and later in this chapter).

Qualitative data analysis is therefore intimately linked to data collection and involves both cogni-tive processes and the application of varying structured techniques. However, several authors identify a number of shared goals, although the terms they use differ. Some of the more commonly cited approaches to analysis are summarised in Table 33.1.

Ritchie et al (2003) argued that two common pro-cesses underlie all qualitative analysis:

- managing the data to reduce it and distil the 'essence';
- making sense of the data and generating either descriptive or explanatory accounts.

Descriptive accounts are closer to the data and would be readily recognised by participants in the research. Later these descriptive accounts may be 'classified' into more abstract ideas that retain the original meaning of the data but use more complex language. More sophisticated explanatory accounts seek to find links and connections between two or more phenomena, in order to generate theory.

In taking stock of the various arguments regard-ing the sequencing and purpose of qualitative analysis, it seems to me that these might be sum-marised using an 'alliteration' of C's. These are briefly outlined in Table 33.2.

This format captures, hopefully in an easily re-membered fashion, the way in which data analysis

Table 33.1 – *Some frequently cited strategies for qualitative analysis*

Framework – Ritchie and Spencer (1994)	Miles and Huberman (1994)	Grounded theory (simplified)
This comprises 5 stages which occur in the following order: Familiarisation – provides an overview of the issues by immersion in the data and identification of recurrent themes Identify a thematic – (coding) framework that crystallises key concepts that can be applied to the rest of the data Indexing – the systematic application of the coding framework to the data Charting – the abstraction of themes using headings from the framework. This produces a 'picture' of the data analysis that can be viewed by others to demonstrate themes and links Mapping and interpretation – a description of the findings in the form of typologies, concepts, associations and explanations	These authors recommend a 3-stage analysis process comprising: Data reduction – this involves coding and processing, requiring a detailed reading and rereading of transcripts and then coding the data to identify key issues Data display – recognising and re-presenting codes now allows the scrutiny of texts and the display of data in tables, charts or matrices to facilitate comparison. This enables a fuller thematic description to emerge Conclusion drawing – further analysis and theorising – this involves further interrogation of data and the identification of links between themes and categories resulting in the formation of possible theories that explain relationships in the data	Described by Bryman and Teevan (2005) as 'by far the most widely used framework for analysing qualitative data'. They provide a simplified description of the process as comprising: Coding – breaking data into component parts and giving them names. May involve different levels of coding, which proceed sequentially as follows: (a) Open – keeping close to the data and identifying initial concepts (b) Axial – creating categories or higher-order concepts that further reduce the data (c) Selective – identifying the main or core category and looking for relationships with other categories in the data Constant comparison – maintaining a close link between data and conceptualisation, comparing concept with concept, concept with category, and category with context in an iterative fashion Theoretical sampling – whereby further data are collected to inform the emerging theory and to achieve theoretical saturation when no new themes or ideas emerge

moves from the 'raw data' and generates ever more abstract ideas that are however still connected with, and are traceable back to, the data. Depending on their purpose, studies may stop at any point along this continuum. So, for example, using Ritchie

et al's (2003) suggestions, studies that are primarily descriptive and exploratory might go no further than the creation of concepts. At a slightly higher level of abstraction, studies that wished to 'classify' concepts would aim for the creation of categories. Researchers

Table 33.2 – *The sequencing of qualitative analysis – the 5 C's*

Codes	Following an initial immersion in the data, numerous preliminary ideas, thoughts and feelings begin to emerge*	↑ Higher level of abstraction/fewer, more complex ideas
Concepts	Following further consideration of the data and/or more data collection, codes that reflect common trends are identified and named	
Categories	More detailed interrogation and/or further data collection allows categories of concepts to emerge, further reducing the data	
Connections	Links between similar categories are identified, suggesting recurrent connections within the data; initial 'hypothesis' may be formulated, suggesting the conditions necessary for links between categories.	
Conclusions	Typologies, explanatory accounts or tentative theories are described	↓

*These may be used to inform future data collection.

who wanted to provide more sophisticated explanatory accounts would need to find connections and draw conclusions from their work. Of course, in qualitative work, 'conclusion' does not signal some ultimate or final result but rather indicates that this is the furthest point it is possible to teach with the data available.

Once again an example from the respite care study mentioned earlier might help to illustrate how this process works. One major component of this study was to understand the respite care experience from the older person's perspective, as initial data analysis had clearly indicated that carers got most benefit from respite care when the older person had a positive experience. The service in question worked on a rota basis in which the older person spent two weeks in hospital, followed by six weeks at home, with this cycle being repeated over a number of months, or even years. It therefore seemed very important to find out why some older people seemed to enjoy their stay, whereas others found it extremely distressing. In order to appreciate this, interviews were conducted with the older people themselves, and extensive periods of observation were undertaken in the hospitals concerned. Staff and carers were also interviewed about

their views on respite care. This generated masses of data, detailed analysis of which identified a 'typology' of differing types of respite user in which three main groups, one with a number of subgroups, were identified (Nolan & Grant 1992b).

The three main groups were the:

- Beneficiaries – these older people really enjoyed their stay, were active throughout, and looked forward to their next period of respite.
- Tolerators – these older people 'put up' with the respite care because they knew their carer needed the break, but they did not enjoy their stay, nor did they look forward to it. There were three subgroups identified here: the endurers, the disillusioned and the martyrs.
- Abandoned – these older people could see no purpose at all for their respite stay, and deeply resented the fact that they had to spend time in hospital.

Underpinning this typology were differing 'connections' between a number of main categories of data. The main categories were:

- Reason for coming – this was concerned with how the older person explained to themselves and others why they were using respite care.

- Being active – what the older person did during their respite stay.
- Impact on relationships – the impact of respite on the relationships older people had with other patients, staff and their family carer.
- Effect on self-esteem – the impact that the respite care admission had on the older person's view of themselves.

The way in which these 'categories' of data 'connected' to shape the typology is summarised in Table 33.3.

If we take the analysis back a stage further using the category of 'keeping active' as an example, this was generated following the merging of several concepts, including: basic care; therapy and assessment; treatment; social interaction; group activity; individual activity; disengaged. These concepts in turn were the result of bringing together a greater number of less abstract codes which included: washing; dressing; feeding; walking; bathing; exercising; playing games; talking; reading; watching the TV; seeing the doctor; receiving visitors; doing nothing; staring into space, and so on.

Hopefully, starting from the final typology and disaggregating data in this way, is helpful in understanding how the typology itself was constructed.

Table 33.3 – *A typology of respite care users (adapted from Nolan and Grant 1992b)*

Typology/ Category	Reason for coming	Being active	Impact on relationships	Effect on self-esteem
Beneficiaries	Because they enjoyed it and saw a personal benefit/ gain. Benefit to carer was secondary. Looked forward to next stay	Highly active and engaged throughout their stay, socially, physically, and they believed, therapeutically. Received frequent visitors	Forged good relationships with staff, other respite users on the same rota, and other patients. Had an improved relationship with their family carer	Positive effect on self-esteem, and reinforced their view of themselves as a person of value and worth
Tolerators Endurers	Because their carer needed and deserved a break	Less active and engaged, tended to engage in solitary as opposed to group activity. Fairly long periods of inactivity	Relatively superficial relationship with staff, other users and patients. No real impact on relationship with carer	Managed to sustain self-esteem. They 'put up and shut up', 'making the most of a bad job'
Disillusioned	Had been told they were coming for 'therapy' but rarely received any. Therefore became disillusioned. Believed carer needed and deserved break	As above	As above	Realisation that they were not considered to need or benefit from therapy, tended to reduce self-esteem

Table 33.3. *A typology of respite care users (adapted from Nolan and Grant 1992b) Cont'd*

Typology/ Category	Reason for coming	Being active	Impact on relationships	Effect on self-esteem
Martyrs	Believed their carer needed a break, but did not necessarily deserve it	As above	Very limited relationships with staff, users, patients. Damaging to relationship with family carers, as voiced their discontent upon return to home, causing friction and tension	Mainly negative effect on self-esteem, as they felt 'martyred' to the family carer's needs
Abandoned	Could see no good reason for coming. Did not believe the family carer either needed or deserved a break	Inactive for most of their stay, generally refused or resisted attempts to get them to participate	Forged no relationships with staff, patients and users. Very poor and deteriorating relationships with family carer, who saw the older person as manipulative, domineering or unappreciative	Very low self-esteem, but also very angry

Morse (1994) might argue that the above example uses three of the four 'cognitive' processes that, for her, underpin all qualitative research. These are: comprehending; synthesising; theorising, and recontextualising. I personally have always found Morse's approach very useful and so it is described in greater detail below.

Resolving methodological and conceptual conflict – the views of Janice Morse

Concerned that despite the 'proliferation' of qualitative method texts there remained a lack of clarity about analysis, and alarmed by the 'internal conflicts' amongst qualitative researchers themselves, Morse (1994) argued that qualitative research had reached a crisis point that could no longer be ignored. In an attempt to find some common ground within disparate methodological traditions Morse (1994) suggested that there are four cognitive processes that, to a greater or lesser extent, underpin all qualitative analysis. She acknowledged that these processes might be 'weighted' differently according to a given tradition, for example grounded theory or phenomenology, but nevertheless believed that they all played a part. As noted above, she termed these four processes: comprehending; synthesising; theorising and recontextualising. Each of these is now considered in turn.

Comprehending

For Morse the process of comprehending begins before data collection has started because for her the longstanding debate in qualitative research about whether or not to use existing literature is largely redundant; she puts her view as follows:

The debate about how much the researcher should learn about the setting before beginning the study is not difficult to resolve. The researcher should learn everything possible if he or she is to avoid re-inventing the wheel. (Morse 1994, p. 26)

This would include consulting the literature, and identifying already existing theories or themes. However, Morse cautions that this prior knowledge should not dominate the study but rather result in 'wise and smart researchers' who are able to 'recognise leading without being led'.

Having gained a good overview of the field, data collection then begins and Morse advocated that researchers need, as far as possible, to:

- enter the field as a stranger;
- be capable of passive learning, of absorbing non-judgementally everything remotely relevant;
- adopt a stance of active inquiry, asking questions such as what?, when?, where? and why?
- make notes (memos) frequently and as completely as possible;
- keep literature and non-research data separate.

Morse advocated that comprehension has been reached when 'the researcher has enough data to be able to write a complete, detailed, coherent and rich description' of the area of study.

Synthesising

For Morse synthesising is the process whereby stories, experiences and accounts are brought together to identify composite patterns. This represents the 'sifting' part of analysis that provides an aggregate account, allowing a better understanding of shared experiences to emerge, along with the potential identification of significant factors that may help to account for variation in the data. At this stage the data have been 'decontextualised' from individual experiences and the search for linkages and relationships has commenced.

Theorising

Morse argued that theory is what gives qualitative research its structure and facilitates its application to the world of practice. Such theory does not come in a flash of insight but involves a constant process of speculation and conjecture until a 'best fit' model between data and theory is created. This should be the most comprehensive, coherent and simplest account that links the data in a useful way. This search for the simplest or most parsimonious account is the hallmark of a good theory. Morse described this as follows:

Theorising is the process of constructing alternative explanations and of holding these against the data until a best fit that explains the data most simply is obtained. (Morse 1994, p. 33)

This process cannot be rushed and takes time as it represents the 'real work' of qualitative research.

Recontextualising

Although qualitative research does not generate findings that can be 'generalised' in a statistical sense, several authors argue that findings or theories should be of relevance beyond the particular context in which they were generated. Several terms are used for this. For example, Guba and Lincoln (1989) talked of findings being 'transferable' to other settings, contexts or groups; Bassey (1984) coined the term 'relatability', whereas for Morse this process is captured by the phrase 'recontextualising'. She believes that this is the 'real power' of qualitative research and it is here that already existing theory plays a greater role. So, for example, the emerging theory derived from a particular study would now be compared more systematically and fully with existing literature on the same or related topics, so that the potential explanatory power of the theory may be extended.

In this way qualitative research can generate insights that are relevant to settings and contexts beyond the study itself. For some qualitative researchers who do not believe in the generation of theory this is irrelevant, but for those operating within a broadly defined 'sociological' tradition it is essential. Generally speaking, theories vary depending upon two main characteristics – scope and abstraction. Scope is concerned with the range of phenomena that the theory attempts to explain, and abstraction relates to how abstract ideas within the theory are. Often within the nursing literature there is talk of several kinds of theory, frequently termed 'practice' theory, 'mid-range' theory and 'grand' theory. Practice theories deal with a relatively limited range of issues and the concepts used are closely tied to the empirical world. Mid-range theories attempt to explain a wider range of phenomena, using ideas that are more abstract, whereas 'grand' theories seek to explain as many phenomena as possible using-highly abstract ideas. The relationship between these two characteristics is illustrated in Figure 33.1.

Qualitative research usually generates 'mid-range' theories and by a process of 'recontextualising' and comparing newly developed theories with existing work the 'scope' or number of phenomena that the theory can explain is extended, and knowledge is built in an incremental fashion. For example, the 'mid-range' theory of respite users described above built on earlier work by Chenitz (1983) who was looking at older people's reactions to relocation from home to a nursing home. Later the ideas from Chenitz's work and the adaptations made during the respite study were used to define a typology of nursing home admissions (see Nolan et al 1996). More recently these ideas have been extended to explore nursing home admission in other countries such as Sweden (see Sandberg et al 2002). I would therefore agree with Morse (1994), that recontextualisation represents the 'real power' of qualitative research.

Future challenges for qualitative research in health care: enabling user and carer involvement

As noted earlier, the field of qualitative research has expanded considerably over the last 15 years, and in many respects is now unrecognisable from what it was a couple of decades ago. With regard to research in the field of health and social care, one of the most significant challenges has been the increasing emphasis placed on user and carer involvement in research. As Grant and Ramcharan (2006, p. 54) note, this trend has emerged as a result of the growing political movement towards consumerism and is in part recognition of the fact that 'those best placed to inform service development are those on the receiving end of such services'. Realising the ideals of user and carer involvement in research poses several significant challenges and raises fundamental issues of power and control that impact not only on analysis but on the entire research process.

In considering the challenges that greater user involvement poses, Grant and Ramcharan (2006) argued that this can be seen as a continuum, at one end of which is consultation, moving through collaboration and finally to complete user control. For me the most appropriate way forward is to think of research as a collaborative endeavour based on a partnership model in which users and carers have important roles to play in:

■ determining which research questions/issues are important;

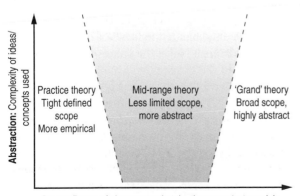

Scope: Range of phenomena that the theory seeks to explain

Figure 33.1 – *Scope and abstraction as properties of theory.*

- deciding which methods or approaches to use;
- designing relevant questionnaires, instruments, or interview schedules;
- taking part in data collection and analysis;
- contributing to the writing up and dissemination of results.

Working in such a way challenges existing thinking about what 'research' actually is, and about the 'rules' for undertaking research studies. It means in particular that we need to rethink what counts as 'evidence' and accept a wider, more holistic definition.

With respect to nursing research, the above developments have coincided with the movement away from research-based practice to evidence-based practice (EBP) (Rolfe 1999). However, some argue that there are distinct tensions between EBP and initiatives promoting user and carer involvement (Kitson 2002), with Humphries suggesting that, whilst concepts such as user participation are 'part and parcel' of a more inclusive social policy agenda, EBP is a 'practitioner engineered movement', incompatible with the rhetoric of participation.

Consequently, rather than users and carers being 'active shapers of knowledge and subsequent action' (Clough 2005, p. ix), it is contended that EBP has resulted in a biasing of research towards a professional's view of the world, rather than a user's (Kitson 2002), with users still being seen primarily as sources of data, which are subsequently used to develop professionally dominated services and outcomes (Humphries 2003).

Such debates raise fundamental issues of power, expertise and evidence (Owen 2005), and beg the question as to 'what counts as research, and whose research counts?' (Nolan 2005). If current and emerging initiatives such as the 'expert patient programme' (Donaldson 2003), and the identification of 'expert family carers' (Scottish Executive 2005) are to stand any chance of being maximally successful, then mechanisms have to be devised that enable all forms of evidence to 'come equally to the table' (SCIE 2003). This will mean bringing together the varying but potentially complementary forms of evidence generated by researchers, practitioners and users/carers.

Recently there have been calls for a more inclusive definition of evidence-based practice so that decisions about services are primarily made by those receiving care, informed by the tacit and explicit knowledge of those providing it, within the context of available resources (Dawes et al 2005). However, if this is to be achieved, then in terms of research at least, there is a need to 'transform the rules by which the game is played' (Barnes 2002), so that users and carers can be genuinely involved in generating new knowledge for:

> *Knowledge, as much as any resource, determines definitions of what is considered important, as possible, for, and by whom. Through access to knowledge and participation in its production, use and dissemination, actors can affect the boundaries, and indeed the conceptualisation of the possible. (Gaventa & Cornwall 2001)*

If users and carers are to participate genuinely in the production, use and dissemination of knowledge and extend the boundaries of the possible then, as Seale et al (2004) suggested, there is a pressing need to challenge the increasingly abstract and possibly irrelevant debates that have resulted in qualitative analysis becoming 'fragmented and hyper-specialised' (Atkinson & Delamont 2005). In particular, the language we use as researchers and practitioners needs to change, as do the means by which we disseminate the fruits of our efforts. At a more fundamental level the values and motivations we bring to the research endeavour must be questioned. Do we follow the path urged by authors such as Fawcett (2003) whereby nurse researchers are mandated only to undertake studies that are explicitly underpinned by a nursing conceptual model and nothing else, or do we heed the advice of Whall (1999) who cautioned that we should focus on 'what is good for clients rather than what is good for the discipline'? If we are to realise the potential of user and carer involvement the answer should be self-evident.

Dedication

This chapter is dedicated to the memory of Will Nolan (1955 2006) who, as a gifted engineer, relied on absolute precision in his work and would have smiled wryly at the arguments advanced above. As we struggle to understand the chaos that surrounds his loss, we can only hope that order, and eventually peace, will be achieved.

References

Atkinson P, Delamont S 2005 Analytic perspectives. In: Denzin N K, Lincoln Y S (eds) The Sage Handbook of Qualitative Research, 3rd edn. Sage, Thousand Oaks, CA: 821–840

Barnes M 2002 Bringing differences into deliberation? Disabled people, survivors and local governance. Policy and Politics 20(3): 319–331

Bassey M 1984 Pedagogic research: on the relative merits of search for generalisation and study of single events. In: Bell J, Bush T, Fox A, Gooday J, Goulding S (eds) Coordinating Small Scale Investigations in Educational Management. Harper and Row, London: 103–122

Bryman A, Teevan J J 2005 Social Research Methods. Oxford University Press, Ontario

Chenitz W C 1983 Entry into a nursing home as status passage: a theory to guide nursing practice. Geriatric Nursing 4(2): 92–97

Clough E 2005 Foreword. In: Burr J, Nicolson P (eds) Researching Health Care Consumers, Critical Approaches. Palgrave (Macmillan), Basingstoke: ix–xi

Creswell J W 1998 Qualitative Inquiry and Research Design, Choosing Among Five Traditions. Sage, Thousand Oaks

Dawes M, Summerskill W, Glasziou P, et al 2005 Sicily statement on evidence-based practice. BMC Medical Education 5: 1

Denzin N K, Lincoln Y S 2005a Preface. In: Denzin N K, Lincoln Y S (eds) The Sage Handbook of Qualitative Research, 3rd edn. Sage, Thousand Oaks: ix–xix

Denzin N K, Lincoln Y S (eds) 2005b Introduction. In: Denzin N K, Lincoln Y S (eds) The Sage Handbook of Qualitative Research, 3rd edn. Sage, Thousand Oaks: 1–32

Donaldson L 2003 Expert patient ushers in a new era of opportunity for the NHS. British Medical Journal 326(7402): 1279

Donovan J, Sander C 2005 Key issues in the analysis of qualitative data in health services research. In: Bailey A, Ebrahim S. (eds) Handbook of Health Research Methods: Investigation, Measurement and Analysis. Open University Press, Berkshire: 515–532

Fawcett J 2003 On bed baths and conceptual models of learning. Journal of Advanced Nursing 44(3): 229–230

Gaventa J, Cornwall A 2001 Power and knowledge. In: Reason P, Bradbury H (eds) Handbook of Action Research: Participative Inquiry and Practice. Sage, London: 70–80

Guba E G, Lincoln Y S 1989 Fourth Generation Evaluation. Sage, Newbury Park

Humphries B 2003 What else counts as evidence in evidence-based social work? Social Work Education 22(1): 81 91

Kitson A 2002 Recognising relationships: reflections on evidence-based practice. Nursing Inquiry 9(3): 179–186

Lathlean J 2006 Qualitative analysis. In: Gerrish K, Lacey A (eds) The Research Press in Nursing. Blackwell, Oxford: 417–433

Liamputtong P, Ezzy D 2005 Qualitative Research Methods, 2nd edn. Oxford University Press, Melbourne

Miles M, Huberman A 1994 Qualitative Data Analysis, 2nd edn. Sage, Thousand Oaks

Miller W L, Crabtree B F 1992 Primary care research: a multi-method typology and qualitative road map. In: Crabtree B F, Miller W L (eds) Doing Qualitative Research. Sage, Newbury Park: 3–28

Morse J M 1994 'Emerging from the data': The cognitive processes of analysis in qualitative inquiry. In: Morse J M (ed) Critical Issues in Qualitative Research Methods. Sage Thousand Oaks: 23–43

Nolan M R 1990 Timeshare beds: a pluralistic evaluation of rota bed systems in continuing care hospitals. PhD thesis, University of Wales, Bangor

Nolan M R 2005 What counts as research and whose research counts? Towards 'authentic' participatory inquiry. Plenary paper given at the RCN 2005 International Nursing Research Conference. Spires Conference Centre, Belfast, Northern Ireland, 8–11, March 2005

Nolan M R, Grant G 1992a Regular Respite: an Evaluation of a Hospital Rota Bed Scheme for Elderly People. Ace Books, Age Concern Institute of Gerontology Research Papers Series No 6, London

Nolan M R, Grant G 1992b Mid-range theory building and the nursing theory practice gap: a respite care case study. Journal of Advanced Nursing 17(2): 217–223

Nolan M R, Grant G, Keady J 1996 Understanding Family Care: A Multidimensional Model of Caring and Coping. Open University Press, Buckingham

Owen J 2005 Users, research and 'evidence' in social care. In: Burr J, Nicolson P (eds) Researching Health Care Consumers, Critical Approaches. Palgrave (Macmillan), Basingstoke: 155–179

Ritchie J, Spencer L 1994 Qualitative data analysis for applied policy research. In: Bryman A, Burgess R (eds) Analysing Qualitative Data. Routledge, London. Reported in Huberman, A M, Miles M B (eds) The Qualitative Researchers Companion. Sage, Thousand Oaks: 305–331

Ritchie J, Spencer L, O'Conner W 2003 Carrying out qualitative analysis. In: Ritchie J, Lewis J (eds) Qualitative Research Practice: A Guide for Social Science Students and Researchers. Sage, London: 219–262

Rolfe G 1999 Insufficient evidence: the problems of evidence-based nursing. NET 19: 433–442

Ryan G W, Bernard H R 2000 Data management and analysis methods. In: Denzin N K, Lincoln Y S (eds) The Sage Handbook of Qualitative Research, 2nd edn. Sage, Thousand Oaks: 769–802

Sandberg J, Nolan M R, Lundh U 2002 Entering a New World: empathic awareness as the key to positive family/staff relationships in care homes. International Journal of Nursing Studies 39(5): 507–516

Schwandt T A 1997 Qualitative Inquiry: A Dictionary of Terms. Sage, Thousand Oaks

SCIE 2003 Media Release 25/3/03

Scottish Executive/Office of Public Management 2005 The future of unpaid care in Scotland: headline report of recommendation. Report of the Care 21 Unit. Scottish Executive/OPM, London

Seale C, Gobo G, Gubrium J F, Silverman D (eds) (2004) Qualitative Research Practice. Sage, London

Whall A L 1999 Bridging the gap between nursing and gerontology: an epistemological view. In: Gueldner S H, Poon L W (eds) Gerontological Nursing Issues for the 21st Century. Center Nursing Press, Sigma Theta Tau International, Washington DC: 29–34

Chapter 34

Descriptive Statistics

Ian Atkinson

Introduction

Quantitative research often involves the collection of very large amounts of numerical data. To make sense of numerical data we need to apply methods to summarise numbers into a format which is easy to assimilate. This is known as descriptive statistics. Once data are described, a further range of inferential statistics remains to be applied before a full understanding of the data can be achieved (Chapter 35).

The nature of numerical data

Information obtained as part of quantitative research is stored and analysed in numerical format. Sometimes information is directly recorded as numbers, for example age, blood pressure and body weight. Information which is not numerical can be changed by using systems of data coding. For example, a person's gender could be recorded as '1' for a man and '2' for a woman. The actual numbers used are not important so long as we use a different number for each category. For example, suppose a surgical patient's experience of pain is assessed using the terms 'no pain', 'mild pain', 'severe pain' and 'very severe pain'. These categories have an obvious logical order in terms of pain severity and coding should involve ascribing the lowest number to the lowest level of pain and the highest number to most severe pain. Consequently the codes would be as follows, 1 = no pain; 2 = mild pain; 3 = severe pain; and 4 = very severe pain.

Already it can be seen that numbers are used in rather different ways. Those used to record age or weight can quite properly be added, subtracted, multiplied and divided. On the other hand, in the case of gender, it would be completely meaningless to add the above. The above measurement of pain allows us to place values in an orderly fashion but if we attempted to subtract severe pain from mild pain then our answer would have no meaning. The different ways in which numbers have been used in these examples can be referred to as different levels of measurement.

Levels of measurement

There are four different levels of measurement and these include, in order of increasing precision, nominal, ordinal, interval, and ratio levels. Each level of measurement can be defined in terms of the properties shown in the first column of Table 34.1. The different levels of measurement appear in the first row. The nominal level is the lowest level of measurement and is more a system for classification, its single property being that we can distinguish different categories. For example, information about gender falls into two different categories, i.e. men and women. These differences cannot be measured numerically nor can the categories be ranked.

At the ordinal level of measurement we distinguish different categories and also place them in ascending order. An example of this type of measurement can be seen in grades of medical staff, i.e. junior house officer, senior house officer, registrar and consultant. We know there are differences between the grades and they can be meaningfully ranked in terms of seniority. However, the differences between the grades cannot be quantified.

The interval level of measurement has one additional property to the ordinal level, i.e. there are equal differences between the categories. This means that we are able to subtract one category from another to give a result which has a meaning. A very commonly used example of this is the measurement of temperature in degrees Celsius. Here there is an equal distance of one degree of heat between every point on the scale. What this scale lacks is a fixed zero point which means that, for example, 10°C is not double 5°C. In this case zero has only been set at a point where water freezes and not where there is a complete lack of heat. Examples of interval levels of measurement can be seen in visual analogue and interval scales for the measurement of attitudes (Oppenheim 1992).

The highest or most precise measurement is at a ratio level. This has all the properties associated with the interval level only this time zero is fixed. Examples of characteristics which can be measured at this level include weight, length and capacity. These scores can be added, subtracted, multiplied and divided.

Another important characteristic of a variable is whether or not it is 'discrete' or 'continuous' in nature. The so-called discrete variable can only be expressed as a whole number, for example the number of nurses or the number of beds on a ward. On the other hand, interval and ratio levels of measurement can be expressed as a fraction and in such cases data are referred to as continuous. For example, patients are weighed in kilograms expressed with one or two decimal places following the whole number, e.g. 78.63 kilos. Where measurements are continuous, the last decimal point has to be rounded off.

Table 34.1 – *Different levels of measurement and their properties*

	Nominal	Ordinal	Interval	Ratio
Different categories	Yes	Yes	Yes	Yes
Categories can be ranked	–	Yes	Yes	Yes
Equal distances between categories	–	–	Yes	Yes
Fixed zero	–	–	–	Yes

Numerical data

Once data from a quantitative study are obtained, descriptive methods are applied as a first stage of interpreting their meaning and obtaining answers to the research questions. Imagine we have conducted a survey of 80 people recently discharged from hospital. These people are our study 'sample' and have been selected from the study 'population' of all people discharged from the hospital. The methods of sample selection are very important but these cannot be fully discussed in this chapter and readers are advised to consult alternative texts, for example Bland (2000).

From our sample of 80 we have collected information that among other things, includes their gender, length of inpatient stay (in days), and route of admission (i.e. waiting list, emergency, transfer, outpatient department (OPD) referral and GP referral). These three recordings from each patient are referred to as variables. Examination of these variables shows that gender is recorded at a nominal level, length of stay is recorded at a ratio level and route of admission is also at a nominal level. Length of stay is recorded in actual number of days but gender is coded as 1 = man and 2 = woman. The route of admission is also coded into a number format where: 1 = waiting list, 2 = emergency, 3 = transfer, 4 = OPD referral, and 5 = GP referral.

Table 34.2 shows the data that were obtained on these variables from 80 discharged patients. It can be seen that four columns have been allocated to hold these data. The unshaded columns contain unique case identity numbers which should be linked to every person's information for ease of data management. The second columns contain information on gender and one labelled 'Sex'. The columns headed 'LoS' (length of stay) contain the number of days the person was in hospital. The fourth columns labelled 'Route' contain a code for the route by which each patient was admitted. Now we can see, for example, that case number 22 was a man, in hospital for 20 days after having been admitted to hospital as an emergency. The information held in Table 34.2 may be very useful but in this format visual examination tells us very little.

To gain further insight the frequency of occurrence of the different values must be ordered and grouped. In this chapter, the modes of data presentation are only described rather than detailing the different procedures which must be gone through to construct them. These procedures are most often performed by specialist computer software, for example the 'Statistical Program for the Social Sciences' (SPSS). Those readers who wish to achieve a fuller understanding of the methods involved are referred to Watson et al (2006).

Presentation of numerical data – tables

The most common way of presenting data in research papers is in the form of tables. The method allows data from a number of different variables to be presented in an easily understood format. Tables can also illustrate associations between the variables presented. Many formats can be used but certain features should always be present.

A basic principle is to present data in a way which fully meets the needs of the reader. A second general principle should be to maintain transparency of what is presented. This means making it absolutely clear how the numbers presented are derived; for example, if percentages are used the actual number of cases must be shown, otherwise transparency will be lost. A good principle when referring to a table in accompanying text is to ensure the text could still be understood even if the table could not be seen.

Table 34.3 summarises and presents the information on gender and route of admission collected in our example survey data set. It is a cross-tabulation of two variables. The title generally includes a table number which is essential for indexing. Then a full description of the variables presented is required. Should this mean the caption is going to be very long then it is acceptable to summarise and put a note with an additional explanation at

Table 34.2 – Data collected on sex, length of inpatient stay and route of admission on 80 patients discharged from hospital

Case No.	Sex	LoS	Route	Case No.	Sex	LoS	Route	Case No.	Sex	LoS	Route	Case No.	Sex	LoS	Route
1	2	3	1	21	2	6	2	41	2	3	1	61	1	1	1
2	1	10	1	22	1	20	2	42	2	4	5	62	2	4	4
3	2	5	1	23	2	11	1	43	1	4	4	63	2	4	2
4	2	6	2	24	1	6	1	44	1	6	1	64	1	19	2
5	2	5	1	25	1	5	4	45	1	1	1	65	2	2	1
6	1	4	1	26	2	3	1	46	2	4	1	66	2	5	1
7	1	5	2	27	2	28	1	47	2	4	1	67	2	3	1
8	1	13	2	28	1	3	2	48	2	4	1	68	2	5	2
9	2	6	1	29	1	3	5	49	1	1	5	69	1	4	2
10	2	3	1	30	1	5	3	50	1	5	1	70	1	4	5
11	2	6	1	31	2	19	1	51	2	3	2	71	2	31	3
12	1	5	3	32	2	12	2	52	1	5	1	72	2	7	1
13	2	5	2	33	2	6	3	53	2	6	1	73	2	20	5
14	1	4	1	34	2	4	5	54	1	3	5	74	2	5	2
15	2	16	4	35	2	14	2	55	2	10	5	75	1	2	2
16	2	11	1	36	1	4	2	56	2	3	1	76	1	4	1
17	1	3	2	37	2	6	1	57	1	3	5	77	2	7	1
18	1	9	2	38	1	4	2	58	1	2	2	78	2	4	3
19	2	4	4	39	2	4	5	59	2	12	2	79	1	4	1
20	1	3	1	40	2	13	3	60	1	4	1	80	2	5	2

Table 34.3 – *Patients discharged from hospital, route of admission by gender* (n = 80)

	Gender		
Route of admission	*Men*	*Women*	*Total*
Waiting list	13	23	36
Emergency	12	11	23
Transfer	2	4	6
OPD referral	2	3	5
GP referral	5	5	10
Total	34	46	80

*All patients discharged during January 2005.

and all the categories of the variable follow in the cells below. Should there be any natural ranking within the categories they must be placed in order. In Table 34.3 the top cell of the stub contains the variable name 'route of admission' and in the cells beneath are the different ways in which patients are admitted.

The first rows of a table contain headings for each of the columns. In Table 34.3 they refer to the variable gender and contain the labels 'Men' and 'Women'. The last column to the right is labelled 'Total' as the cells below are used to show the sum of each row. In this way each of the cells in the body of the table has a clear meaning and the number contained within it refers to the number of individuals in the sample who satisfy its conditions. The cell which falls where the column labelled 'Men' and the row labelled 'Emergency' cross contains the number 12. This means that in our sample 12 men were admitted as emergency cases. At the end of this row we can see that in the entire sample 23 people were emergency admissions and at the bottom of the column it can be seen that there were 34 men in the sample.

the foot of the table. In Table 34.3 a short footnote is included to specify the month and year when the patient discharges took place. An asterisk is used to draw the attention to this. Notes underneath the table should be used to explain aspects of the presentation which may not be immediately obvious to the reader.

It is good practice to include the sample size in the caption and here it appears in brackets at the end. The first column in a table is referred to as the 'stub' and contains names or labels for each of the rows. The variable name appears in the top cell

In Table 34.4 the columns representing gender have been split into four columns representing length of stay grouped into different bands,

Table 34.4 – *Patients discharged from hospital, route of admission, length of inpatient stay by gender* (n = 80)

Route of admission	**Gender** Men				Women				Total
	Length of inpatient stay (days)				Length of inpatient stay (days)				
	<10	10–19	20–29	30–39	<10	10–19	20–29	30–39	
Waiting list	12	1	0	0	19	3	1	0	36
Emergency	9	2	1	0	8	3	0	0	23
Transfer	2	0	0	0	2	1	0	1	6
OPD referral	2	0	0	0	2	1	0	0	5
GP referral	5	0	0	0	3	1	1	0	10
Total	30	3	1	0	34	9	2	1	80

*All patients discharged during January 2005.

i.e. fewer than 10 days, 10–19 days, 20–29 days, 30–39 days. Here the table contains more information, although grouping the cases into bands of length of stay means the data shown are not entirely precise. A further problem is the large increase in the number of cells in the body of the table.

In both Tables 34.3 and 34.4 it would be useful to include the percentage of cases falling in each cell. This allows the reader to see the differences in proportions rather than just the crude differences in numbers. To do this a decision has to be taken as to how the percentage will be calculated, i.e. which numbers to use as the denominator in the percentage fraction. It is possible to use the number in the sample for this purpose, the row totals or the column totals. Whichever of these is used it must be made clear on the table.

Presentation of numerical data – charts

If we want to present data in a way that will have an immediate visual impact then we need to use charts. Here we look at three charts: the bar chart, the histogram and the pie chart. The bar chart is used for presenting information taking a lower level of measurement. To illustrate this the data on 'route of admission' taken from our sample survey are shown as a bar chart in Figure 34.1.

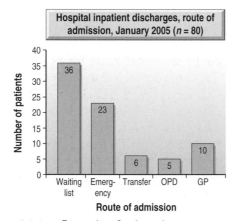

Figure 34.1 – *Example of a bar chart.*

Compared with the numbers in Table 34.2, the bar chart in Figure 34.1 has instantaneous impact on the reader, conveying a good deal of information about the variable called 'route of admission'. It can be seen that the most commonly occurring route is admission from the waiting list and the second most common are emergencies. It is also obvious that very few patients come from the outpatient department or are transferred from other wards.

The bar chart is plotted on two axes, the horizontal or 'x' axis shows the different values for the nominal variable 'route of admission'. The vertical or the 'y' axis is scaled to show number of patients. In this example the scale goes from zero to 40. The height of the vertical bars above each label represents the number of patients in each of the different categories. At the top of each bar is shown the number of patients represented. Inserting this number is optional but they make identifying the actual number easier than looking at the scale to the left. All tables and charts should have a clear caption and each axis must be given a title and labels when necessary.

The visual structure of the bar chart can be varied in a number of ways but the bars must be separated by a gap, preferably half the width of a bar. More information could be incorporated into this chart by adding another variable and Figure 34.2 provides an example of this. Here the bars have been divided to show the number of men and the number of women contained within each route of admission. The pairs of bars are shaded and a legend is added to indicate which bar refers to each of the sexes. This time the numbers on top of the bars have been omitted but horizontal gridlines have been added to guide the eye from the bars to the scale. The amount of information provided is effectively doubled in comparison with Figure 34.1. We can see very distinct differences between the numbers of men and women admitted from the waiting list but in other categories almost equal numbers of men and women fall into the different categories.

A further way of charting data that uses a lower level of measurement is the pie chart: dividing a

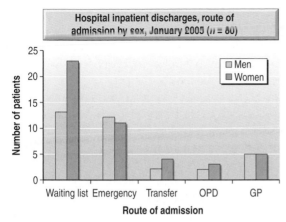

Figure 34.2 – *A bar chart with pairs of bars to indicate numbers of men and women in each category.*

circle into sectors which are proportionate in size to the number of cases in each category. Figure 34.3 shows the route of admission data presented in the form of a pie chart. Computer software can be used to produce these charts but if this is not available then the number of degrees to include in the angle forming each sector is easily calculated. In the example shown in Figure 34.3 there are 10 cases referred by GP, divided by 80 makes 0.125 then multiplied by 360 gives 45. Therefore, the angle

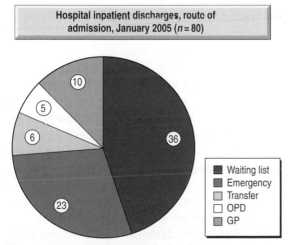

Figure 34.3 – *Example of a pie chart.*

of the sector illustrating the proportion of GP referrals is 45 degrees.

The pie chart is most useful for comparing proportions of each category to the whole and to other categories. This is in comparison to the bar chart where the length of the bars are the key feature, allowing ease of comparison between the numbers within each category but not in relation to the whole sample. In Figure 34.3 it is instantly obvious that almost half of the total discharges were admitted from the waiting list and that just a little over a quarter were emergency admissions.

The last type of chart to consider here is called the histogram and this is used for data using an interval or ratio level of measurement. The main difference between the histogram and a bar chart lies in the property that the former has a scaled variable on both of the axes. As a consequence the area of a bar chart has a meaning. This property is used extensively for the conduct of inferential statistics and readers are recommended to consult Watson et al (2006) for a more detailed discussion. At first glance the two types of chart are very similar except that the bars of the histogram are positioned side by side. The only variable in the example survey data set which can be used to construct a histogram is length of hospital stay and this is shown in Figure 34.4.

The axes of this chart both have values measured at a ratio level, i.e. the number of patients and the number of days. It can be seen that most of the area of the bars are grouped at the left hand end of the horizontal axis with far fewer patients having long hospital stays as shown at the right hand end. Figure 34.4 presents the length of every patients' stay in hospital and as a result many bars have to be included on the axis. For some lengths of inpatient stay, gaps between the bars must be left as there are no patients in the sample with those values. Also the horizontal axis has to be long and few cases appear at the far right hand end. To avoid this we can group the data into classes. In Figure 34.5 values along the horizontal scale have been grouped into bands of five days. Reducing the number of bars to six results in the

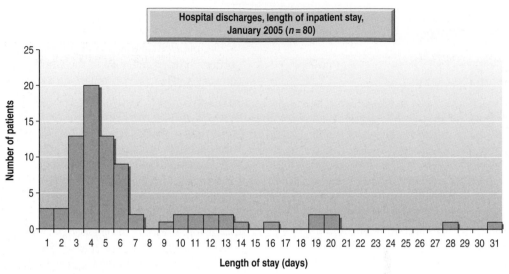

Figure 34.4 – *Example of a histogram.*

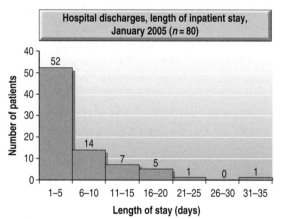

Figure 34.5 – *A histogram with the data grouped into classes on the horizontal axis.*

loss of some detail but the chart becomes easier to read.

The bar chart, pie chart and histogram are excellent ways to present data and provide an immediate visual impact but they are not much help if we want to compare sets of data. For example, imagine we have two groups of patients each receiving a different form of treatment and we want to compare the lengths of stay to find which treatment was most effective. The histogram would be of little help in this comparison. To make comparisons we need to have ways to summarise our data in a numerical format. To do this, we use statistics which reflect two properties of data. These properties are first, how the data spread out along the horizontal axis and second, how they cluster together between the two ends of the axis. These are known as the statistics of dispersion and central tendency.

Measures of central tendency and dispersion

The measures of central tendency and dispersion are summarised in Table 34.5. There are three main measures of central tendency and four of dispersion. The definitions of each are shown in the second column from the left. Some of these measures can only be applied to data at higher levels of measurement and this is shown in the four columns to the right.

Many readers will already be familiar with the arithmetic mean, commonly referred to as the average. Its formula uses every value included in a series. It is determined arithmetically and consequently can be built into further calculations. The mean balances the values in a data set on either side of it. It is easily distorted by extreme scores

Table 34.5 – *Measures of central tendency and dispersion*

Measure	Definition	Nominal	Ordinal	Interval	Ratio
Measures of central tendency					
Mode	The most frequently occurring value in a series of numbers. Where more than one value equally shares the highest number of frequencies then the data are said to be multi-modal	Yes	Yes	Yes	Yes
Median	The central value in a series of numbers arranged in ascending order. If there are two central values then it is the average of the two		Yes	Yes	Yes
Arithmetic mean	All the numbers in a series added together and divided by the number of numbers in the series			Yes	Yes
Measures of dispersion					
Range	Difference between the highest value and the lowest in a series of numbers			Yes	Yes
Inter-quartile range	In a set of ordered numbers in a series it is the difference between the number at the 25th percentile and the number at the 75th percentile			Yes	Yes
Standard deviation	Calculated by subtracting the mean from each number in a series. The standard deviation is the mean of the remaining values			Yes	Yes
Variance	The standard deviation multiplied by itself			Yes	Yes

so, for example, say the maximum value for the variable length of stay is 31 and the arithmetic mean is 7. If the longest length of stay happened to be 100, then the mean would increase from 7 to 10.45 with the change of a single value in the series.

The median is a fairly weak measure of central tendency but it can be incorporated into more detailed calculations and confidence limits can be determined (Altman et al 2000). One of its main characteristics is its insensitivity to extreme values in a set of data. For example, for length of stay in our survey data, the values range from 1 to 31 and the median is 4. If the highest value of 31 increased to 100, the value of the median would remain unaffected, i.e. it would still be 4.

The mode in a series of numbers is the category in which the largest number of observations falls. In the example data set for the variable 'route of admission', the mode, or the modal class is 'waiting list admission'. This is because more patients fall into this category than any other. For the variable length of stay the mode is four days. The mode can be applied at all levels of measurement but is probably most useful at the lowest levels. It is not an especially strong measure of central tendency as it is determined by inspection rather than by calculation. This is because it is based on only part of the series of numbers or set of different categories and can be manipulated by combining categories (Watson et al 2006).

The simplest and most crude measure of dispersion is the range or the distance along the scale which data spread themselves. As the range is determined by the two most extreme values in a data set it is quite unstable and consequently of little use. Sometimes its instability is dealt with by calculating the inter-quartile range, which in effect removes the measurements at the extreme ends of the scale.

The standard deviation statistic is defined in Table 34.5 and is a very commonly-used measure of dispersion for data at an interval or ratio level of measurement. Its main strengths are that it is determined mathematically and every number in a set of data is used in its calculation. The standard deviation allows us to make comparisons between data sets and is widely used in inferential statistics. The variance, which is the standard deviation multiplied by itself (i.e. squared), is largely used for purposes of reference rather than for data description.

Using measures of central tendency and dispersion

Of the three measures, the mode and the median are not extensively used whereas the mean is applied in many statistical calculations. We can already see from Table 34.5 that it plays a major part in calculating measures of dispersion.

In descriptive statistics the mode, median and mean are used together to describe distributions of data (Watson et al 2006). Figure 34.6 shows three different shapes of distribution. Figure 34.6A is a symmetrical distribution where the mode, median and mean are all equivalent and are all in the exact centre of the curve. This type of curve is commonly found to exist in data relating to naturally occurring characteristics. For example, the height and weight of people have this type of distribution.

The curve shown in Figure 34.6B has a negative skew, which means that the left hand tail stretches out much further from the centre than does the right hand tail. We can see that in such a situation the three measures of central tendency all take on different values with the mode being greater than the mean. In Figure 34.6C the right hand tail is stretched out further than the left so this curve is positively skewed. In this case the mode is less than the mean.

Measures of central tendency used in combination with measures of dispersion, e.g. the mean and standard deviation, provide two very useful tools for summarising data distributions and form the foundation stones of inferential statistics to be considered in Chapter 35.

Conclusion

The above discussion covers the ways numbers are used to measure phenomena and outlines several different ways in which numerical data can be presented which can be easily assimilated by an audience. Methods for summarising the properties

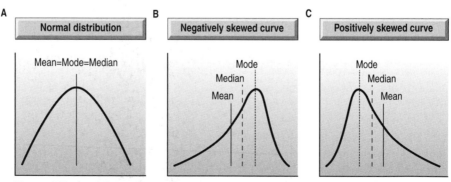

Figure 34.6 – *Three different distributions of data: A, normal; B, negatively skewed; C, positively skewed*

of sets of numbers, i.e. central tendency and dispersion, have been presented and the first principles of applying them to describe sets of numbers have been introduced. The chapter on inferential statistics (Chapter 35) introduces the next stage of statistical analysis for which the ideas presented here provide the key for a full understanding.

EXERCISES

1. At what levels of measurement could the following variables be measured?

   ■ Annual income
   ■ Gender
   ■ Marital status
   ■ Ability to walk up stairs
   ■ Social class
   ■ Blood glucose
   ■ Pulse rate
   ■ Eye colour
   ■ Temperature
   ■ Limb movement

2. Which of the above variables are continuous and which are discrete in nature?
3. Some of the variables in the above list can be measured at more than one level. Specify which these are and the different levels of measurement which could be appropriately used.
4. Which measures of central tendency (i.e. mode, median and mean) and dispersion (range, standard deviation and variance) could be applied to each of the variables listed in question 1?
5. Using your answers to the above questions, identify associations between the continuous or discrete nature of these variables and the following factors:

   ■ the number of different levels of measurement which can be applied to the variable
   ■ the different measures of central tendency which can be applied
   ■ the measures of dispersion which can be applied.

References

Altman D, Machin D, Bryant T, Gardener M 2000 Statistics with Confidence: Confidence Intervals and Statistical Guidelines. BMJ Books, London

Bland M 2000 An Introduction to Medical Statistics, 3rd edn. Oxford Medical Publications, Oxford

Oppenheim A N 1992 Questionnaire Design, Interviewing and Attitude Measurement, 2nd edn. Pinter, London

Watson R, Atkinson I, Egerton P 2006 Successful Statistics for Nursing and Healthcare. Palgrave Macmillan, Basingstoke

Chapter 35

Inferential Statistics

Roger Watson

What is inferential statistics?

Inferential statistics is concerned with applying conclusions to something wider than the observation at hand due to some properties of that observation. For example, if we met a group of people – men and women – and the women earned more than the men, we could infer that women, generally, earned more than men. What inferential statistics allows us to do is make that inference (or not) with some degree of certainty that what we are inferring from the sample applies to a wider group of men and women, i.e. the population of men and women (Swinscow & Campbell 2002).

Confidence

One of the first concepts to understand in inferential statistics is that of confidence, which means the confidence with which we can make an inference about a population based on a sample (Gardner & Altman 2000). For example, if we wished to study the patients on a medical ward, all of whom were admitted with a diagnosis of either heart disease or another diagnosis, and to find out how many of each there were, then this can be used to illustrate confidence. In a ward with a limited number of beds we can easily check the patient records or ask the nurse in charge and we will have an answer. However, suppose that you wish to know how many people in the general population with a medical diagnosis have either heart disease or another diagnosis, then we cannot simply ask someone to check all their records – there are too many of them to make this practical. If we consider all the patients on our ward to be the population and there are 20 beds on the ward, then we can start by finding out the diagnosis of one patient; if this patient's diagnosis is not heart disease then we know that the number of patients with heart disease lies between 0 and 19. If we find out the diagnosis of a second patient is heart disease then we know, with a greater degree of confidence, that the number of patients with heart disease lies between one and 18. The more patients whose diagnosis we discover, the nearer we get to the true figure for those with heart disease until we sample them all. In reality, it is very rare to be able to obtain the whole population for any study; we almost always work with samples and inferential statistics is concerned with drawing conclusions about the population based on a sample.

Confidence intervals

The example above, where we considered the concept of confidence, leads us naturally to the first concept in inferential statistics: the confidence interval. A confidence interval is a range of values between which a population statistic is thought to lie, with a particular degree – usually 95% – of confidence (Watson et al 2006).

Taking the example of a mean value for a population parameter, for example height, we can take a sample and, as described in the previous chapter, calculate a mean for the sample. We can also calculate a standard deviation of the mean for that sample, the standard deviation being a measure of the spread of the data. The standard deviation is related to the normal distribution, mentioned in the previous chapter, and describes a set proportion of the sample. One standard deviation either side of the mean includes 68% of the sample; two standard deviations 95% and three standard deviations 99% and so on as shown in Figure 35.1.

If we wanted to go beyond simply calculating a set of sample statistics and wanted to know about the true mean value in the population – without having access to the whole population – we could take repeated (and different) samples from the first

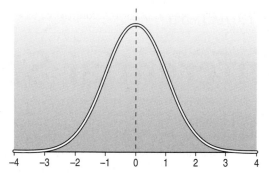

Figure 35.1 – *Normal distribution showing standard deviations.*

one we used and, for each of these, calculate a sample mean and standard deviation. Clearly, not all the means will be the same: they will be distributed about the population mean and it is this distribution from which we obtain the standard error of the mean. We do not have to carry out the tedious procedure of taking repeated samples; using our sample statistic, the standard deviation, we can calculate the standard error of the mean as shown:

$$\text{Standard error} = \text{Standard deviation}/\sqrt{(N-1)}$$

where N = number of subjects.

It should be noted that the standard deviation and the standard error are different statistics with different properties; the easiest level at which to differentiate them is that the standard deviation refers to a sample – unless you have the whole population available – and the standard error refers to the population – they are often confused (Altman & Bland 2005).

The standard error of the mean is used to calculate confidence intervals, which are usually quoted at 95% indicating that 95% of all the calculated sample means will fall within the range of the confidence interval. We know that the sample means are normally distributed; therefore, we can use this property to find the correct number from a table of values for the normal distribution corresponding to 95% confidence. The number is 1.96 (for the purposes of this chapter you do not need to know more about how this number is obtained) and this is used in the calculation of the confidence interval as shown.

$$\text{Confidence interval} = \text{Sample mean}$$
$$- (\text{Standard error} \times 1.96) < \text{Population mean}$$
$$< \text{Sample mean} + (\text{Standard error} \times 1.96)$$

Therefore, taking the example of blood glucose, if we sample a group of 20 people and calculate their mean blood glucose to be 5 mmol/l with a standard deviation of 1 mmol/l, we can calculate the standard error of the mean to be:

$$0.23$$

and enter this into the equation for calculating the confidence interval at 95%, thus:

$$\text{Confidence interval (CI)} = 5 - (0.23 \times 1.96)$$
$$< \text{population mean} < 5 + (0.23 \times 1.96)$$

That is:

$$\text{CI} = 5 - 0.45 < \text{population mean} < 5 + 0.45$$
$$\text{CI} = 4.55 < \text{population mean} < 5.45$$

which gives a 95% confidence interval of 4.55 to 5.45 mmol/l blood glucose, meaning that 95% of the samples we take will have a mean within that range.

If we want to be more confident, say 99% confident, we can calculate 99% confidence intervals and find the value in our tables of the normal distribution relating to 99% probability (this value is 2.58). Entering this into the equation for calculating confidence intervals gives us a 99% confidence interval from 2.42 to 7.58 mmol/l blood glucose. We see that the confidence interval is wider; i.e. the more confident we are about where the mean lies the less certain we know precisely what it is, i.e. the less accurate we are. This seeming paradox can be illustrated by asking someone to estimate the distance between their head and the ceiling. They may be able to give the distance to the nearest metre with a high degree of confidence but if you then ask them to estimate the distance to the ceiling to the nearest centimetre they will be less confident in their estimation – the more accurate they are required to be, the less confident they are in their estimate.

Confidence intervals can also be calculated for differences between means and for statistical tests such as odds ratios (Gardner & Altman 2000). This takes us beyond the scope of the present chapter but you are advised to consider the use of confidence intervals whenever possible as they are more informative than just the mean value (Watson et al 2006).

Statistical significance

In statistical terms, to say that something is significant has a particular meaning. For instance, if the outcome of a clinical trial is that one drug is statistically significantly better than another, this means there is a difference in their performance and that this is known at a particular level of statistical significance, usually $p < 0.05$. What we are doing is ascribing a level of probability to the outcome, which means the extent to which that outcome has happened by chance; in the case of $p < 0.05$ this means that there is a probability of less than one in 20 that the observed result has happened by chance (Hinton 1995). In other words, the result that we are observing is likely to have happened as a result of the phenomenon that we are measuring. In the example of the drug trial above we are stating how likely we think it is that the difference in the performance of one drug over another happened by chance and not as a result of some property of the drug. If the result were significant at $p < 0.1$ it would mean that there was a 1 in 10 probability that this would have happened by chance and if the result were significant at $p < 0.01$ it would be one in 100. The application of the concept of statistical significance will be exemplified in the inferential statistical tests described below.

The use of statistical significance enables us to avoid something called type I error and this means that we do not ascribe statistical significance to a result too readily (Watson et al 2006). We will meet another concept, type II error, towards the end of the chapter.

Statistical significance does not, necessarily, indicate that a result is clinically significant. It is possible to obtain statistical significance, for example, in a study of the action of two drugs, where the actual difference between the effectiveness of the drugs is very small and would, in fact, not confer any clinical advantage. Therefore, the actual size of the difference needs to be calculated. In the case of tests of association between two variables – to be described below – the same thing applies and how to do this will be described. Confidence intervals for the difference between two means is also useful in showing how big a difference really is (Gardner & Altman 2000). Clinical judgement is always required in conjunction with statistical tests.

Differences between means

One of the common uses of inferential statistics is in the study of differences between means as exemplified by the study of the effect of drugs in a clinical trial described above. There are three ways in which the difference between means can be tested and these involve:

- the difference between a mean value obtained from a study and the population mean for the same measurement;
- the mean difference between two independent groups;
- the difference in means before and after an intervention.

The statistical test commonly used in such studies is the t-test, so called because statistical significance is obtained by calculating a value which, arbitrarily, has been labelled 't'.

Population mean

If you wished to study the effect of a drug on a particular group of people, for example older people, and compare this with the effect of the same drug on the general population, then this could be done using a single sample t-test (Swinscow & Campbell 2002). For example, you may wish to study by how many millimetres of mercury (mmHg) a drug lowers blood pressure. The drug could be administered to a sample of older people and, if a value could be obtained for the action of the same drug on lowering blood pressure in the general population, then the two values could be used in a single sample t-test. In the single sample t-test the population parameters such as the standard deviation and the standard error have to be estimated for the sample; they are already known for the population, and these estimates are used in calculating a value of 't' from which the statistical significance of the test is obtained.

Differences between groups

The independent t-test is applied when the difference between the means of two independent groups is being tested (Swinscow & Campbell 2002); for example, if the mean blood pressure is being compared between men and women or young and old or between two groups in a clinical trial where one has received the treatment being tested and one is being used as a control. In this case, either no population mean value for the alternative treatment is available or, more likely, both treatments have to be compared under the same conditions and at the same time on comparable groups of participants. This independent t-test, therefore, is based on the sample statistics and uses these to estimate population parameters such as the standard deviation and the standard error for both samples and these are used in calculating 't' for the test from which the statistical significance is obtained.

Before and after

Finally, the t-test can be used to compare the means of a single group before and after treatment and this is called a related or dependent t-test (Swinscow & Campbell 2002). This could be applied to studies of the effect of a treatment such as a sedative on hours slept in hospital or of a session of hypnotherapy in improving quality of life in irritable bowel syndrome. In these studies there is no control group and the participants are being used as their own controls. For the related t-test the relevant population parameters have to be estimated, as in the tests above, and the related t-test enables the calculation of a value of 't' from which the statistical significance of the test can be obtained.

How is 't' used to obtain statistical significance?

't' is really a set of values with their own distributions – similar to the normal distribution – from which a probability for a statistical test can be obtained. The shape of a particular 't' distribution is determined by the degrees of freedom. It is beyond the scope of this chapter to explain what degrees of freedom mean and you are referred to a dedicated statistical text to seek this explanation if you wish (Hinton 1995). However, degrees of freedom can be approached pragmatically by considering them to be essential to the use of statistical tests (Swinscow & Campbell 2002). In the single sample t-test and the related t-test, degrees of freedom are obtained by subtracting 1 from the size of the sample (i.e. $n - 1$); in the independent t-test, degrees of freedom are obtained by subtracting 2 from the size of the combined samples (i.e. $n - 2$), which is the same as subtracting 1 from the size of the samples in each group. The practical application of degrees of freedom is in the use of statistical tables which are used to find the probability of a result from a calculated value, such as 't'. For example, taking our independent t-test described above, say we calculate the value of 't' to be 2.3. We have already decided the level of probability at which we will accept the difference to be statistically significant and say we set this at the conventional level of 0.05. If the number of people in the control group was 11 and the number in the intervention group was 31, then we know that the degrees of freedom are $(11 + 31) - 2 = 40$. Turning to Table 35.1, we find a table of values of 't'. Such tables are commonly found appended to statistical textbooks and these have been created by statisticians to save us having to produce our own each time we perform a test. The value of 't' we need is

Table 35.1 – Critical values of 't'

df	0.05 Level of significance		0.01 Level of significance	
	One-tailed test	Two-tailed test	One-tailed test	Two-tailed test
1	6.314	12.706	31.821	63.657
2	2.920	4.303	6.965	9.925
3	2.353	3.182	4.541	5.841
4	2.132	2.776	3.747	4.604
5	2.015	2.571	3.365	4.032
6	1.943	2.447	3.143	3.707
7	1.895	2.365	2.998	3.499
8	1.860	2.306	2.896	3.355
9	1.833	2.262	2.821	3.250
10	1.812	2.228	2.764	3.169
11	1.796	2.201	2.718	3.106
12	1.782	2.179	2.681	3.055
13	1.771	2.160	2.650	3.012
14	1.761	2.145	2.624	2.977
15	1.753	2.131	2.602	2.947
16	1.746	2.120	2.583	2.921
17	1.740	2.110	2.567	2.898
18	1.734	2.101	2.552	2.878
19	1.729	2.093	2.539	2.861
20	1.725	2.086	2.528	2.845
21	1.721	2.080	2.518	2.831
22	1.717	2.074	2.508	2.819
23	1.714	2.069	2.500	2.807
24	1.711	2.064	2.492	2.797
25	1.708	2.060	2.485	2.787
26	1.706	2.056	2.479	2.779
27	1.703	2.052	2.473	2.771
28	1.701	2.048	2.467	2.763
29	1.699	2.045	2.462	2.756
30	1.697	2.042	2.457	2.750
40	1.684	2.021	2.423	2.704
60	1.671	2.000	2.390	2.660
120	1.658	1.980	2.358	2.617
∞	1.645	1.960	2.326	2.576

located by locating the appropriate degrees of freedom on the left margin of the table and the appropriate probability on the top margin (using the two-sided test columns) and finding the value of 't' where these intersect, which we see is 2.021. If our calculated value of 't' exceeds the tabulated value, which in this case it does, then we can consider that the difference between the two means in the control and intervention group is statistically significant. We could write this result as: the result for the test was statistically significant (t = 2.04; df = 40; $p < 0.05$).

One- or two-sided test?

The difference between a one- and a two-sided test is that, in the former, we can predict the direction in which any difference is likely to lie and use a particular set of 't' values; in a two-sided test we do not know in which direction the difference will lie, i.e. we do not know which mean will be larger than the other, and we use a set of 't' values related to two-sided t-tests. In most situations you do not know the direction in which the difference will lie and it is wiser to use a two-sided test. In fact, the commonly used computer program for statistics, SPSS, by default provides two-sided tests and it is generally considered prudent to use these at all times as they are more conservative – they are less likely to lead to you making a type I error – explained earlier in the chapter.

ANOVA

Sometimes we wish to compare more than two means. For example, we may wish to test two treatments against a control or to compare means in three age groups: children, adolescents and adults. While it would be possible to conduct a series of t-tests, in the case of three means, three t-tests would be required; in the case of four means, six t-tests would be required (Watson et al 2006). You can imagine, beyond four means, that this becomes very complex and time-consuming. Therefore, we use a single test called ANOVA (analysis of variance), strictly speaking a one-way ANOVA (there are other ANOVAs), to test for the difference between more than two means. It should be noted that if ANOVA is applied to two means then the outcome is identical to an independent t-test; therefore, the t-test is a special case of ANOVA. The details of the test are not important but ANOVA provides a value, called F, which can be used to find the statistical significance of the test in a way that is very similar to the use of 't'; the desired level of significance and the degrees of freedom are required and you are referred to a more advanced text to find out how the degrees of freedom are calculated. The usual level of significance for ANOVA is 0.05 and it is important that you realise what this is telling you: it indicates that at least two of the pairs of means in the test are significantly different. You are then required to t-test the pairs of means (luckily statistical packages will do this for you) to see precisely which pairs differ and you should note that you do not apply the level of significance for the whole test to each of the pairs – otherwise it is easy to make a type 1 error. It is conventional to reduce the statistical significance and one way in which this is done (post hoc testing) is to divide the initial level of significance by the number of means being tested. Therefore, for three means, you would divide 0.05 by 3 (0.05/3 = 0.017) to find out at what level of probability you would accept the pairs of means as being significantly different; this process is called the Bonferroni procedure (Watson et al 2006).

Correlation

In addition to examining differences between groups, inferential statistics can also be used to examine relationships between variables and this is know as correlation. An example of a correlation would be the increase in mobility of an injured joint with increasing hours of physiotherapy or the decrease in pain with increasing dose of an analgesic drug. What correlation allows us to do is to calculate the strength of a relationship and to test its statistical significance. Please note, however, that while correlation can test such a relationship between two variables is does not, necessarily, indicate causation. For example, when we increase the dose of a drug and measure an effect we are reasonably sure that the drug is causing the effect. However, if we look at the correlation, for example, between income and social class we cannot say that one causes the other: a causal effect either way between income and social class could be proposed.

The best way to consider correlation is graphically as shown in Figure 35.2. The figures represent plots of the relationships between two variables, P and D, measured in a group of people. For example, P and D could be length of physiotherapy session and distance walked without pain after an injury. For each person in the group the two values are plotted on the graph; therefore, each point on the graph represents the point at which the two variables for one person meet on the two axes of the graph. Figure 35.2A shows the plot when there is no correlation between the variables, in other words, length of physiotherapy session has no relationship to the length of time walked without

pain. Figure 35.2B shows the plot when there is a relationship between the two variables. However, this is a weak relationship; if we compare Figure 35.2B with Figure 35.2C we can see that the points in Figure 35.2C approximate more to a straight line and this indicates a strong relationship. Figure 35.2D shows a negative correlation between the two variables, in other words, the greater the length of the physiotherapy session, the shorter the distance walked without pain.

In the relationship between the variables, therefore, we are interested in three things: the direction of that relationship, the strength of that relationship and the probability that the relationship has occurred by chance. Correlation allows us to analyse all of the above by finding the straight line that best fits the plot, giving the direction in which it slopes (positive or negative), providing a number (the correlation coefficient) which tells us how close

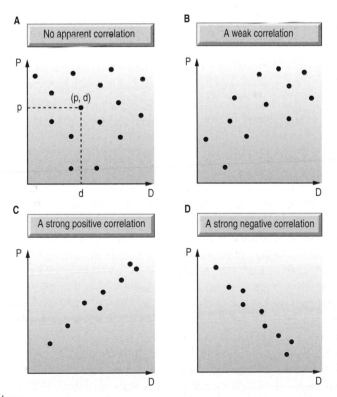

Figure 35.2 – *Correlations.*

the points in the graph are to that straight line. Correlation also provides us with a level of statistical significance for the test and there are tables of correlation coefficients for specific levels of probability, whether or not the test is one- or two-sided and at specific degrees of freedom. The correlation coefficient (r) ranges from -1 to 1; 0 represents no relationship and -1 or 1 represents perfect negative or positive correlation respectively. It would be unusual to get a perfect negative or positive correlation, or 0; the values usually lie somewhere in between. For example, Table 35.2 shows two sets of values for a group of 10 people who have received physiotherapy for an injury with the hours shown and the distance walked without injury. If we use these values to calculate a value for the correlation coefficient (known as r) then we get a value of 0.78. Note that the value is positive, indicating that the relationship between the two variables is positive (like Figures 35.2B and 35.2C); therefore, we have the size and the direction the correlation. To find the statistical significance we need the degrees of freedom and these are obtained by subtracting 2 from the number of subjects. Therefore, the degrees of freedom equal 8. Turning to a table (Table 35.3) of correlation coefficients and using the column for $p < 0.05$ for a two-sided test we can locate a value of r, using degrees of freedom 8. If the calculated value of r (0.78) is greater than

the tabulated value (0.63), then the correlation is statistically insignificant – which it is. Correlation is said to be weak, moderate or strong if the correlation coefficient (r) is less than 0.3; 0.3 to 0.7, or greater than 0.7 respectively.

How many subjects?

One of the issues for all studies using statistics is how many subjects should be included in the study. Statistics can help us and this is called power analysis. Expert statistical help is usually required to carry out power analysis and some software can also be obtained. Power analysis is necessary to avoid type II error whereby a statistically significant result is missed because too few subjects were included in the study (Watson et al 2006). Power analysis also helps us to avoid using too many subjects as this adds time and expense to a study. Power analysis can be applied to all statistical tests and this emphasises the need to know, in advance of your analysis – i.e. at the design stage of a study – how you are going to analyse your data. The essential piece of information that is required for power analysis is the likely effect size; in other words, if you are looking at a difference between means, how large do you expect that difference to be or, if you are looking at a relationship between two means, how strong do you expect the correlation to be. It is common simply to estimate the effect size, which can be described as being small, medium or large (Cohen 1992). Large effect sizes are very rare; small effect sizes are of little interest clinically; therefore, it is common in clinical research to use medium effect sizes. The other information required for a power analysis is the statistical significance you require, and this is conventionally set at 0.05, and the power you require from the test, in other words, the ability of the test to avoid type II error. The power of the test is usually set at a value of 0.8.

Conclusion

Inferential statistics allow us to work with samples but to apply the results of our analysis to the

Table 35.2 – *Length of physiotherapy after injury and distance walked*

Hours of physiotherapy	Distance walked (m)
1	10
3	50
2	10
5	30
4	60
6	40
7	50
9	70
2	15
3	35

Table 35.3 – *Critical values of 'r'*

df	0.05 Level of significance		0.01 Level of significance	
	One-tailed test (directional)	*Two-tailed test (non-directional)*	*One-tailed test (directional)*	*Two-tailed test (non-directional)*
1	0.9877	0.9969	0.9995	0.9999
2	0.9000	0.9500	0.9800	0.9900
3	0.8054	0.8783	0.9343	0.9587
4	0.7293	0.8114	0.8822	0.9172
5	0.6694	0.7545	0.8329	0.8745
6	0.6215	0.7067	0.7887	0.8343
7	0.5822	0.6664	0.7498	0.7977
8	0.5494	0.6319	0.7155	0.7646
9	0.5214	0.6021	0.6851	0.7348
10	0.4973	0.5760	0.6581	0.7079
11	0.4762	0.5529	0.6339	0.6835
12	0.4575	0.5324	0.6120	0.6614
13	0.4409	0.5139	0.5923	0.6411
14	0.4259	0.4973	0.5742	0.6226
15	0.4124	0.4821	0.5577	0.6055
16	0.4000	0.4683	0.5425	0.5897
17	0.3887	0.4555	0.5285	0.5751
18	0.3783	0.4438	0.5155	0.5614
19	0.3687	0.4329	0.5034	0.5487
20	0.3598	0.4227	0.4921	0.5368
25	0.3233	0.3809	0.4451	0.4869
30	0.2960	0.3494	0.4093	0.4487
35	0.2746	0.3246	0.3810	0.4182
40	0.2573	0.3044	0.3578	0.3932
45	0.2428	0.2875	0.3384	0.3721
50	0.2306	0.2732	0.3218	0.3541
60	0.2108	0.2500	0.2948	0.3248
70	0.1954	0.2319	0.2737	0.3017
80	0.1829	0.2172	0.2565	0.2830
90	0.1726	0.2050	0.2422	0.2673
100	0.1638	0.1946	0.2301	0.2540

general population. However, this can only be done within the bounds of statistical significance and confidence, and both concepts have been explained. Inferential statistics covers the difference between means, the relationship between variables (both covered in this chapter) and a great many other statistical tests not covered in this chapter. It is also possible to use some of the concepts in inferential statistics to estimate the sample size required for a study.

EXERCISE

Find three nursing research papers, one each using: descriptive statistics – including confidence intervals, differences between means, and correlation. Read them and, in each case, make notes and ensure that you understand what the tests tell you about the results of the study.

References

Altman D G, Bland J M 2005 Standard deviations and standard errors. BMJ 331: 903

Cohen J 1992 A power primer. Psychological Bulletin 112: 155–159

Gardner M J, Altman D G, Gardner M J 2000 Means and their differences. In: Altman D G, Machin D, Bryant T N, Gardner M J Statistics with Confidence, 2nd edn. BMJ Books, London: 28–35

Gardner M J, Altman D G 2000 Estimating with confidence. In: Altman D G, Machin D, Bryant T N, Gardner M J Statistics with Confidence, 2nd edn. BMJ Books, London: 3–5

Hinton P 1995 Statistics Explained. Routledge, London

Swinscow T D V, Campbell M J 2002 Statistics and Square One. BMJ Books, London

Watson R, Atkinson I, Egerton P 2006 Successful Statistics for Nursing and Healthcare. Palgrave, London

Chapter 36

Interpretive Phenomenological Analysis

Catherine Quinn and Linda Clare

Introduction

Interpretive phenomenological analysis (IPA) explores lived experience and how people assign meanings to make sense of their experience (Smith 2004). IPA attempts to make sense of the participant's subjective world through a process combining descriptive and interpretive activity (Willig 2001). IPA is descriptive in that it attempts to present an account of subjective experience; however, it is also acknowledged that such experience is never directly accessible. Thus, IPA is also interpretive as it acknowledges the researcher's role in creating a thematic account (Smith et al 1997). IPA is not a hypothesis-driven approach, but rather answers broader research questions. IPA can be used to question or further explore knowledge gained from the existing literature (Smith 2004) by focusing primarily on participants' accounts of their experiences. It is only at the end of an IPA that the findings are then integrated with existing research.

This chapter will explore the theoretical background of IPA and how it differs from other qualitative approaches. It will provide an outline of how to conduct IPA research and a practical illustration of how to analyse an interview transcript using IPA. The final sections of this chapter will focus on the use of IPA in health research, focusing in particular on how IPA has contributed to the field of dementia research.

What is IPA?

The origins of IPA can be found in philosophical traditions of phenomenology, in theories developed within the social sciences, and in social cognitive psychology. From the social sciences, IPA has been influenced by concepts derived from phenomenology and symbolic interactionism (see Chapters 21 and 22 for additional information on these approaches). Moreover, both symbolic interactionism and phenomenology contribute to the foundations of IPA through their emphasis on the importance of how events are perceived and on the meanings that people attribute to events (Smith 1996). IPA also shares with social cognitive approaches a conviction that there is a link, albeit an imperfect one, between verbal accounts, underlying cognitive processes and behaviour (Smith et al 1997). The accounts people present in interviews are understood as relating to internal psychological meanings and experience. This is particularly relevant when considering the applicability of IPA in health research (Smith & Osborn 2004) and may help to account for the frequent focus in IPA findings on psychological issues relating to self and identity.

IPA aims to explore subjective experience (Smith 2004, Willig 2001). IPA proposes that people will experience the same event differently because of the different meanings they attribute to the event (Willig 2001). IPA, although expressly 'interpretive', incorporates elements drawn from both descriptive and interpretive phenomenology. The descriptive phenomenological aspects of IPA are concerned with the aim of identifying the individual's personal perceptions of the phenomenon under investigation (Smith et al 1999) and developing a credible account of these. However, IPA recognises that insight into the personal world is elicited only through a dynamic, interactive research process involving interpersonal engagement which brings with it an inevitable element of interpretation. Thus, an IPA is always an interpretation of the participant's experience, and is dependent upon, and complicated by, the researcher's own beliefs, assumptions and understandings (Smith 2004), which operate both within the interview context and subsequently as the researcher engages with the interview transcripts. This interpretive activity distinguishes IPA from the purely descriptive phenomenological approach. IPA researchers must therefore attempt to acknowledge pre-existing values, assumptions and beliefs that may affect the interpretation of data, and to reflect on factors that may influence their interactions with the participant or the text. Through acknowledging these influences and possible biases, the researcher attempts to reduce their impact on the analysis.

Some of the assumptions underlying IPA have been challenged. In particular, researchers have questioned the extent to which IPA can explain, rather than simply describe, the nature of individual experience (Willig 2001). Of course, description may itself be valuable, especially in the case of poorly understood phenomena, and this kind of information can contribute to enhancing clinical practice. Arguably, this criticism can be countered by the observation that many IPA studies do move beyond simply describing themes in order to build dynamic and interactive models – or process-based accounts – as part of the interpretive element within this approach (as an example, see Clare 2003). Unlike grounded theory, the main aim of IPA is to provide an account of participants' experience with regard to a particular phenomenon, rather than developing a theory of that phenomenon. IPA in contrast to grounded theory is more concerned with answering specific research questions and providing an account of participants' experiences (Brocki & Wearden 2006), and the data collection and analysis phases are usually conducted sequentially. The resulting account is necessarily a thematic one, presenting key elements that are shared across the accounts of a group of participants. It has been noted that focusing on identification of themes across accounts is likely to imply a lack of attention to narrative elements. IPA does not generally focus on narrative, story or plot and is suitable for use when the primary aim of the research endeavour is to find the key thematic components of a particular phenomenon, or experience.

From a social constructionist perspective, there has been some critique of the reliance in IPA on participants' use of language to communicate their experiences. Willig (2001) commented that since people can describe an event in different ways, IPA may be examining how people talk about experiences in a given context rather than the nature of the experiences themselves. However, as previously noted, IPA is based on the assumption that what people have to say about their experience does reflect something of their 'inner world'. While both IPA and discourse analysis recognise the importance of language in describing people's experiences, these two approaches differ with regard to the link between behaviour and underlying cognitions (Smith et al 1999). Discourse analysis interprets verbal responses as behaviours and minimises the link between overt behaviour and underlying cognitions. IPA, on the other hand, with its links to social cognitive psychology, proposes that there is a link, be it direct or indirect, between people's verbal responses and their underlying thoughts and feelings (Smith 1996). Therefore, IPA endeavours to study the cognitions underlying these verbal responses. Again, this may help to account for the widespread application of IPA in clinical and health research since it is typically through talk that individuals and practitioners negotiate the meaning of, and responses to, physical symptoms or psychological states.

Conducting an IPA

The following section will explain some of the factors to consider when planning a research project using IPA, such as sample characteristics and data collection. This section will also explain, step-by-step, how to analyse interview transcripts using IPA.

Research question

The choice of an appropriate form of qualitative analysis for any project depends on the nature of the research question to be addressed. IPA can be most appropriately used to answer questions concerning how people make sense of a particular phenomenon that they are experiencing. IPA studies have explored a range of issues, such as the experience and meanings attributed to:

- caring for stroke survivors (Hunt and Smith 2004)
- living with Parkinson's disease (Bramley & Eatough 2005)
- aggressive behaviour in adult slot machine gamblers (Parke & Griffiths 2005)
- women's self-injury in the context of lesbian or bisexual identity (Alexander & Clare 2004).

Researchers typically attempt to address the implications of their analyses for clinical practice, service development or social policy, highlighting the relevance of IPA research to practical concerns of social and clinical importance.

Participants

As IPA is concerned with answering specific research questions, the sample chosen should have the potential to generate an answer to this question. A homogeneous sample is considered most likely to offer the opportunity to identify common themes and issues effectively, especially given the generally small sample sizes employed in this kind of study, which means that careful selection of participants is essential. Small sample sizes reflect the detailed and systematic nature of the approach, in which often lengthy interview transcripts are subjected to micro-analysis in a process extending over several stages. Smith (2004) recommended between five and 10 participants. However, IPA can also be used effectively with larger sample sizes, given appropriate time and resources (Reynolds & Prior 2003).

Data collection

Data are usually gathered through face-to-face semi-structured interviews. Semi-structured interviews allow flexibility in coverage, enabling the researcher to follow up interesting topics that emerge in the interview as well as ensuring that all key areas are addressed. The use of semi-structured interviews is described by Smith (1995). Other data collection techniques can involve focus groups (Flowers et al 2003) or interviewing participants via email (Murray 2004).

Analysis of transcripts using IPA

This section will provide an outline of how to analyse an interview transcript using IPA. Analysis using IPA can be done either by hand with or without the assistance of a basic word-processing package, or through using computer-assisted qualitative data analysis software such as NVivo. The example presented in this chapter was analysed by hand in order to illustrate the various stages of IPA. When learning to use IPA we would suggest that it is advisable to begin analysing transcripts in this way, in order to become fully familiar with the method, before progressing to the use of data analysis software.

IPA methodology

IPA involves a thorough and meticulous examination of transcripts in order to identify themes. IPA can be viewed as a cyclical method in which the quality of the analysis can be improved by continuously going back to the original transcripts and checking the fit of emerging themes. IPA uses an idiopathic approach in which each interview is analysed individually before proceeding to the group-level analysis in which themes are identified across transcripts for the group as a whole. There is no rigidly defined way of conducting an IPA; here we present the method that we use in our own research.

The process of conducting IPA is illustrated by an extract from an interview with a partner of a person with early stage dementia. The extract shown in Box 36.1 is taken from an interview with

Box 36.1 – *Extract from interview transcript*

'You know, it just seems so cruel after all that effort that he is being robbed of this good retirement; however, we are going to try and do some of the things we want to do more quickly. The first week I walked around this flat feeling like I had a stake in my heart because I didn't know he could be so ... well composed about it in terms of the diagnosis because I just felt so heartbroken for him. I did not know how he would come to terms with something like that being told to you and I would get into bed at night and my heart would pound ... and I feel that we are doing the best we can and we are trying to make strategies for coping with things ... we are finding that the more people we tell the more support we have got.'

a female caregiver describing her initial reactions to her partner's diagnosis.

Analysis of individual interviews
Stage 1: Reading the transcript

In order to become familiar with the text, the first stage of the analysis involves reading and re-reading the interview transcript.

Stage 2: Making margin notes

Once familiar with the transcript, the researcher inserts notes about key points into one of the margins – the right hand margin has been used here. These notes should be very similar to the participant's own words; this ensures that the analysis is grounded in what the participant actually says. Notes should be made throughout the transcript and it is a good idea to read the transcript a few more times as it is likely that more key points will be identified during this process. It can also be helpful to write memos of any points that seem particularly relevant and/or reflect general thoughts about the interview. Box 36.2 shows our extract with the margin notes made by the researcher.

Box 36.2 – *Extract with initial margin notes*

'You know, it just seems so cruel after all that effort that he is being robbed of this good retirement; however, we are going to try and do some of the things we want to do more quickly. The first week I walked around this flat feeling like I had a stake in my heart because I didn't know he could be so ... well composed about it in terms of the diagnosis because I just felt so heartbroken for him. I did not know how he would come to terms with something like that being told to you and I would get into bed at night and my heart would pound ... and I feel that we are doing the best we can and we are trying to make strategies for coping with things ... we are finding that the more people we tell the more support we have got'.	It just seems so cruel He is being robbed of his retirement Try and do some of the things we want to do more quickly The first week I walked around this flat Felt like I had a stake in my heart I didn't know how he could be so composed I just felt so heartbroken for him I did not know how he would come to terms with it Something like that being told to you I would get into bed at night and my heart would pound We are doing the best that we can We are trying to make strategies for coping The more people we tell the more support we have got

Stage 3: Summary list of margin notes

Once the whole interview has been analysed, the margin notes can then be compiled into a list. This helps to ensure that all aspects of the interview have been covered. The list for our extract is shown in Box 36.3.

Stage 4: Grouping of margin notes into thematic areas

In this stage the margin notes are grouped into initial thematic areas. This involves close examination of the margin notes, and is a gradual cyclical process of clustering together similar items often involving several revisions. These clusters can be viewed as initial themes, which encompass similar items. Each theme should be given a heading which encapsulates the tone of theme, and wherever possible the participant's own words should be used

Box 36.3 – *Summary list of margin notes*

It just seems so cruel
He is being robbed of his retirement
Try and do some of the things we want to do more quickly
The first week I walked around this flat
Felt like I had a stake in my heart
I didn't know how he could be so composed
I just felt so heartbroken for him
I did not know how he would come to terms with it
Something like that being told to you
I would get into bed at night and my heart would pound
We are doing the best that we can
We are trying to make strategies for coping
The more people we tell the more support we have got

in the creation of the headings in order to ensure that the analysis remains close to the text, reflecting the participant's experiences, rather than imposing predefined constructs.

The themes can then be further organised into groups. This involves clustering together themes which seem to be related to each other. The groups containing these themes, now called sub-themes, can be organised under a thematic heading, or superordinate theme. As with the theme headings, it is helpful wherever possible to use the participant's own words for the superordinate theme headings. The example presented in Box 36.4 includes two superordinate themes which encompass the sub-themes identified from the transcript.

Stage 5: Left margin codes

Having identified and organised the themes, the next stage involves coding the themes on the left hand side of the transcript. This ensures that every instance of each theme occurring in the transcript is identified. It also provides the opportunity to re-examine the 'fit' of the themes. The themes can then be compiled into a final list of themes for the individual interview.

Analysis across interviews

Once each interview has been analysed individually, the process is then extended to look across the full set of transcripts.

Stage 6: Full listing of theme summaries

All the themes and sub-themes identified from each of the interviews are compiled into a single list.

Stage 7: Grouping of theme summaries

The themes from the individual interviews are reviewed and grouped together with similar themes from other interviews to form new clusters of themes, each of which may comprise a number of sub-themes. This process may involve separating the sub-themes from the superordinate themes to which they originally contributed in the individual analysis. The themes used for the final overall

Box 36.4 – *Example of two superordinate themes containing sub-themes*

Just seems so cruel

I just felt heartbroken for him
The first week I walked around this flat
Felt like I had a stake in my heart
I would get into bed at night and my heart would pound
I just felt so heartbroken for him
It just seems so cruel
He is being robbed of his retirement

Did not know how
I didn't know how he could be so composed
I did not know how he would come to terms with it
Something like that being told to you

Strategies for coping

To make strategies for coping
We are trying to make strategies for coping

Doing the best that we can
We are doing the best that we can
Try and do some of the things we want to do more quickly

The more people we tell the more support we have got
The more people we tell the more support we have got

account need to reflect the experiences of the participants as a whole, and so should occur in most of the transcripts. As a general rule, to be included in the final account, themes should appear in at least two-thirds of the transcripts, depending on sample size. Infrequently occurring themes are usually removed from the final analysis, although they may still provide some useful information about individual differences, and may therefore be an important topic for discussion. Equally, there may be instances where different stances are observed

Box 36.5 – *Example of a higher-order theme encompassing superordinate themes and sub-themes*

You cope in different ways	Higher-order theme
Get on and cope with it	Superordinate theme
Nothing I can do about it	Sub-themes
You have to cope	
Copes as we are going along	
Doing the best that we can	
We must do the best we can	
You adjust your mind to it.	
You cope in different ways	
Yes we are coping, we're coping	
We have to tackle our problems	
It's in my interest – learn to develop strategies	
I keep everything straightforward	
I try to get him to think for himself more	

within the participant group, suggesting a range of responses, and in such cases less frequently occurring themes may form part of an interpretive model (e.g. Clare 2003). The result of this stage will be a list of themes with associated sub-themes. In a further level of analysis, some of the themes may cluster together under the heading of a higher-order theme. Box 36.5 shows an example of the final list of themes to which our original extract contributed.

Stage 8: Recoding transcripts with overall themes

All transcripts should be recoded with the finalised theme headings identified in stage 7. This again provides the opportunity to check the 'fit' of the themes and ensure that all relevant aspects of the participants' experience are covered.

Stage 9: Final list of themes with extracts

All relevant extracts from each transcript should be entered under the appropriate headings on the final list of themes, providing a complete account of the group-level thematic analysis. At this stage it is also useful to create a summary table of the themes, indicating which themes were identified from which interviews, showing the distribution of themes across individual transcripts.

Stage 10: Writing up the findings

The final list of themes with associated extracts forms the basis of the results sections. The themes are described and illustrated with extracts from the participants' accounts.

Credibility and trustworthiness

Due to the interpretive nature of the analysis, the researcher's own preconceptions and knowledge about the topic could bias their approach to, interaction with, and account of, the participants' experiences. Whilst this interpretive activity is accepted as an integral part of IPA, it is important to address and minimise possible sources of bias. At the outset, and during the research process, the researcher should consider his or her own feelings and reactions to the participants and their accounts. Involving other researchers in the analysis process can help the researcher to identify any instances of specific personal bias and any ways in which the researcher is influencing the content of the accounts being presented. To take an overly simplistic example, a young researcher interviewing older people in a care home about perceptions of dependency and death may be viewed as someone lacking life experience and in need of 'protection' from difficult emotions. In contrast, a researcher nearer in age to the participants may find it much easier to 'open up' such discussion and facilitate more sensitive and meaningful accounts. Identifying and discussing such effects can help researchers to develop their interviewing skills further so as to address issues effectively.

In order to ensure the credibility of the research, the researcher needs to show that the results are grounded in the text (Whitemore et al 2001). In the example presented above, the participant's own words were used as theme headings to ensure that we did not try to impose pre-existing theoretical concepts and thus pre-empt a credible and unclouded description of the participant's experience. In writing up the research, descriptions of the themes must be illustrated with extracts from the interviews. Another very important strategy used to maximise credibility is to go back to the original participants with the themes identified and request their comments, which can then be used to enhance the credibility of the account. For example, in one of our recent studies, one participant commented that while the themes seemed appropriate there was one issue that she felt was important that had not been highlighted. On examination of the data it was evident that, while this point had in fact been mentioned, it could have been given a stronger emphasis, and the account was adjusted accordingly.

IPA and health research

Whilst IPA has emerged mainly from social and cognitive psychology, its most extensive application has been in physical and mental health research. The majority of research using IPA has involved people who are dealing with issues surrounding health and illness (Smith 2004). Qualitative research, in general, has become more popular in health research as it allows the exploration of patients' beliefs and experiences without the need to quantify them. This can provide valuable information for practitioners, enabling them to become more sensitive to the concerns of clients and their families. Subjective experience has tended to be a neglected area in biomedical research, but there is an increasing acknowledgement that the interaction between biological, psychological and social factors is crucial in determining health outcomes. IPA is valuable in health research because it is underpinned by an understanding that there are links between a person's physical condition, their underlying cognitive processes and their verbal response (Smith 1996). IPA furthers this by focusing on the links between these three factors, discovering the influence of the subjective nature of experiences and therefore helping to explain why people with the same condition can respond to it differently (Chapman & Smith 2002). Models of participants' experiences can be created through an IPA analysis, and while IPA does not seek or claim to identify specific predictors of particular health outcomes, these models can illuminate some of the processes underlying different health behaviours and outcomes (van Dijkhuizen et al 2006). IPA can also be used to identify differences in the experiences and perspectives reported by the patient and practitioner (e.g. Dean et al 2005). An additional, emerging advantage of IPA with its focus on subjective experience is that it can be used effectively with a range of groups who may in the past have tended to be excluded from opportunities to have a voice and present their own subjective experience, including for example people with learning disabilities or with cognitive impairments due to dementia or acquired brain injury.

Case study: The contribution of IPA to dementia care research

In order to illustrate how IPA can contribute to and develop existing knowledge and practice, this section will provide examples from the field of dementia research. Clare (2002, 2003) used IPA to develop a model of the experience of early-stage dementia. In this model, people with dementia engage in five interrelated processes as they respond to the changes that are experienced through the progression of the disorder: registering the changes, reacting to the changes, explaining the changes, experiencing the emotional impact of the changes, and adjusting to the changes. Themes relating to each of the five processes demonstrate that responses for each individual fall somewhere along a continuum ranging between self-maintaining and self-adjusting stances. A self-maintaining stance consists of attempting to normalise the situation and minimise difficulties, thus maintaining continuity with the prior sense of self, while a self-adjusting stance consists of attempts to confront difficulties head on and incorporate them into an adjusted sense of self. While this model holds for both women and men, there appear to be some gender differences in the way they are expressed, with men focusing more on their abilities in practical tasks (Pearce et al 2002) and women placing more emphasis on the extent to which they feel connected with and supported by others (van Dijkhuizen et al 2006). Coping styles appear to polarise somewhat over time, with individuals responding more consistently in either a self-maintaining or self-adjusting style (Clare et al 2005). Understanding where a given individual falls on this continuum of responses can help in identifying how best to support that individual. For example, someone who is using a self-adjusting style is more likely to engage in cognitive rehabilitation interventions aimed at maximising coping and well-being (Clare 2003).

The continuum of responses is also evident in accounts of the shared experience of couples where one partner has a diagnosis of dementia. Robinson et al (2005) found that couples engaged in a process of negotiation as they tried to make sense of what was happening to them, with both partners engaging in self-maintaining and self-adjusting responses both individually and in relation to the spouse. Couples seemed to oscillate between an overwhelming sense of loss and difficulty on the one hand and a sense that they can move on, adapt and adjust to living with dementia on the other. Again, this provides valuable pointers for those supporting couples where one partner has dementia; both partners must be taken into consideration as the level of well-being for each partner will reciprocally influence that of the other.

The important role of 'explaining' in the model outlined above acknowledges that the way in which people understand and make sense of their condition crucially affects the way in which they cope and adjust, both individually and as part of a couple. Harman and Clare (2006) investigated how people who had received, and were willing to acknowledge, a diagnosis of dementia understood their condition, and how this affected their everyday experience. Most participants spoke of difficulties with memory and forgetfulness, and only a few used terms such as 'dementia' or 'Alzheimer's', but all understood that the condition would get worse over time. This created a conflict with the desire to retain sense of self and social roles, and gave rise to a series of personal and interpersonal dilemmas. Personal dilemmas centred around ways of responding to dementia, for example the question of whether to carry on or attempt to put an end to one's life, while interpersonal dilemmas reflected the perception that as a person with dementia one was treated differently by others and accorded less respect by health professionals. This is a stark reminder to practitioners of how people with dementia may experience even essentially well-meaning interactions as unhelpful, and a strong motivation to consider how to improve clinical practice in this respect.

Conclusion

The aim of this chapter was to explore IPA and its contribution to health research. Having reviewed the theoretical background of this approach, the chapter provided a practical framework for analysing interview transcripts using IPA. A case study was used to illustrate the applicability of this approach in clinical and health research. This showed how IPA can be used to derive a model that is directly relevant to clinical practice and that offers avenues for further research. By focusing on subjective experience, IPA research can provide a new and different perspective on familiar topics and an excellent starting point for exploring new issues and questions. It should be evident that this approach has considerable potential utility for nurse researchers wishing to research aspects of nursing practice and to understand more about the experiences of those they seek to help and support.

Acknowledgements

We would like to thank Jonathan Smith for his support, encouragement and advice on understanding and using IPA.

References

Alexander N, Clare L 2004 You still feel different: The experience and meaning of women's self injury in the context of a lesbian or bisexual identity. Journal of Community and Applied Social Psychology 14: 70–84

Bramley N, Eatough V 2005 The experience of living with Parkinson's disease: an interpretative phenomenological analysis case study. Psychology and Health 20: 223–235

Brocki J M, Wearden A J 2006 A critical evaluation of the use of interpretative phenomenological analysis (IPA) in health psychology. Psychology and Health 2: 87–108

Chapman E, Smith J A 2002 Interpretative phenomenological analysis and the new genetics. Journal of Health Psychology 7: 125–130

Clare L 2002 We'll fight it as long as we can: Coping with the onset of Alzheimer's disease. Aging and Mental Health 3: 179–183

Clare L 2003 Managing threats to self: awareness in early stage Alzheimer's disease. Social Science and Medicine 57: 1017–1029

Clare L, Wilson B A, Carter G, et al 2004 Awareness in early-stage Alzheimer's disease: relationship to outcome of cognitive rehabilitation. Journal of Clinical and Experimental Neuropsychology 26: 215–226

Clare L, Roth I, Pratt R 2005 Perceptions of change over time in early-stage Alzheimer's disease: implications for understanding awareness and coping style. Dementia 4: 487–520

Dean S G, Smith J A, Payne S, Weinman S 2005 Managing time: an interpretative phenomenological analysis of patients' and physiotherapists' perceptions of adherence to therapeutic exercise for low back pain. Disability and Rehabilitation 27: 625–636

Flowers P, Duncan B, Knussen C 2003 Re-appraising HIV testing: An exploration of the psychosocial costs and benefits associated with learning one's HIV status in a purposive sample of Scottish gay men. British Journal of Health Psychology 8: 179–194

Harman G, Clare L 2006 Illness representations and lived experience in early-stage dementia. Qualitative Health Research 16: 484–502

Hunt D, Smith J A 2004 The personal experience of carers of stroke survivors: an interpretative phenomenological analysis. Disability and Rehabilitation 26: 1000–1011

Murray C D 2004 An interpretative phenomenological analysis of the embodiment of artificial limbs. Disability and Rehabilitation 26: 307–316

Parke A, Griffiths M 2005 Aggressive behaviour in adult slot machine gamblers: an interpretative phenomenological analysis. Journal of Community and Applied Social Psychology 15: 255–272

Pearce A, Clare L, Pistrang N 2002 Managing sense of self: coping in the early stages of Alzheimer's disease. Dementia 1(2): 173–192

Reynolds F, Prior S 2003 'A life-style coat-hanger': A phenomenological study of the meanings of artwork for women coping with chronic illness and disability. Disability and Rehabilitation 25: 785–794

Robinson L, Clare L, Evans K 2005 Making sense of dementia and adjusting to loss: psychological reactions to a diagnosis of dementia in couples. Aging and Mental Health 9: 337–347

Smith J A 1995 Semi-structured interviewing and qualitative analysis. In: Smith J A, Harré R, van Langenhove L (eds) Rethinking Methods in Psychology. Sage, London

Smith J A 1996 Beyond the divide between cognition and discourse: using interpretative phenomenological analysis in health psychology. Psychology and Health 11: 261–271

Smith J A 2004 Reflecting on the development of interpretative phenomenological analysis and its contribution to qualitative research in psychology. Qualitative Research in Psychology 1: 39–54

Smith J A, Osborn M 2004 Interpretative phenomenological analysis. In: Breakwell G M (ed) Doing Social Psychology Research. Blackwell, Oxford

Smith J A, Flowers P, Osborn M 1997 Interpretative phenomenological analysis and the psychology of health and illness. In: Yardley L (ed) Material Discourses of Health and Illness. Routledge, London

Smith J A, Jarman M, Osborn M 1999 Doing interpretative phenomenological analysis. In: Murray M, Chamberlain K (eds) Qualitative Health Psychology: Theories and Methods. Sage, London

van Dijkhuizen M, Clare L, Pearce A 2006 Surviving for connection: appraisal and coping among women with early-stage Alzheimer's disease. Dementia 5: 73–94

Whitemore R, Chase S K, Mandle C L 2001 Validity in qualitative research. Qualitative Health Research 11: 522–537

Willig C 2001 Introducing qualitative research in psychology: adventures in theory and method. Open University Press, Buckingham

Index

Notes: Page numbers in *italics* refer to boxed material, figures and tables.

testing, 305
validity, 305

R

randomised controlled trials (RCTs), 190–194
  access tools, *77*
  bias issues, 190–191, 193–194
  control, 192–193
  data collection, 266
  double-blind techniques, 193–194
  evaluation, complex interventions,
    59–60, *60*
  limitations, 90, 194, 196, 199–200
  publication format, *77*
  purpose, 55, 58
  rigour, 60–61
  strengths, 194
  variables, 8, 10
  Zelen design, 194
range, descriptive statistics, *361*, 362
rating scales, questionnaire construction,
  302–303
rationales, research proposals, 139
R&D (research and development)
  departments, 150–151
realist synthesis, systematic review
  methodology, 93
reciprocal translational analysis (RTA), 92
RECs (Research Ethics Committees), 149
references, research proposals, 143–144
referencing, literature evaluation, 118
reflective cycles, 57
reflexivity
  action research, 214
  ethnography, 245, 246–247
  feminist research, 37
  participatory research, 27
  qualitative research, 9, 327
  student researchers, 158
refutational synthesis, meta-ethnography, 92
relative risk, definition, 105
relevance trees, research topic selection,
  68–69, *69*
reliability
  definition, 121
  Delphi technique, 256
  observation schedules, 312
  research tools, 9, 305
research, 13–21
  collaboration *see* collaboration
  data analysis *see* data analysis
  data collection *see* data collection
  definition, 6–7, 57, 350
  dissemination *see* dissemination/
    publishing

emancipatory, 24
evaluation *see* evaluation research
feminist *see* feminist research
historical *see* historical research
language use, 6–10
participative *see* participatory research
primary, 14, 15
project management *see* project
  management
secondary, 14
theoretical frameworks *see* theoretical
  frameworks
theory generation *see* theory generation
research and development (R&D)
  departments, 150–151
research culture, 128, 151
research design, 167–168, *168–170*
  action research *see* action research
  choice, 14, 18
  definition, 70–71
  Delphi studies *see* Delphi technique
  ethical issues, 168
  ethnography *see* ethnography
  evaluation, 116, 117
  experiments *see* experiments
  grounded theory *see* grounded theory
  longitudinal studies *see* longitudinal
    studies
  phenomenology *see* phenomenology
  surveys *see* surveys
  triangulation *see* triangulation
  see also specific designs
Research Ethics Committees (RECs), 149
research governance, 125–129, *126, 128, 129*
research papers *see* dissemination/
  publishing
research partnerships *see* collaboration
research proposals, 137–145, 286–287
  abstracts, 138
  appendices, 143–144
  data analysis, 142
  elements, 138–144
  ethical issues, 142–143
  functions, 137–138
  funding, 68, 143, 144–145, 153–154
  hypotheses, 140–141
  references, 143–144
  resource issues, 143
  sampling, 141
research questions, 67–73, *166*
  action research, 215–216
  development, 67–68, 116
  equilibrium/equipoise, 72
  evaluation research, 62
  formulation, 69–72
    resource issues, 71

historical research, 48
Interpretive phenomenological analysis,
  377
participatory research, 25–26
phenomenological research, 236
Q methodology, 321–322
questionnaire development, 300
research proposals, 139
surveys, 180
topic selection, 68–69, *69*
research supervision, 157–164
  authorship issues, 162
  codes of good practice, 157, 158
  ethical issues, 162
  examination process, 162–163
  feedback, 159–160
  intellectual property, 162
  learning plans, 160–161
  roles and responsibilities, 161–162
  standards, 158–159, 160, 162, 163–164
  student-supervisor relationship,
    159–162
research support office, 153
research tools/instruments, 167–168, *169*
  psychometric properties, 9
  purpose, 9
  qualitative methods, 9, *169*
  quantitative methods, 9, *169*
  reliability, 9, 305
  researchers as, 282
  validity, 9–10, 305
researcher(s)
  participatory research roles, 27, 28
  as research instrument, 282
resource issues
  participatory research, 28–30, *29*
  Q methodology, 328
  research proposals, 143
  research question formulation, 71
  see also funding/finance
respiratory nurse specialists (RNSs), 315,
  316
respite care services, qualitative research,
  343, 345–346, *346–347*
retrospective studies, 14, 120
risk ratios, 106, *106*
RNSs (respiratory nurse specialists), 315,
  316
Royal College of Nursing, *84*
RTA (reciprocal translational analysis), 92

S

sampling, 167
  Delphi technique, 252–254
  event, 312